Natural Health
COMPLETE GUIDE TO
INTEGRATIVE MEDICINE

Natural Health

COMPLETE GUIDE TO

INTEGRATIVE
MEDICINE

*The Best of Alternative and
Conventional Care*

DR. DAVID PETERS &
ANNE WOODHAM

A Dorling Kindersley Book

Dorling DK Kindersley

LONDON, NEW YORK, SYDNEY, DELHI, PARIS,
MUNICH and JOHANNESBURG

Natural Health magazine is the leading publication in the field of
natural self-care. For subscription information call 800-526-8440 or
visit www.naturalhealthmag.com. Natural Health® is a registered
trademark of Weider Publications, Inc.

Editor David Summers
Art Editor Emy Manby
Designer David Ball
Senior Editor Penny Warren
Managing Editor Susannah Marriott
Managing Art Editors Clare Shedden, Tracey Ward
DTP Designer Conrad van Dyk
Production Controller Martin Croshaw
US Consultant David S. Riley, M.D.
US Editor Constance M. Robinson

For Ben, Theo, Sam and Lilah, Tamsin and Jonty

AUTHORS' NOTE
The authors strongly recommend that you consult a conventional
medical practitioner before following any complementary
therapies if you have any symptoms of illness, any diagnosed ailment
or are receiving conventional treatment or medication for any condition.
Do not cease conventional treatment or medication without first consulting
your doctor. Always inform your doctor and your complementary
practitioner of any treatments, medication or remedies that you are
taking or intend to take. See also page 21.

First American Edition, 2000
2 4 6 8 10 9 7 5 3 1

Published in the United States by
Dorling Kindersley Publishing, Inc.
95 Madison Avenue
New York, New York 10016

Dorling Kindersley Publishing, Inc. offers special discounts for bulk
purchases for sales promotions or premiums. Specific, large-quantity needs
can be met with special editions, including personalized covers, excerpts of
existing guides, and corporate imprints. For more information, contact
Special Markets Department, Dorling Kindersley Publishing, Inc.,
95 Madison Avenue, New York, NY 10016 Fax: 800-600-9098

Library of Congress Cataloging-in-Publication Data
Peters, David, 1948–
   The complete guide to integrative medicine / by David Peters and Anne
Woodham. p. cm. Includes index.
ISBN 0-7894-5177-8 (alk. paper) 1. Alternative medicine.
2. Health. 3. Self-care, Health. I Woodham, Anne. II. Title.
R733.P426 2000
615.5--dc21   99-050060

Reproduced in Italy by GRB Editrice, Verona
Printed and bound by Sun Fung Offset Binding Co., Ltd., China

See our complete catalog at
www.dk.com

CONTENTS

INTRODUCTION

As fast as medical science forges ahead into a future of online diagnosis, gene therapy, and laser surgery, older, gentle modes of healing are acquiring renewed appeal. In many countries that boast state-of-the-art medicine, for example, nearly half the population claims to be using some form of non-conventional therapy, such as acupuncture, herbal medicine, or massage – healing techniques that are hundreds or even thousands of years old.

HOLISTIC HEALTH

Many reasons are suggested for the popularity of non-conventional therapies. Most persuasive, perhaps, is the desire in a computerized impersonal world to exert a measure of control over well-being. At the same time, researchers are confirming what traditional healers have always known: There is a constant interplay between our emotions, thoughts, and actions and our body systems. It seems that our food, the air we breathe, the exercise we get, how much we laugh or cry, and our feelings about family, friends, and colleagues all have a direct bearing on health. This interaction is played out at every level of our being and affects all biochemical, structural, and psychosocial systems. Clearly more is involved in health care than practitioners of high-tech medicine could possibly hope to deliver on their own.

BEST OF BOTH WORLDS

Of course it would be foolish to ignore the lifesaving achievements of modern medicine, and many of us have cause to be grateful for the latest drugs and skills of medical specialists. But the future of health care involves practitioners of all approaches working hand in hand. While the surgeon repairs organs and tissues and the physician prescribes lifesaving drugs, the naturopath, herbalist, and homeopath can offer remedies to stimulate natural healing processes, the osteopath can realign the body, the hypnotherapist can teach us calm, and the healer can soothe the spirit. This new approach, known as integrative medicine, is beginning to gain cautious acceptance among some doctors and other health professionals. Meanwhile, with a little knowledge, an intelligent curiosity, an insightful mind, and a seasoning of common sense, you can adopt a more integrative approach to your own health care, drawing on both complementary and conventional methods. It's the aim of this book to show you how.

INTEGRATIVE MEDICINE IN PRACTICE

Here we explore concepts of well-being and healing and reveal how modern medical science and traditional health systems may have more in common than was once thought. We describe how the causes of ailments can be tackled with both complementary and conventional medicine on biochemical, structural, and psychosocial levels, and explain how these three "realms" of the body interact. We show how scientific evidence is accumulating to support non-conventional approaches, and describe the therapies most likely to play a part in integrative health care. Since prevention of disease is as important as treatment, we explain how to make necessary lifestyle changes for optimum health and well-being, from eating a healthy diet to adopting a positive attitude. These steps may help us harness the best of both worlds, surely the way forward for medicine in the 21st century.

chapter

Integrative medicine draws on the lifesaving drugs

and procedures of medical science and on

complementary therapies that relieve stress, stimulate

natural healing processes, and nourish the spirit. It

INTEGRATIVE MEDICINE

addresses the needs of the *whole* person, taking into

account the astonishing subtleties of mind-body

interaction, and seeks to show how structural,

biochemical, and psychosocial health are intimately

entwined. Above all, integrative medicine encourages

patients, doctors, and complementary practitioners

to work as a team for the best possible outcome.

THE INTEGRATIVE APPROACH

Many people already combine conventional and complementary medicine on a self-help basis, in an effort to take the best from both worlds. For example, if you have a cold, you might ease the symptoms with a drug like acetaminophen and take the herb echinacea to boost the immune system. Integrative medicine, however, involves more than just adding together conventional medicine and complementary therapies. It entails thinking about why you might be ill and seeking the kind of treatment – whether conventional, complementary, or both – that is appropriate for your condition, given your situation, beliefs, and temperament. It is also a question of taking charge of your health and, in particular, of making lifestyle changes to promote well-being.

In integrative medicine, doctors and patients work in partnership to improve health.

INTEGRATIVE MEDICINE IN ACTION

A small but growing number of conventional health practitioners and complementary therapists are beginning to explore ways of working together. Such teams offer treatment based on a variety of conventional and complementary options, including psychological care, with an overall emphasis on health education and active self-help. Their aim is to encourage well-being, even in the face of established disease. In this kind of partnership, a doctor might treat migraine, for example, by prescribing medication, but would also look for underlying factors, such as your response to stress, or foods that might be causing or perpetuating the condition. An integrative therapeutic package could include acupuncture to reduce the frequency of attacks and induce relaxation; dietary advice and the keeping of a food diary; the use of the herbal remedy feverfew as a preventive measure (if you were reluctant to rely on the usual drugs); biofeedback to help defuse an attack; and yoga, relaxation, and stress management techniques.

HOLISTIC HEALTH CARE

Since the integrative approach is based on an understanding of the whole person, not just on physical diseases or symptoms, it has come to be known as holistic medicine. This approach is not the exclusive preserve of complementary practitioners. Indeed, some medical doctors have been practicing holistically for years, and it is the accepted aim of both family and internal medicine, obstetrics and gynecology, pediatrics, and psychiatry. Conversely, some complementary therapists stick rigidly to treating physical symptoms, ignoring the psychological dimension of disease. Others attribute even the symptoms of serious conditions such as coronary heart disease exclusively to "blocked energy" rather than to something that is in urgent need of conventional medical attention. Nor do complementary therapists usually have experience of acute disease or necessarily understand the psychological dimension of chronic disease and the often excellent resources afforded by conventional health care. All the more reason, therefore, to bring together the best in every discipline.

At the heart of traditional health systems such as naturopathy and Chinese and Ayurvedic (Indian) medicine is the belief that the body has a natural tendency toward equilibrium. Modern medical science calls this "homeostasis" (*see pages 12–13*), and is increasingly aware that maintaining this internal balance and boosting the body's self-healing powers are crucial to long-term good health and well-being.

Major physical injury, deficiency diseases, severe infection, and even extreme mental illness can overwhelm homeostatic processes, and in these instances modern medicine does its most critical work. In the past, medical science's triumphs have tended to overshadow traditional ideas of homeostasis, but today many doctors agree that it takes more than drugs or surgery to cope with persistent disease or stress-related ailments, and the notion of holistic health is becoming popular once more.

Keeping fit helps the body's self-healing processes work efficiently.

THE MIND-BODY CONNECTION

There is increasing scientific understanding of how mind and body are inextricably intertwined, and evidence to show that the health of one influences the other. Research, for example, reveals that emotional states such as loneliness and grief can depress the immune system, leaving people susceptible to disease. When psychologists, immunologists, and endocrinologists (those who study glands and hormones) began to pool information in the 1980s, they found they could track chemical pathways linking brain activity to physiological processes in the body. It had been understood that the stress hormones epinephrine and cortisol suppress the production of antibodies, the body's defense against disease. But studies in 1977 and 1983 showed precisely how white blood cells (which kill viruses) were temporarily paralyzed in bereaved men – accounting for deaths from the so-called broken-heart syndrome.

In the US, Dr. Candace Pert found that emotions trigger waves of messenger chemicals called neuropeptides, which reach all parts of the body, prompting physical changes that disturb or support homeostasis. Dr. Pert even suggests that these neuropeptides enable different body systems to communicate with each other. Key evidence came in the 1980s when endorphins, which are brain chemicals that enhance mood, were found not only in the brain, but throughout the body, even in the gut and immune system. Even more remarkably, it has now been discovered that messenger chemicals produced in the body, such as hormones, directly affect the workings of the brain.

So in the new scientific view, not only are mind and body one system, but it seems the body may influence the brain as much as the brain affects the body. The body is not just a collection of tissues and cells in a chemical soup, carrying around a detached mind. Rather, it is a moving, pulsing structure that emerges from an ever-changing flow of matter and information. The challenge of integrative medicine is to apply this idea in an intelligent and practical way to health care.

Studying the brain reveals a complex link between body and mind.

THREE-CIRCLE APPROACH TO WELL-BEING

WELL-BEING IS COMPLEX. It depends on body chemistry, on the health of physical structures (for example, blood vessels and muscles), and on how well adjusted you are psychologically. Challenges to health affect all three spheres. On an emotional level, stress can make you anxious, irritable, and depressed, but it has more than just psychological effects. Structurally, stress causes muscle tension, congested circulation, irregular breathing, and raised blood pressure. Biochemically, it has an adverse effect on the messenger molecules in the bloodstream; disturbs the functioning of the gut, circulation, and skin; and undermines the body's repair processes. Unrelenting stress can cause you to succumb to a host of conditions, such as irritable bowel syndrome, eczema, and recurrent viral infections. As homeostasis fails over a long period of biochemical, structural, and pyschosocial strain, the stage is set for chronic inflammatory diseases, coronary heart disease, and even cancer.

The three factors that determine an individual's state of health – biochemical, structural, and psychosocial – are fundamental to homeostasis, disease prevention, and health promotion. How the three realms of the body interact; the reasons why you might become ill; what conventional and complementary treatments you could consider; and how you might prevent illness, maintain well-being, or cope better with established disease are the subjects of this book.

THE THREE REALMS OF THE BODY-MIND

Health depends on the state of three interdependent "realms," which are underpinned by "vital force" or "energy."

BIOCHEMICAL REALM
This is made up of:
- cells
- hormones
- enzymes
- chemical processes
- digestion and respiration
- the chemical environment
- pollution

STRUCTURAL REALM
This is made up of:
- muscles
- bones
- blood vessels and nerves
- movement
- the physical environment

PSYCHOSOCIAL REALM
This is made up of:
- thoughts
- feelings
- relationships
- the social environment
- culture
- family
- community
- workplace

HEALTH IN THE BALANCE

We ought to be more amazed by ourselves. Countless cells in the body, each a miraculous tiny cauldron of chemical processes, perform the intricate chain reactions on which life depends – yet the body does not overheat from the sheer energy involved and copes seamlessly with outside pressures. The body maintains a state of balance, or equilibrium, called *homeostasis*, in which all systems function smoothly. The term implies a stable internal environment, but the very nature of being alive – the continuous generation, growth, and breaking down of cells, and the ever-changing environment and flux of feelings and thoughts – means that homeostasis is a dynamic state.

Well-being of people of all ages depends on staying in healthy homeostasis (balance).

MAINTAINING HOMEOSTASIS

The body is equipped to deal with everyday challenges, perpetually making the adjustments necessary to maintain equilibrium. In order to do this, it draws on resources in each of the three realms of the body and mind – the biochemical realm that fuels body processes; the structural realm that supports the organs and body systems; and the psychosocial realm that governs thoughts, desires, actions, and emotions. For example, after an exhausting and stressful day, a good night's sleep allows the biochemical furnace to cool down, the body's structures to rest and relax, and the mind to assimilate the day's events.

WHEN THINGS GO WRONG

If challenges become intense, unrelenting, or too frequent, the extraordinary capacity of the body and mind to adapt can be overwhelmed. Coping relies on energy and order, but if resources are depleted, the ability to maintain balance is undermined. Defense and repair systems may begin to fail if the integrity of cell chemistry, body structures, and mind are threatened.

So entwined and so intimate is the relationship between the three realms of the body that if a problem develops in one, it can affect the working of the other two. For example, a biochemical disorder such as nutritional deficiency or food sensitivity may have psychological consequences such as depression. Loneliness, bereavement, and inner conflicts can undermine immune defenses, while a structural injury might cause pain that then leads to relationship problems.

The underlying factor upsetting homeostasis might be obvious – a bereavement triggering depression, or a series of rushed working lunches resulting in bouts of indigestion. But sometimes the key cause is more difficult to pinpoint. It may be a combination of daily hassles and unhealthy diet, or the strain may lie in one realm but the effect may manifest in a seemingly unconnected quarter. Eczema, for example, can be provoked by emotional factors.

THE BALANCED BODY	THE BODY OUT OF BALANCE
HOMEOSTASIS IS LIKE A GYROSCOPE, which keeps spinning in the right conditions. Our bodies and minds can cope with change and adapt to challenges if they get what they need and are not pushed too far.	LIKE THE SPINNING GYROSCOPE, which if tilted too far will slow down and fall, homeostasis can be knocked off balance. Susceptibility increases when our needs are not met or if challenges are too great.

What builds up our power to cope and adapt?
- A balanced diet
- Relaxation
- Fresh air
- Regular exercise
- A balance of rest and activity
- Optimism
- Positive relationships
- Knowledge and access to information

What undermines our resilience?
- Poor diet • Unremitting stress
- Environmental pollution and toxins
- Inertia and lack of stimulation
- Low levels of physical activity
- Lack of rest
- Persistent psychological conflicts
- Pessimism and hostility
- Isolation and loneliness

THE RESPONSE TO STRESS

Well-being depends on maintaining a balance in the biochemical, structural, and psychosocial realms of the body, and on the adaptations that each realm must make in order to deal with the stressful demands placed on it. In the 1950s, Dr. Hans Selye first described the effects of stress and explained the three stages of adaptation as follows:

Stage One: The alarm stage, or the "fight or flight" response (*see page 84*). Biochemically, the stress hormones epinephrine and cortisol pour into the body. Structurally, muscles tense, especially around the head, neck, lower back, chest, and abdomen; blood flows to the muscles and away from the gut. Psychosocially, thoughts and feelings focus on escape or attack: The impulse is to fight, flee, or freeze. If the cause of stress is removed, the body returns to normal functioning.

Stage Two: If people remain under stress, their bodies compensate by maintaining these responses. At first this "adaptation" may feel normal, but energy is drained by the continual biochemical, structural, and psychosocial demands, which may produce minor infections, discomfort, or uneasiness.

Stage Three: Long-term biochemical, structural, or psychosocial stress leads to a deeper kind of exhaustion as reserves are depleted. It is harder to recover from even small demands, and severe health problems can develop. Whether this is expressed biochemically (as in a chronic inflammatory disease) structurally (persistent pain), or psychosocially (depression or panic attacks) depends more on the individual than on the stressors.

PREVENTING ILLNESS

The idea that homeostasis or our ability to maintain it depends on how we react to external influences is relatively new to Western medicine. It implies that internal factors may determine an individual's response to external demands. While illness may be triggered by factors such as infections, toxins, and work crises, its outcome is determined by internal resources. These include biochemical factors (diet, genetic constitution), structural factors (fitness, flexibility), and perhaps especially by psychosocial factors (temperament and coping style). Traditional holistic medical systems, such as Traditional Chinese Medicine, have always recognized the interplay between our inner nature and the world we inhabit, which may account for the renewed interest in these medical systems. The key to preventing health problems, increasing the ability to cope with life's demands and recover from illness, lies in mobilizing the natural resources of the body and mind. No matter how or where a health problem first manifests, it helps to tackle it in all three realms; for example, recovery from an infectious illness demands a positive outlook as well as a nutritious diet and plenty of rest.

Homeostasis involves adapting to extremes, such as vigorous exercise and periods of rest.

CHALLENGES TO HOMEOSTASIS

In a healthy person, the body's internal resources can cope with external threats. But if homeostasis is undermined, illness may result.

	BIOCHEMICAL	STRUCTURAL	PSYCHOSOCIAL
External Threats	Infections, pollution, toxins	Physical strain	Work overload, strife, and adversity
Internal Resources	Genetic constitution; good diet	Fitness; grace, flexibilty, strength	Temperament; communication skills; coping style, beliefs
Levels of External Threat			
Small (can be beneficial, helping to strengthen ways of coping, but over time can have cumulative effects)	Infections; environmental pollution	Minor injuries; physical demands and exercise	Deadlines at work; disputes with neighbor or relative
Moderate (can impair the body's ability to cope if internal resources are weak)	Inadequate diet	Persistent poor posture; repetitive occupational strain	Bad relationship; bereavement
Severe (can overwhelm the ability of the body and mind to cope, causing permanent damage or even death)	Poisoning; radiation	Severe injury from an accident or car crash	Suicidal depression; psychosis

TREATING ILLNESS

Illness is not the same as disease. Someone with a headache may feel ill, for example, without having a diagnosable disease. With a diagnosis based on the patient's story and clinical signs, a doctor can prescribe treatment. Complementary practitioners look differently at the symptoms and may suggest treatments to stimulate the patient's self-healing processes. The integrative approach seeks to use conventional treatments if a clear diagnosis and safe, effective treatments are available, and to negotiate complementary treatments with the patient, depending on their appropriateness and availability.

Stimulating the body's self-healing powers is an important part of integrative medicine.

CONVENTIONAL DIAGNOSIS AND TREATMENT

Moments of pain, discomfort, tension, nausea, breathlessness, or weakness are things most of us experience. If they are severe, persistent, or worrisome, we might report them to a doctor, who will ask questions – how long have we had these feelings, perhaps, and what makes them worse or better – and perform an examination to find clinical signs that could indicate the body is working abnormally, such as a raised temperature, rash, lumps, enlarged liver, or alteration in heartbeat. After the examination, the doctor might order blood or urine tests, X-rays, or even scans if a problem is potentially serious. These tests provide clues to the inner workings of the body. Some diseases, like high blood pressure, are detected with tests alone, before feelings of illness become apparent. Others, like depression, are diagnosed by symptoms because there are no relevant physiological tests.

Once a diagnosis is made, the doctor can proceed with suitable treatment. In life-threatening situations, such as appendicitis or a heart attack, medical science's high-tech interventions can be wonderfully effective. Magnetic resonance imaging, laser surgery, computer-targeted radiation therapy, organ transplants, and powerful drugs that fight infection are some of the leading-edge techniques that save lives every day. Gene therapy, with its exciting potential for diseases that are still hard to treat, lies just over the horizon.

DIFFICULT CONDITIONS

Doctors who practice integrative medicine aim to focus not only on symptoms but also on other relevant aspects of the person's life. The approach comes into its own for a number of conditions, including recurring disorders such as arthritis or eczema. For these, conventional

CONVENTIONAL DIAGNOSIS

- A doctor asks you about symptoms.
- You are examined for clinical signs of disease, such as a raised temperature, a rash, lumps, enlarged liver, or abnormal heartbeat.
- You may have blood and urine tests and X-rays.
- Only if concern exists about the possibility of serious illness would you be referred for tests such as magnetic resonance imaging.
- Depending on the diagnosis, treatment might include laser surgery, computer-targeted radiation therapy, organ transplants, and a wide range of drugs.

COMPLEMENTARY DIAGNOSIS

- A practitioner takes a full case history and asks about your lifestyle.
- Depending on the type of therapy, the practitioner might run diagnostic tests.
- The explanation given may bear no relationship to conventional diagnosis.
- The diagnosis will usually imply certain biochemical, structural, or psychosocial causes.
- Treatment is likely to be tailored to suit the individual.

Both conventional and complementary points of view are concidered.

DIFFERENT METHODS OF DIAGNOSIS AND TREATMENT

	CONVENTIONAL MEDICINE	TRADITIONAL CHINESE MEDICINE	INTEGRATIVE MEDICINE
Illness	Recurring headaches	Recurring headaches	Recurring headaches
Physical symptoms	One-sided, with visual disturbance and nausea	In addition, patient looks florid and has a bad taste in the mouth	In addition, patient is eating erratically and overworking
Method of diagnosis	Since onset was recent, full neurological examination to exclude tumor	Note appearance of face and tongue; take pulses	In addition, discuss psychological factors and ways of coping
Diagnosis	Migraine headaches	Stagnant Liver *qi*	Stress-related migraine and poor ways of coping
Treatment	Painkillers and antinausea drugs	Acupuncture and herbal remedy	Possibly medication and acupuncture, and definitely advice about diet, relaxation, and stress management

medicine on its own has no "magic bullet" to offer, and existing pharmaceutical treatments may be unsatisfactory or cause unwanted side effects. Not only are these conditions difficult and uncomfortable to live with, but they frequently require drugs such as anti-inflammatories, painkillers, or antibiotics, which patients are reluctant to take for long periods. For these conditions, other approaches, as well as altering lifestyle, can greatly help to improve well-being.

In chronic fatigue or persistent pain syndromes, for example, a biochemical approach may be unable to offer any effective treatment, since tests will not usually indicate any changes in body tissues. The absence of a specific detectable cause on which to target treatment can be frustrating. Such cases of "undifferentiated" illness pose difficulties for doctors, but those who take a more holistic approach will probe for any factors, such as overwork or poor diet, that might contribute to feelings of illness, and suggest complementary approaches.

Painful, stress-related illnesses that have not responded well to mainstream medicine are the conditions for which integrative medicine is likely to be most relevant. Such an approach might make use of traditional systems, such as herbal medicine or Chinese medicine, when the lack of a set of symptoms or clinical signs recognizable to Western medicine presents a problem. Language and concepts can be an obstacle to cooperation, however. Complementary therapies, which base diagnosis on a different interpretation of information about the patient's body and experiences, express ideas about causes that are incomprehensible to a conventional doctor. For example, an acupuncturist might attribute a certain type of headache to "stagnant Liver *qi*."

WHY TRY INTEGRATIVE MEDICINE?

Surveys show that between one-third and one-half of people in industrialized countries are using complementary therapies, which is perhaps evidence of the gap between people's expectations of conventional medicine and what it can actually provide. In particular, mainstream medicine's poor track record with chronic disorders (*see Glossary, pages 177–78*) and stress-related illnesses could be one of the

reasons for the growing popularity of non-conventional medicine. Even where conventional medicine is successful, the hope of avoiding unpleasant side effects has led to a growing public skepticism and even suspicion of the medical profession. Ironically, orthodox medicine could be a victim of its own success. Better housing, nutrition, and public health

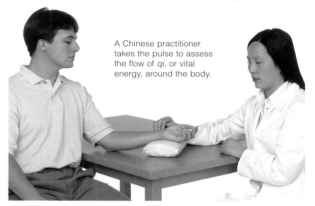

A Chinese practitioner takes the pulse to assess the flow of *qi*, or vital energy, around the body.

have overcome the much-feared infectious diseases of the 19th century, and in wealthy countries, child mortality has fallen and people live longer than ever before. As our expectations of well-being have risen, it is perhaps inevitable that we hope for too much from medical science.

However unrealistic these expectations, disappointed people are now also less inclined to accept that "doctor knows best," and we all are less prepared to tolerate paternalistic or authoritarian attitudes.

The integrative approach to health, with its emphasis on active self-help and on making use of complementary approaches, is especially relevant for chronic illnesses and stress-related conditions. If a doctor or a complementary therapist spends an hour or more asking detailed questions about our lifestyle, feelings, and experiences, we are likely to find this personally validating. It may also give us room to consider the emotional aspects of illness and even to explore a spiritual dimension. On a more mundane level, time spent working out how to become more healthy is time well spent.

IMPROVING RESILIENCE

Health and well-being are too important and too complex to be simply a medical matter. Ultimately they depend on the ability to adapt to challenges and to maintain homeostasis (*see pages 12–13*). In all three realms of the "body-mind" there are aspects of life that build us up and break us down. If we are under strain in one realm, strengthening the others may compensate. For example, playing tennis releases "feel-good" chemicals (endorphins) that can offset the damaging effects of emotional stress. The likelihood of becoming ill, which increases if body and mind fail to adapt to outside pressures, depends on factors that influence *susceptibility* and *resilience*.

Practicing yoga regularly helps improve resilience, raising resistance to disease.

ADAPTING TO PRESSURES

Some aspects of life are more controllable than others. It is possible to modify our diet, the amount of exercise we get, and our ways of coping with stress, for example, more readily than our workload or environment; our genetic inheritance and past medical history, on the other hand, are totally beyond our control. Optimum well-being involves learning to minimize factors that increase susceptibility to challenges and increase resilience.

"Susceptibility" is determined by factors that undermine well-being and make us more likely to become ill. Factors can be biochemical (inadequate diet, a genetic tendency toward certain diseases), structural (lack of exercise, unsanitary living conditions), or psychosocial (job loss, hostility). They may be one-time traumatic structural events, such as deprivation of oxygen at birth, or a major, hurtful psychological event in childhood. Alternatively they may be cumulative negative influences, for example, an overcritical parent or a chronically curved spine (scoliosis).

Resilience in one realm can be undermined by weakness in another. Even the sturdiest genetic constitution can be sabotaged by childhood malnutrition, for example, or by a disabling injury. However, it is often possible to learn to cope with factors that could sabotage health, and sometimes

susceptibility can even be a spur for personal growth. Fortunately human beings are remarkably resilient. Factors that promote health can be biochemical (good diet, protective genes), structural (regular exercise, clean airy accommodations), and psychosocial (high self-esteem, community, supportive friends and family, a culture of openness). We are creative and responsive by nature, and given the chance will naturally move toward well-being.

PROMOTING GOOD HEALTH

There is a direct relationship between susceptibility and disease; low susceptibility implies a high resilience. This equation varies enormously according to an individual's ability to cope, and obviously some people have more to work on in some areas than in others. Health promotion means building up what is good rather than only changing what is bad. It is important to aim for optimum health in all realms: biochemical, structural, and psychosocial (*see pages 138–75*). The great majority of diseases may be preventable if resilience is improved. In the early stages, if mind and body are not functioning well, but there are no obvious signs of disease, improving diet, lifestyle, and outlook will encourage the body's natural health-restoring processes to work effectively.

Eating antioxidant fruit and vegetables protects against cell damage.

SUSCEPTIBILITY AND RESILIENCE

	CAUSES OF SUSCEPTIBILITY	AIDS TO RESILIENCE
Biochemical	Hereditary tendencies	Antioxidant- and fiber-rich low-fat diet
Structural	Poor environment (overcrowding, pollution)	Appropriate exercise
Psychosocial	Poor coping skills; pessimism and hostility; poverty	Social support; sense of humor; self-esteem

BECOMING INVOLVED IN YOUR CARE

We have a lot to thank modern medicine for. Drugs or surgery can be lifesaving, even life-enhancing. At the same time, if you are ill, you should try to become involved in your care, building yourself up as much as possible to counteract any side effects of orthodox treatment or to maximize postoperative recovery as well as to help the body's self-healing powers do their work. You may need drugs for high blood pressure, for instance, but a healthy diet that includes foods high in potassium, such as fresh fruit and vegetables, combined with appropriate exercise and relaxation and stress management techniques, could forestall an increase in the dosage.

Becoming involved in your health care leads to a greater sense of control – what some experts have called "health empowerment." For example, an international program known as the Arthritis Self-Help Course teaches people with arthritis to manage their own disease. They learn how to design their personal exercise regimes, improve their nutrition, and master pain management techniques such as relaxation. They are also shown how to fight depression and fatigue, how to solve problems created by their condition, and how to communicate better with their doctors. The result is that participants report a dramatic decrease in pain, experience less disability than other people with arthritis, and need fewer visits to the doctor.

The trend toward consulting people as experts about their condition is part of a welcome change in doctor-patient partnerships. It promises a new science of well-being in which people help to shape the health care system to meet their real needs.

Learning how to relax can help the body's self-healing powers.

BENEFITS OF FITNESS

AEROBIC EXERCISE CAN HELP people cope with stress, depression, and other types of psychological strain. It releases "feel-good" chemicals (endorphins) and improves resilience in other ways (see pages 152–53).

STRUCTURAL
- Stretches soft tissues
- Improves muscle tone
- Makes the heart work harder
- Expands lung capacity
- Helps muscles relax (after exercise)

BIOCHEMICAL
- Produces "feel-good" chemicals
- Boosts metabolic rate
- Burns off stress chemicals

PSYCHOSOCIAL
- Provides companionship
- Releases aggression
- Encourages pride in athletic skills
- Promotes calmness (after exercise)

STEPS TO IMPROVE RESILIENCE

Efforts to improve resilience and maintain homeostasis should be made in all three realms of body and mind.

Biochemical Good nutrition (see pages 158–59) helps build and nourish cells and tissues, protects against disease, and counters premature aging. Avoiding pesticides, additives, and environmental chemicals may help counter cell damage.

Structural Exercise has far-reaching effects (see left) and generates a sense of well-being (see pages 152–53). Massage and other touch therapies, yoga, and qigong induce the "relaxation response" (see pages 170–71) that reverses the "fight or flight" response (see page 168).

Psychosocial Helpful techniques include behavioral methods (biofeedback, relaxation, and breathing) and cognitive approaches (meditation, guided imagery). These also induce the relaxation response (see page 172). Psychotherapy may counteract a tendency toward anxiety or depression. Positive thinking can help raise self-esteem and increase a sense of control, enabling people to communicate better and develop social support networks.

INTEGRATIVE CARE IN ACTION

Combining conventional and complementary medicine is more common than most people realize. In the US, a recent survey of family doctors found that more than half regularly prescribe complementary treatments or have tried such therapies themselves. When properly organized, the integrative approach can benefit all those involved – practitioners as well as patients. Most frequently integrated into family practices are those therapies with which doctors are most comfortable. These tend to be manipulation, acupuncture, stress management techniques, dietary advice, and counseling. Herbal medicine and meditation are sanctioned, though less frequently provided. Massage therapy, aromatherapy, and reflexology have been introduced into hospitals largely by nurses.

After diagnosis, patient and doctor agree on a treatment plan.

PIONEERING INITIATIVES

A number of programs around the world have pioneered the use of integrative medicine. In the US, for example, Dr. Dean Ornish has devised a program to reverse coronary heart disease without recourse to surgery or drugs. Patients follow a high-fiber diet, of which only 10 percent of daily calories come from fat. They exercise regularly, practice yoga and other stress management techniques, and attend group therapy sessions. It's an exacting regime – but it gets results.

The benefits of innovative programs are far-reaching. A California psychiatrist, Dr. David Spiegel, found that women with advanced breast cancer who attended weekly support groups and also used relaxation techniques and self-hypnosis survived twice as long as those who did not. His study, published in *The Lancet* in 1989, has encouraged thousands of similar support groups around the world – not only for breast cancer patients but for those with other life-threatening diseases, adding immeasurably to their quality of life.

INTEGRATIVE CARE IN HOSPITALS

Pain clinics, cancer treatment centers, and hospices are at the forefront of integrative health care, in which doctors and therapists cooperate to provide all-around care. Cancer patients at London's Hammersmith and Charing Cross Hospitals are routinely offered massage, aromatherapy, reflexology, and relaxation, as well as art therapy for those who prefer an alternative to "touch and talk" therapies. The service has the enthusiastic support of doctors, radiation therapists, and nurses; one noticeable effect is that patients with cancer of the head and neck require less Valium when undergoing claustrophobic radiation therapy.

INTEGRATIVE MEDICINE CENTERS

Centers for integrative medicine are flowering in the US. In Lyme, New Hampshire, for example, Dr. Robert Rufsvold, a holistic family doctor, merged practices with naturopath Maureen Williams to found the New England Center for Integrative Health, Inc. The two practitioners have regular case conferences to discuss shared patients and to tap into each other's expertise. Also working at the Center are a nutritionist, massage therapist and other body workers, two counselors, a chiropractor, and a Traditional Chinese Medicine practitioner, as well as yoga and t'ai chi instructors. Patient care is "relationship-centered," meaning that the alliance of patient and practitioner is central to all treatment and healing – a key element in integrative medicine.

London's Marylebone Health Centre, which opened in 1987, was the first UK National Health Service practice to employ complementary therapists and it is the subject of a long-term research study into the effectiveness of integrative medicine. The team comprises three full-time and two part-time family doctors, an osteopath, homeopath, naturopath, acupuncturist, massage therapist, and counselor. Conventional medicine is still the foundation of the practice, but doctors have the option of suggesting a therapy if they consider it appropriate for the patient's condition. Dr. Sue Morrison, who is in charge of the practice, says that she could not now imagine working without complementary therapies. "We have found we can contain problems – emotional as well as physical – that are usually difficult to look after in normal practice." Integrative medicine may also be part of the reason why Marylebone Health

Acupuncturists increasingly work in tandem with conventional doctors.

Centre has a low rate of referral to specialists and a drug-prescribing rate that is half the national average.

THE FUTURE OF INTEGRATIVE MEDICINE

Integrative medicine centers occasionally come under the umbrella of a hospital or university. Most of these centers, such as Dr. Herbert Benson's Mind/Body Medical Institute at New England's Deaconess Hospital and Harvard University Medical School, focus on research. Dr. Jon Kabat-Zinn's Center for Mindfulness in Medicine, Health Care and Society at the University of Massachusetts Medical Center is at the forefront of patient care as well.

"What are the common elements that allow a healing interaction to take place?" is a question that the planned Osher Center for Integrative Medicine at the University of California, San Francisco, seeks to answer. It hopes to offer patients complementary approaches of proven value and to provide information about integrative medicine to both the public and medical communities. Of course there are many questions and

difficulties in the path of integration. More research is needed to provide evidence that complementary therapies are safe and effective. Safety and efficacy themselves depend on a practitioner's skills, which is why education and training need to be improved and regulation introduced.

The US National Institutes of Health National Advisory Council for Complementary and Alternative Medicine now spends many millions of dollars a year on research and disseminating information. In the UK, the Foundation for Integrated Medicine, whose president is the Prince of Wales, is focused on resolving issues of safety, efficacy, and training.

Communication between doctors and different therapists can still be difficult. Even finding a common language is problematic. "Energy," "vital force," and "*qi*" are concepts that conventional medicine stumbles over, while some therapists abhor medical science's impersonal language of drugs and procedures. Nevertheless, the popularity of complementary medicine and the scale of public interest in health is a powerful driving force for change. A new type of medicine is definitely evolving for the 21st century.

Therapies such as reflexology are currently being evaluated and integrated into mainstream medicine.

THE POWER OF THE THERAPEUTIC RELATIONSHIP

THE TRUST BETWEEN PATIENT AND PRACTITIONER is a powerful force for healing, as demonstrated in the so-called placebo response. (A placebo is a chemically inert substance given in place of a drug.) It shows the power of relationships and expectations, and is one explanation of why a medication or treatment that should have no effect can actually make someone feel better.

If a group of people is given a placebo treatment, 30 percent – and, according to some researchers, as many as 90 percent – will report improvements. In clinical research trials, one half of a patient group is given placebo pills, while the other receives the active drug. Any treatment must outperform the placebo to be considered effective. Researchers have shown that expectation can actually change immune responses, even in

animals. Some experts say this shows that the mind can trigger our natural healing processes.

PATIENT-PRACTITIONER TRUST
According to Professor Herbert Benson, of Harvard Medical School, the essence of this healing depends on three elements:
• The patient's belief in or expectation of a good outcome.
• The caregiver's belief in and expectation of a good outcome.
• A relationship between the patient and the caregiver that generates positive belief and expectations.

Perhaps the special relationship between the patient and the practitioner is the most important fuel for this expectation of healing. In a famous study at Boston's Massachusetts General Hospital in 1964, patients undergoing

surgery who received a preoperative visit from a warm and sympathetic anesthetist recovered more quickly than other patients undergoing similar surgery who did not.

It also seems that the patient has responsibilities to cultivate a good relationship with caregivers. In another Boston study, patients with chronic illnesses such as diabetes, rheumatoid arthritis, and high blood pressure were coached to ask relevant questions of their doctor. Afterward they reported more satisfaction with their visit and even enjoyed better health than those who were not coached.

However, expectation can also work against healing. People experiencing insensitive treatment from practitioners often complain that they feel worse. This is known as the "nocebo" effect – the opposite of the placebo.

YOUR HEALTH CARE STRATEGY

Health is defined as the ability to adapt to change. The capacity to adapt depends on three interdependent realms: biochemical, structural, and psychosocial (*see right*). Disease, or simply feeling ill, is more likely if the body or mind is under strain. While factors that make illness more likely are found in all three realms, so too are the means of healing. In Treating Ailments (*pages 22–113*), various conditions and the different options for treatment, both conventional and complementary, are described, while Your Health Care Plan (*pages 138–75*) explains health skills that help you maintain well-being and build up resilience in all realms of body and mind.

THE THREE REALMS

BIOCHEMICAL REALM
Consists of cells, hormones, and enzymes; body systems such as digestion and respiration; the chemical environment and pollution; nutritional factors

STRUCTURAL REALM
Consists of muscles, bones, blood vessels, nerves, organs, and tissues; movement and posture; the physical environment

PSYCHOSOCIAL REALM
Consists of thoughts, feelings, and relationships; the social environment, culture, family, the community, and the workplace

TAKING CHARGE OF HEALTH

Becoming involved in your own health care, working with your practitioners and caregivers, and taking charge of your health destiny is empowering. Research shows that when people take responsibility for their health care, symptoms often improve and quality of life is enhanced. Responsibility, however, depends on knowledge and resources, so it is important to learn as much as possible about all the factors that influence your health. If you are prone to or already have a health problem, understanding that you need to compensate for this susceptibility is a necessary start. Knowing about causes, symptoms, and the range of available treatment options is obviously empowering. Knowledge about healthy eating, exercise, relaxation, and stress management techniques is essential for everyone who wants to build good health.

Certain attitudes of mind improve your chances of well-being, while others, such as poor self-esteem, high anxiety, not feeling in control of your life, pessimism, and hostility can make you more susceptible to illness. The relationship you have with health professionals, including complementary therapists, may determine whether you forge a "therapeutic alliance" (*see page 19*), potentially a key to unlocking the healing process. As in any good partnership, trust, communication, and mutual respect are vital (*see Working with Your Doctor, pages 146–47 and Finding a Practitioner, page 180*). To make best use of this book, follow the route below.

THE ROUTE TO BETTER HEALTH

1. SELF-ASSESSMENT
Which approaches best suit your personality, situation, and lifestyle?
• Fill out the questionnaire (*pages 140–43*) and see Finding the Right Therapy (*pages 144–45*).

2. ASSESSING YOUR PROBLEM
• Find out about particular health problems in Treating Ailments (*pages 22–113*).
• Any treatment should be safe and effective. Although research on complementary therapies is limited, it is growing. The "evidence of efficacy" ratings for each therapy in Treating Ailments indicates how effective the therapy is likely to be for that specific ailment.
• Research your ailment using the Bibliography (*pages 182–85*) and Finding Out More (*page 181*).

4. MAKING PROGRESS
• Keep a symptom diary (*page 147*) to monitor the success of your integrative health program.
• Fill out the questionnaire How Healthy Are You? (*pages 140–43*) again to compare your progress.

3. FINDING INFORMATION AND SUPPORT
• To find out how to improve your health, see Your Structural Health (*page 148–57*); Your Biochemical Health (*pages 158–67*), and Your Psychosocial Health (*pages 168–75*).
• To access the help you need, see Working with Your Doctor (*page 146*); Finding a Practitioner (*pages 180–81*), Finding Out More (*page 181*), and Useful Addresses (*pages 186–87*).

GENERAL PRECAUTIONS

• Do not attempt to diagnose a health problem yourself. Always consult your doctor.

• Consult a doctor immediately if you have any of the warning signs (*see page 147*).

• Check with a doctor if there is no improvement within 2–3 weeks (48 hours in children under five) or if symptoms get worse.

• Do not stop taking any prescribed medication without first consulting your doctor.

• Tell your complementary practitioner about any prescription medication you are taking, as well as any other complementary remedies you are taking.

• Tell your doctor about any complementary treatments you are receiving.

• Always check with a doctor before embarking on any complementary treatment if you have any serious medical condition.

• Do not begin a vigorous exercise program without first consulting a doctor if you have serious back pain, high blood pressure, or heart disease, or if you are pregnant.

• People with persistent mental illness may be disturbed by hypnosis, visualization, and meditation.

• Advise your practitioner if you have any sexually transmitted disease.

• Do not begin a course of complementary therapy without first consulting your doctor if you are pregnant or trying to conceive.

• Do not take or use any herbal or aromatherapy products or nutritional supplements during pregnancy or if breast-feeding unless supervised by an experienced practitioner.

• Consult your doctor before allowing either babies or infants to receive long-term complementary treatments.

• Enemas and certain herbal remedies are unsuitable for small children.

• Children under 12 should receive complementary treatments only with professional supervision, a doctor's consent, and parental involvement.

• Children under 16 should not fast.

• Do not take supplements of iron or vitamin A without first consulting your doctor. Do not exceed the recommended dosage of other supplements unless directed by a qualified practitioner.

• Do not take high doses of nutritional supplements without professional supervision.

• Do not embark on fasts lasting longer than two days without professional advice.

HERBAL REMEDY PRECAUTIONS

SOME HERBAL REMEDIES can interfere with the action of conventional drugs or heighten their effect. Consult a pharmacist, doctor or medical herbalist.

Echinacea can affect the liver if used for more than eight weeks, especially if taken with liver-toxic drugs, e.g. anabolic steroids.

Evening primrose oil and **borage oil** can lower the seizure threshold if taken with anticonvulsants.

Feverfew, **ginkgo biloba**, **garlic** and **Chinese angelica** (dong quai) can interfere with warfarin.

Ginseng can interfere with digoxin, increase the effect of estrogens and corticosteroids, and cause manic side effects with antidepressants.

Licorice can increase side-effects of corticosteroids.

St John's wort can increase side effects of antidepressants.

Do not take without medical advice if prescribed cyclosporin, warfarin, digoxin, theophylline or oral contraceptives.

Senna, **cascara** and **psyllium** can decrease drug absorption.

Valerian may increase the sedative effects of barbiturates.

Yohimbe can increase hypertension if taken with tricyclic antidepressants.

A partnership of trust between patient and practitioner is key to the success of integrative health care.

POINTS TO REMEMBER

• Sharing ideas and working together to address different aspects of a patient's health is a bold new step for many practitioners, both conventional and complementary. If you are not fortunate enough to be in an integrative practice, expect to find that YOU are the one orchestrating any integration of health care approaches.

• Not all orthodox practitioners are knowledgeable about non-conventional therapies and few can offer expert advice about procedures, benefits, or even risks.

• Many complementary practitioners know little about other therapies and tend to believe that the one they practice will suit you best.

• Find out as much as you can about

(a) your illness

(b) your practitioner and/or therapist

(c) treatments available

chapter

2

Drugs and surgery are essential for life-threatening

conditions and can ease many symptoms, while

complementary therapies may alleviate some of their

side effects and tackle underlying causes of illness.

TREATING AILMENTS

Here we describe over 40 ailments that especially

benefit from integrative medicine. We explain the

best treatment options, suggest self-help strategies,

and offer case studies of the integrative approach in

action. To help you evaluate the efficacy of a therapy

in relation to a particular ailment, we give ratings

based on the available evidence (*see pages 182–85*).

HEADACHES

Most adults suffer from tension headaches at some time, and about 2–3 percent of adults get chronic tension or muscle contraction headaches more than 15 days a month. "Tension headache" is the conventional diagnosis when there is no vascular cause, as in a migraine (*see page 26*).

The exact cause is poorly understood, but factors include disorders of the joints and muscles of the neck and jaw, and psychological strain. The site of the pain may vary and the pain can range from a dull thudding to sharp intensity. A doctor will try to identify and treat the root cause of a severe, unusual nontension headache.

CASE STUDY

Mark, an osteopath, saw Simon, 32, a journalist, who often suffered from neck pain and headaches. Mark found tender points in the back of Simon's neck and restricted upper-neck movement. "Simon is a tall guy and, as I discovered, he often sat hunched over his keyboard. His screen was set to one side of his desk, with glare from a window, and his office chair was difficult to readjust." After stretching and manipulating Simon's neck joints, Mark gave him advice about posture and a booklet explaining how to position his work station correctly. Simon also persuaded his employer to buy him a better chair. After three sessions, his neck pain eased. "The headaches were slow to get better, but moving the computer screen has made a big difference."

BIOCHEMICAL FACTORS

Headaches can be a sign of drinking too little water or too much caffeine or alcohol. They may also be a side effect of a drug or a symptom of a fever. Headaches that occur daily, soon after waking, may be due to low blood-sugar levels. If painkillers are taken daily for months, they lose their effect and actually cause more headaches. Withdrawal headaches can also result if painkillers are stopped suddenly.

BIOCHEMICAL TRIGGERS

• Low blood-sugar levels (hypoglycemia)
• Mild dehydration • Excess caffeine or sudden withdrawal • Excess alcohol • Food additives • Premenstrual tension and other hormonal changes • Medication such as oral contraceptives or HRT • Overuse of painkillers, especially codeine • Constipation or fever

PSYCHOSOCIAL FACTORS

Stress, fatigue, and depression account for the tension that produces most headaches, especially those located in the back of the head or behind the forehead.

PSYCHOSOCIAL TRIGGERS

• Anxiety • Lack of sleep • Overwork
• Emotional trauma • Depression • Personality traits (such as difficulty expressing anger)

STRUCTURAL FACTORS

Conditions such as high blood pressure and sinusitis can give rise to headaches. However, tension in the muscles of the shoulders, neck, and around the eyes and jaw is probably the most usual cause. This structural tension builds up gradually and eventually becomes persistent, with the muscles prone to irritability and spasm.

STRUCTURAL TRIGGERS

• Poor posture • Working too long at a computer • Neck injury (such as whiplash)
• Wear and tear on neck joints • Bright sunlight, wind, or changes in atmospheric pressure • Sinusitis • High blood pressure

PRECAUTIONS

Consult a doctor about any unusual, severe, one-sided, or persistent headache, especially if it is accompanied by drowsiness, nausea, vomiting, intolerance of light, stiff neck, or a rash. Also see a doctor after a head injury and if self-help treatments for minor headaches do not work within 3–7 days.

Realms of the Body *(see page 20)*

● **BIOCHEMICAL**
Body systems,
such as digestion

● **STRUCTURAL**
Muscles, bones,
joints, and nerves

○ **PSYCHOSOCIAL**
Thoughts, feelings,
and relationships

Key: Evidence of Efficacy *(see page 182)*

❶ ❷ ❸ ❹ ❺

least evidence ◀────────▶ most evidence

BIOCHEMICAL TREATMENT OPTIONS

CONVENTIONAL MEDICINE
Painkillers such as acetaminophen, aspirin, or ibuprofen *(see Drugs Glossary, page 179)* help relieve occasional headaches. Some drugs have a muscle relaxant. Amitriptyline can help chronic tension headaches.

COMPLEMENTARY THERAPIES
Western Herbalism ❷ *(see page 127)*
A practitioner may recommend a calming herb such as valerian, kava, or chamomile. These help calm the mind,

reduce stress, and encourage sleep.
Caution: Do not take valerian with sleep-inducing drugs.
Nutritional Therapies ❷
(see pages 128–29)
Practitioners seek to address the cause, such as constipation or low blood sugar, and try to boost general health. This might involve detoxification to support the liver, short fasts, and antioxidant vitamins.

Valerian

Homeopathy ❷ *(see page 130)*
Nux vomica may be worth trying for chronic tension headaches, although there is little research to support its use.

SELF-HELP TECHNIQUES
• Eat sensibly and make time for regular meals and snacks if you are prone to low blood-sugar levels
• Drink plenty of fluids but limit tea, coffee, cocoa, and cola, which contain caffeine • Do not smoke or drink excess alcohol.

STRUCTURAL TREATMENT OPTIONS

CONVENTIONAL MEDICINE
If headaches are severe, unusual, or persistent, a blood test, X-rays, and even a brain scan may be advised. Physical-therapy can help ease muscle tension.

COMPLEMENTARY THERAPIES
Chiropractic ❸ *(see page 118)* and
Osteopathy ❸ *(see page 119)*
Treatment aims to help the muscles relax and the joints to move more freely. Cranial osteopathy uses delicate manipulation to ease tension.

Alexander Technique ❷ *(see page 121)*
This can help prevent tension headaches by correcting poor posture.
Hydrotherapy ❷ *(see page 126)*

Cold water relieves symptoms.

Splashing your face with cold water before lying down for an hour eases a headache. Alternate hot and cold showers dilate, then constrict blood vessels, stimulating circulation. An ice pack on the back of the head may help.

Caution: Avoid alternate hot and cold showers if you have a heart condition.

SELF-HELP TECHNIQUES
• Exercise improves cardiovascular function, reducing stress and releasing endorphins, the body's painkillers
• With your fingertips, massage up the back of your neck, around the base of your skull, over your scalp, and around your ears • Pressing acupressure points Colon 4 and Liver 3 may help *(see page 125)*.

PSYCHOSOCIAL TREATMENT OPTIONS

CONVENTIONAL MEDICINE
Clinical depression should be treated. Cognitive behavioral therapy might be advised if headaches are chronic and severe.

COMPLEMENTARY THERAPIES
Visualization ❸ *(see page 134)*
Learning this technique, which shows you how to harness the power of your imagination, can enable you to relax tense muscles and calm your mind at will, which relieves stress.

Biofeedback ❹ *(see page 136)*
Techniques that train you to control muscle tension may relieve headaches.

SELF-HELP TECHNIQUES
• Keep a symptom- and stress-trigger diary *(see pages 147 and 175)* • Examine the causes of stress in your life and be prepared to make some changes • Make sure you get adequate sleep
• Practice relaxation and

breathing techniques *(see pages 170–71)* and use stress management techniques *(see pages 168–69)* • If you feel a headache coming on, a therapy such as meditation *(see page 135)* or autogenic training *(see page 136)* may help prevent it. Alternatively, follow the self-help relaxation sequence on page 171.

Autogenic training can allow you to relax at will.

MIGRAINE

About 10 percent of people suffer from migraine, with three times as many women affected as men. An intense, throbbing pain is felt, usually on one side of the head, with nausea, vomiting, and sensitivity to sound, light, and smells. Before an attack, about 25 percent of sufferers have visual disturbances such as zigzag lines, blind spots, and flashing lights, known as an aura. Migraine is caused by a spasm of large blood vessels in the brain. Blood vessels constrict, which can bring about the hallucinatory aura, and then dilate, causing the throbbing pain. Attacks vary in severity and frequency and can last for up to 72 hours.

CASE STUDY

John, who runs a hatha yoga class, helped Angie control the migraines that had plagued her for years. Angie, a 40-year-old manager with two children, had suffered a major migraine almost every week. After trying painkillers and other treatments, her doctor recommended the yoga class. John suggested that Angie do a series of neck-stretching exercises, the Cobra, the Pose of the Child, and alternate nostril breathing. After her first class, Angie had her best night's sleep for a long time. Angie now practices yoga daily. She concludes, "Calm, deep breathing helps me recognize when I am tense; I can relax my mind and body, and I feel in control. Now months go by without a migraine."

BIOCHEMICAL FACTORS

Migraine tends to run in families, so there may be a genetic predisposition. Certain chemicals found in food or made by the body raise levels of the chemical serotonin, which constricts blood vessels in the brain. When these vessels widen again, they release prostaglandins, causing pain, nausea, and vomiting.

BIOCHEMICAL TRIGGERS

• Intolerance of certain foods, especially of tyrosine-rich foods, such as aged cheese, red wine, and pickled herring, and of preservative nitrates, found in processed meats
• Chemicals such as caffeine and alcohol
• Hormonal swings caused by the Pill, menstruation, pregnancy, or menopause

STRUCTURAL FACTORS

Musculoskeletal disorders sometimes cause migraines possibly because a spasm in the arteries that supply the brain is triggered by misalignment of the neck vertebrae. This seems more likely to happen if there are tender points in the upper back or neck. Tension in the muscles of the neck and shoulders makes the problem worse.

STRUCTURAL TRIGGERS

• Physical tension caused by emotional stress such as anxiety or overwork • Poor posture • Injury to the neck • Lack of exercise and fitness • Hyperventilation

PSYCHOSOCIAL FACTORS

Lifestyle and stress can contribute to migraine attacks. Personality is also a factor. Ambitious, intelligent, extroverted, or obsessive people are more likely to be sufferers. Even childhood experiences and relationships can influence a person's reaction to emotional or environmental triggers.

PSYCHOSOCIAL TRIGGERS

• Emotional stress such as anxiety, excitement, anger, or shock • Loud noises, strong smells, bright or flickering lights • Travel, weather changes • Lack of, or too much, sleep

Realms of the Body (see page 20)

● **BIOCHEMICAL**
Body systems,
such as digestion

● **STRUCTURAL**
Muscles, bones,
joints, and nerves

○ **PSYCHOSOCIAL**
Thoughts, feelings,
and relationships

Key: Evidence of Efficacy (see page 182)

❶ ❷ ❸ ❹ ❺

least evidence ◄————————► most evidence

BIOCHEMICAL TREATMENT OPTIONS

CONVENTIONAL MEDICINE

A doctor may prescribe painkillers, such as acetaminophen, aspirin, or codeine; antinausea drugs such as metoclopramide or ergotamine (these are now used less since they can cause side effects); or serotonin-inhibiting drugs such as sumatriptan, zolmitriptan, or naratriptan (see Drugs Glossary, page 179). Severe migraine attacks can be halted with injectable medicines.

COMPLEMENTARY THERAPIES

Western Herbalism ❹ (see page 127)
Regular intake of fresh feverfew leaves may prevent attacks. Parthenolide, the key ingredient in feverfew, can inhibit the release of serotonin. Feverfew tablets are available over the counter, but check that the parthenolide content in them is high.
Caution: Do not take feverfew if you are pregnant or if mouth ulcers appear.

Fresh feverfew

Nutritional Therapies ❹
(see pages 128–29)

Short fasts are recommended to clear toxins, and elimination and rotation diets to avoid trigger foods. Nutritional supplements such as evening primrose oil and bioflavin (vitamin B_2) may be recommended.

SELF-HELP TECHNIQUES

• Avoid foods high in tyrosine (see opposite) and preservatives • Do not skip meals.

STRUCTURAL TREATMENT OPTIONS

CONVENTIONAL MEDICINE

You may be prescribed beta blockers or a serotonin blocker to prevent the dilation of blood vessels (see Drugs Glossary, page 179).

COMPLEMENTARY THERAPIES

Chiropractic ❸ (see page 118) and
Osteopathy ❸ (see page 119)
Manipulation of the neck or cranial osteopathy may be used to correct misalignments of the vertebrae that can cause migraines.

Shiatsu ❷ (see page 125)
A combination of massage and pressure aims to restore "energy balance" and induce relaxation.
Acupuncture ❹ (see page 125)
Practitioners seek to restore "energy balance". Needling may ease pain by stimulating endorphins, or natural painkillers.

SELF-HELP TECHNIQUES

• Massage your neck, scalp, and face (see page 116) • Soothing aromatherapy

oils include lavender, peppermint, eucalyptus, and chamomile essential oils (see page 117) • Apply pressure to acupressure points Liver 3, Liver 4, Gallbladder 14, and Gallbladder 20 (see page 125) • Helpful yoga postures are neck stretches and breathing exercises.

Massage away the pain of a migraine.

PSYCHOSOCIAL TREATMENT OPTIONS

CONVENTIONAL MEDICINE

Your doctor may advise you to learn to recognize and avoid potentially stressful situations.

COMPLEMENTARY THERAPIES

Hypnotherapy ❸ (see page 134)
Experiencing trance-induced relaxation during hypnosis may help you to relax at will.
Meditation ❸ (see page 135)
Relaxation techniques such as meditation can help you recognize signs of

stress in your body, and let you calm the mind and relax muscles.
Biofeedback ❹ (see page 136)
By using a sensory device you can learn to control spasms in the arteries that supply the brain.

Biofeedback can aid relaxation.

SELF-HELP TECHNIQUES

• Keep a diary of your migraine attacks, noting any triggers to avoid
• Techniques that lower stress can be learned as part of a therapy such as autogenic training (see page 136)
• Learn relaxation and breathing techniques by following the self-help sequence on pages 170–71. The diaphragmatic breathing and relaxation these techniques encourage can relax muscle tension, and may help prevent a migraine attack in its early stages.

ACNE

For a number of reasons, the sebaceous (oil) glands at the base of hair follicles in the skin can become blocked, resulting in acne – an unsightly skin disorder that includes pimples, blackheads, whiteheads, and, if the oil gland becomes inflamed, pustules and cysts. The most common form, *Acne vulgaris*, affects the areas of the body with high concentrations of sebaceous glands: the face, neck, upper chest, shoulders, and upper back. A tendency toward acne may be hereditary and the condition is linked to hormonal activity – some women are prone to outbreaks in the days before their periods, for example, and outbreaks commonly occur at puberty, affecting as many as seven out of ten adolescents.

CASE STUDY

Karen, a nutritionist, treated Matt, 13, for acne. A fast-growing boy, he ate a typical teenage diet of junk food and sugary drinks. His doctor had prescribed low-level antibiotics and Karen suggested "live" yogurt and *lactobacillus* supplements to restore friendly gut bacteria. Matt agreed to reduce his intake of sweet and fatty foods, to eat three pieces of fruit and a green vegetable every day, and to drink at least a quart of water.
"Zinc is a vital nutrient for skin health and is often depleted as the body's demand increases during growth spurts," said Karen. She recommended taking 15 mg of zinc daily and advised Matt to wash only with natural, unperfumed soap. Six months later Matt's acne had diminished and his skin looked better.

BIOCHEMICAL FACTORS

At puberty, testosterone production increases in both sexes, which stimulates overproduction of sebum (the skin's natural oil) in some people. Most doctors say there is no evidence that diet and stress play a part, but many complementary therapists think that a high-fat, sugary diet can aggravate acne.

BIOCHEMICAL TRIGGERS

• Increase in testosterone production at puberty • Midcycle female hormonal fluctuations • Family history • Certain drugs such as corticosteroids, androgens, barbiturates, and anticonvulsants • Oral contraceptives • Contact with cooking oils, greasy cosmetics, and industrial pollutants • High intake of junk food and sodas

STRUCTURAL FACTORS

A plug of sebum can form in a hair follicle, creating a blackhead. If the opening to the hair follicle is blocked, the sebaceous gland enlarges, turning into a whitehead. Bacteria multiply, infecting the blocked follicle, which becomes inflamed, forming a pimple. This fills with pus and eventually bursts. Infection can spread, particularly if hygiene is poor, so that as one pimple heals, others appear.

STRUCTURAL TRIGGERS

• Poor skin hygiene • Irritation from backpack or helmet straps

PSYCHOSOCIAL FACTORS

Although acne is not a serious complaint, and certainly not infectious, the emotional impact can be considerable, particularly on self-conscious teenagers. Some practitioners believe that the stress resulting from the psychological effects of acne, which can include embarrassment, lack of confidence, anxiety, and even depression, make the condition worse.

PSYCHOSOCIAL TRIGGERS

• Stress and fatigue

Realms of the Body (*see page 20*)

● **BIOCHEMICAL**
Body systems,
such as digestion

● **STRUCTURAL**
Muscles, bones,
joints, and nerves

● **PSYCHOSOCIAL**
Thoughts, feelings,
and relationships

Evidence of Efficacy (*see page 182*)

❶ ❷ ❸ ❹ ❺
least evidence ◄――――――――► most evidence

BIOCHEMICAL TREATMENT OPTIONS

CONVENTIONAL MEDICINE

If topical preparations (*see below*) do not clear up acne, a doctor may prescribe long-term courses of antibiotics, usually tetracycline or erythromycin (*see Drugs Glossary, page 179*), to kill bacteria and reduce inflammation. Your doctor may also prescribe retinoid drugs to reduce production of sebum and to promote skin regrowth. Hormones might be prescribed to treat women with cyclical acne.

COMPLEMENTARY THERAPIES
Western Herbalism ❷ (*see page 127*)
Practitioners may recommend blood-cleansing herbs such as red clover and dandelion, and immunity-enhancing remedies, including echinacea.
Nutritional Therapies ❸
(*see pages 128–29*)
Practitioners see acne as a sign that the digestion and/or hormonal systems are unbalanced. They may recommend an elimination diet and a short fast or a raw food diet, with supplements of zinc,

beta carotene, and other antioxidants including selenium; vitamin E; evening primrose oil; and, for menstrual-related acne, vitamin B_6. Long-term use of antibiotics can affect well-being, so if you are taking these a nutritionist may treat you for dysbiosis (*see page 93*).

SELF-HELP TECHNIQUES
• Eat a high-fiber diet and avoid saturated fat (*see page 158*).

Antioxidant fruit
and vegetables

STRUCTURAL TREATMENT OPTIONS

CONVENTIONAL MEDICINE

Your doctor might prescribe topical creams and lotions that contain benzoyl peroxide and retinoic acid (*see Drugs Glossary, page 179*) to reduce sebum and loosen blackheads, and antibiotics to kill bacteria. Controlled exposure to ultraviolet light, in the form of natural sunlight or artificial UVA light, may be recommended. In severe cases, dermabrasion (removal of the top layer of skin) can improve the appearance of the skin.

COMPLEMENTARY THERAPIES
Aromatherapy ❸ (*see page 117*)
A 1990 Australian study found antiseptic essential oil of tea tree to be as effective for acne as benzoyl peroxide. Dab a pimple with one drop, or add 3–4 drops to one teaspoon of witch hazel and use as a lotion. A steam inhalation with 3–4 drops of

Cleansing steam
helps acne.

lavender or chamomile oil can help open pores, reduce inflammation, and aid healing. **Caution:** If you have asthma, use steam inhalations carefully.

SELF-HELP TECHNIQUES
• Do not squeeze pimples, which can make them worse and lead to scarring
• Keep affected areas clean by washing daily with soap or cleansing bars and hot water • Get regular exercise, which stimulates the circulation to the skin and improves immune defenses.

PSYCHOSOCIAL TREATMENT OPTIONS

CONVENTIONAL MEDICINE

A doctor may suggest psychotherapy if lack of confidence and depression are severe.

COMPLEMENTARY THERAPIES
Psychotherapy & Counseling ❷
(*see pages 132–33*)
If the skin condition is severe enough to cause lack of confidence and emotional or relationship difficulties, talking about your feelings with a trained counselor can be useful.

This will help you to put things in perspective, and to restore dented self-esteem and confidence.
Visualization ❷ (*see page 134*)
Biofeedback ❷ (*see page 136*)
Relaxation & Breathing ❷
(*see pages 170–71*)
In a research study a combination of these therapies was found

Diaphragmatic breathing
reduces stress levels.

to be effective in helping to relieve chronic acne.

SELF-HELP TECHNIQUES
• Make sure you get plenty of sleep to help promote skin cell regeneration • Stress management techniques that include regular exercise and relaxation, and limit alcohol, may give your immune system a necessary boost.

PSORIASIS

In psoriasis, raised, rough reddened patches covered with silvery gray scales appear on the skin, accompanied by itching in some cases. They are caused by overproduction of new skin and can occur all over the body but are particularly likely to be found around the elbows, knees, scalp, trunk, and nails. About one person in 50 is prone to psoriasis, which usually appears in late childhood or early adulthood, but can develop at any age. It is hereditary in 30 percent of cases and is not contagious. Psoriasis is a persistent condition, but fluctuates in intensity, tending to be more severe when people are run down or sick, and during the winter.

CASE STUDY

Ling, an herbalist practicing Traditional Chinese Medicine (TCM), treated Alison, 39, who had developed widespread psoriasis following a car accident 11 years previously. Recently the condition had worsened, spreading to her arms, legs, back, and abdomen; it itched intensely at night. Alison had discussed TCM with her doctor because she found conventional ointments messy. He agreed to monitor her progress. Ling examined Alison's skin, tongue, and pulse according to TCM diagnostic methods and then prescribed an herbal remedy with nine ingredients, including rehmannia, red peony root, and licorice. She said t'ai chi would help Alison feel calmer and suggested she decrease her intake of animal fats. In a month, Alison's itching had begun to subside; in four months her skin was much better.

BIOCHEMICAL FACTORS

The cause of psoriasis is unknown, although it tends to run in families. It is thought that an inherited skin defect that allows skin cells to proliferate at many times the normal rate causes psoriasis to develop under certain conditions. Hormonal factors may be involved, since the condition often appears around puberty.

BIOCHEMICAL TRIGGERS

• Family history • Infections, especially strep throat • Certain drugs (chloroquine, lithium, indomethacin, some beta blockers – *see Drugs Glossary, page 179*) • Severe sunburn or irritation • Acute hives (allergic skin rash), especially in children

STRUCTURAL FACTORS

There are three types: discoid or plaque psoriasis with red scaly patches; pustular psoriasis with tiny yellow blisters; and guttate psoriasis in which many small patches develop rapidly. In each case, new skin cells are produced about ten times faster than usual. Live cells pile up, forming thickened patches covered with dead, scaly, flaking skin. One in 20 people develops a painful complication – inflammation of the joints known as psoriatic arthropathy.

STRUCTURAL TRIGGERS

• Skin injury or surgery

PSYCHOSOCIAL FACTORS

Emotional stress and anxiety at home or in the workplace can trigger and aggravate psoriasis. Worry about appearance may also be a contributing factor.

PSYCHOSOCIAL TRIGGERS

• Emotional stress • Embarrassment and lack of confidence if patches are visible and shedding scales • Stress caused by pain and irritation from sore, itchy skin • Interference with work and social life if psoriasis leads to psoriatic arthropathy (*see left*), which can restrict movement • Stress caused by loss of earnings if employers object to time off work for treatment

Realms of the Body (*see page 20*)

● BIOCHEMICAL
Body systems,
such as digestion

● STRUCTURAL
Muscles, bones,
joints, and nerves

○ PSYCHOSOCIAL
Thoughts, feelings,
and relationships

Key: Evidence of Efficacy (*see page 182*)

❶ ❷ ❸ ❹ ❺

least evidence ◄─────► most evidence

BIOCHEMICAL TREATMENT OPTIONS

CONVENTIONAL MEDICINE
Cancer-therapy drugs methotrexate and cyclosporin (*see Drugs Glossary, page 179*) stop cell growth in severe cases but can have unpleasant side effects. Acitretin, derived from vitamin A, reduces the thickness of patches and helps pustular psoriasis, but must not be taken in pregnancy.

Aloe vera

COMPLEMENTARY THERAPIES
Western Herbalism ❸ (*see page 127*)

Natural creams containing beeswax or banana peel extract may help. In German studies, extract of *Mahonia aquifolium* tree bark relieved patients' symptoms. Herbalists may give sarsaparilla to improve elimination, and chamomile, licorice, and aloe vera to calm the nervous system and soothe the skin.
Nutritional Therapies ❸ (*see pages 128–29*)
Practitioners link psoriasis with bowel toxins and impaired liver function, and may advise detoxification and immune-enhancing or elimination diets (*see page 166*). Supplements of vitamin C, zinc, and vitamin A (beta carotene) may be suggested to inhibit excessive skin cell growth. Evidence for benefits of essential fatty acids (fish oils and evening primrose oil) is conflicting.

SELF-HELP TECHNIQUES
• Follow a healthy whole-grain diet with plenty of fruit and vegetables.

STRUCTURAL TREATMENT OPTIONS

CONVENTIONAL MEDICINE
Greasy preparations for the skin, such as soft paraffin, ease dryness. Coal-tar or diflorasone creams (*see Drugs Glossary, page 179*) are helpful but are smelly, messy, and leave stains. Topical retinoid gels inhibit skin cell production and inflammation. Steroid creams are very effective but can thin the skin and are prescribed sparingly. In PUVA (psoralen-ultraviolet A) light treatment, patients take oral psoralen, which sensitizes skin cells to UVA radiation.

Relaxing in a hot bath for 15 minutes each day will help remove skin scales.

COMPLEMENTARY THERAPIES
Hydrotherapy ❷ (*see page 126*)
A hot Epsom Salts bath may help to eliminate toxins through the skin and stimulate circulation.

SELF-HELP TECHNIQUES
• Avoid nylon, leather, and wool
• Moisturize your skin and do not use strong soaps, detergents, shampoos, perfumes, and bubble baths • Exposure to sunlight (for limited periods and with sun protection) may help.

PSYCHOSOCIAL TREATMENT OPTIONS

CONVENTIONAL MEDICINE
Doctors may recommend stress management skills (*see pages 168–69*).

COMPLEMENTARY THERAPIES
Psychotherapy & Counseling ❶ (*see pages 132–33*)
Cognitive behavioral therapy and hypnotherapy can help prevent scratching and improve coping skills.
Meditation ❷ (*see page 135*)
Recent studies have found that meditating "mindfully" while

undergoing controlled exposure to UVA light treatment improved results; patients were asked to become aware of their breathing, and to visualize the light slowing down skin cell growth.
Biofeedback ❸ (*see page 136*)
Learning to lower skin temperature through biofeedback training, plus relaxation techniques, may help.
Relaxation & Breathing ❷ (*see pages 170–71*)
Patients who, while undergoing conventional treatment, learn

relaxation techniques in group therapy improve faster and need fewer drugs.

SELF-HELP TECHNIQUES
• Recording your feelings in a diary (*see page 175*) helps identify and avoid stress triggers
• Avoid overwork. Psoriasis often improves during vacations with plenty of sunshine and relaxation.

Keep a stress diary.

ECZEMA

Also known as dermatitis, eczema is a chronic inflammation of the skin causing itching, blistering, weeping, and scaling. It affects about one in eight children and one in 12 adults. Eczema can occur anywhere, but most commonly appears on the hands, arms, and face, or in skin folds and creases. The most widespread type, *atopic eczema*, runs in families and is associated with asthma and hay fever. *Seborrheic eczema* occurs on the face and head, and is the most common cause of dandruff. It is caused by the overproduction of skin cells and a yeast organism on the skin. *Contact eczema*, as the name suggests, is a localized reaction to irritants.

CASE STUDY

Charles, a homeopath, treated Maria, a hairdresser, 25, for eczema. Maria also complained of a lack of energy, backache, and pains in her hips. "She was charming, quiet, overweight, slightly sweaty, and anxious. When particularly worried – as she was with her wedding coming up – eczema broke out on her face." Charles concluded that Maria was a typical *Calc. carb.* homeopathic type and prescribed a one-time, potent dose of the remedy *Calc. carb. 200c.* For about a month, Maria reported very vivid, anxious dreams, but then her skin improved "about 70 percent," her backache was relieved, and her energy increased. "Once or twice a year she relapses with an outbreak of eczema but another *200c* dose of *Calc. carb.* clears it up," says Charles.

BIOCHEMICAL FACTORS

Eczema is an allergic skin reaction to a wide range of external and internal irritants. In many cases, it can be difficult to identify the exact cause. For some reason, the immune system reacts to an innocuous substance as if it were harmful, triggering inflammation in the skin cells. Food sensitivities can often trigger eczema. Many children with eczema are allergic to house dust.

BIOCHEMICAL TRIGGERS

• Cow's milk • Wheat • Eggs • Peanuts • Citrus fruit • Food addititives and preservatives • Lack of protective proteins acquired during breast feeding • Premature weaning to dairy products and wheat

STRUCTURAL FACTORS

External irritants provoke contact eczema and can work in tandem with internal causes to aggravate atopic eczema. It is possible for some people to become allergic to things they have used for years.

STRUCTURAL TRIGGERS

• Chemicals found in detergent, soap, cosmetics, and perfume • Environmental chemicals and pollutants • Nickel and chrome (found in jewelry and wristwatches) • Adhesive bandages • Wool, leather, and synthetic fibers • Chemicals in rubber • Heat

PSYCHOSOCIAL FACTORS

Stress and emotional tension of any sort can provoke and aggravate eczema. Studies show that people with chronic eczema have higher levels of anxiety, hostility, and neurosis than those without.

PSYCHOSOCIAL TRIGGERS

• Unacknowledged stress • Bereavement • Bullying • Embarassment and lack of confidence

BIOCHEMICAL TREATMENT OPTIONS

CONVENTIONAL MEDICINE

Antibiotics

A doctor will try to identify and remove the cause and may perform allergy tests. Antibiotics (*see Drugs Glossary, page 179*) will be prescribed to clear up infection and antihistamines to reduce itching. Corticosteroid creams reduce inflammation: Hydrocortisone is the weakest and safest. Antifungals help relieve seborrheic eczema.

COMPLEMENTARY THERAPIES
Traditional Chinese Medicine ❹
(*see pages 124–25*)
Traditional Chinese Medicine practitioners regard the occurrence of skin diseases as a failure of digestion and elimination. They treat cases individually, prescribing diets and herbs that reduce toxic buildup and improve excretion. In a 1992 study, a Chinese herbal formula containing licorice was found to be effective in treating atopic eczema.

Nutritional Therapies ❹
(*see pages 128–29*)
Treatments include rotation or exclusion diets to identify food allergies and a detoxifying regime. Supplements of zinc and fish oil may be recommended.

SELF-HELP TECHNIQUES
• Avoid dairy products, citrus fruit, peanuts, eggs, wheat, alcohol, and processed foods • Eat foods rich in essential fatty acids, such as oily fish, plus oats and green leafy vegetables.

STRUCTURAL TREATMENT OPTIONS

CONVENTIONAL MEDICINE
A doctor may use patch-testing to help identify contact allergens. Soothing emollients such as petroleum jelly and preservative-free, unscented moisturizers, which form a protective film over dry, flaky skin, may be suggested. In severe atopic eczema, wet wraps of cotton tubular bandages are soothing and seal in moisture. Tar formulations containing zinc oxide and zinc carbonate soothe the skin, but are messy.

COMPLEMENTARY THERAPIES
Environmental Medicine ❷
(*see page 131*)
A practitioner will run tests to identify irritants so that exposure to them may be avoided or desensitization achieved.

Plenty of moisturizing cream is soothing.

SELF-HELP TECHNIQUES
Give up smoking and avoid smoky atmospheres • Minimize contact with known allergens such as animal dander, house-dust mites, and pollen • Switch to nonenzyme detergent • Bathe frequently and wear cotton • Avoid perfumed detergent, soap, and shampoo • Use only hypoallergenic cosmetics and skin care products • Use emollients continually • Exercise regularly • Consider changing your job if conditions cause contact eczema.

PSYCHOSOCIAL TREATMENT OPTIONS

CONVENTIONAL MEDICINE
Patients are encouraged to learn how to resist the urge to scratch – a habit that makes eczema worse. The itch-scratch-itch cycle is exacerbated by stress and anxiety. Techniques include aversive conditioning, methods of relaxation and stress management, and training in social skills to boost self-esteem.

Stress and anxiety can be relieved by counseling.

COMPLEMENTARY THERAPIES
Psychotherapy & Counseling ❸
(*see pages 132–33*)
Ways are found to express unacknowledged anxiety and emotional tension. Cognitive behavioral therapy and autogenic training (*see page 136*) can relieve symptoms and lessen the need for steroid creams.
Hypnotherapy ❸ (*see page 134*)
Studies have shown that hypnotherapy can be effective in controlling itching.

SELF-HELP TECHNIQUES
• Keep a stress-trigger diary (*see page 175*) • Practice relaxation and breathing techniques (*see pages 170–71*) and stress management skills such as time management and prioritizing.

HERPES

The herpes viruses cause several conditions characterized by small, painful blisters on the skin and mucous membranes. There are two kinds of the *herpes simplex* virus. Type 1 (HSV1) usually causes cold sores (blisters on the lips and mouth) and type 2 (HSV2) causes genital herpes. However, both types can lead to either problem. The virus lives in the nerves and can also inflame the eyes and even the brain. The related *herpes zoster* virus causes chickenpox. This can reemerge as shingles, causing mild, flu-like symptoms, a localized rash and blisters, and pain that settles in one place. Intense pain, known as postherpetic neuralgia can persist longterm.

CASE STUDY

Christine, a homeopath, saw George, 23, who had genital herpes and was anxious about infecting his fiancée. Conventional drugs seemed to clear up an attack, but after a few days he was run down and fed up. "From his answers to my questions, I concluded his constitutional type was *Sulfur*," said Christine, who prescribed a single dose of *Medorrhinum 200c*, a "nosode" designed to counteract his susceptibility to *herpes simplex*. She suggested a high-lysine, low-arginine diet (*see Nutritional Therapies, opposite*). They talked about stress management. He was advised to avoid sex at the first sign of an attack. George says, "In the first four months I had a few mild attacks, and for the last nine months I've had none at all."

BIOCHEMICAL FACTORS

By adulthood, most people have been exposed to HSV1, which is transmitted by touching and kissing. Most either become immune or prone just to cold sores. HSV2 is sexually transmitted. The first attack of HSV2 may pass unnoticed or seem like a mild dose of flu, while further bouts cause genital blisters. The *herpes zoster* virus remains dormant in the nerve cells after chickenpox. Once in the body, all the herpes viruses remain for life and can be activated by a number of different triggers.

BIOCHEMICAL TRIGGERS
• Other infections • Lowered immunity
• Inadequate diet • Hormonal changes, such as those during menstruation

STRUCTURAL FACTORS

It is not clear why some people get recurring severe episodes of herpes. A patient is infectious just before the blisters appear, when the telltale tingling in the lips or genitals heralds the appearance of a sore. In genital herpes, there may be some local pain. Swollen and painful lymph nodes disappear along with the blisters after about a week. A shingles rash lasts about 2–3 weeks, but in a third of cases, pain continues for months or even years because of damage to the nerves. In general, the older you are, the more badly shingles affects you.

STRUCTURAL TRIGGERS
• Heat, fever, sun, and cold winds (cold sores)

PSYCHOSOCIAL FACTORS

Stress is linked to an increased susceptibility to viral infections because it depresses the immune system. One of the triggers below may be responsible for a herpes outbreak.

PSYCHOSOCIAL TRIGGERS
• Anxiety • Overwork and lack of adequate sleep • Depression • Traumatic events, such as bereavement or divorce

Realms of the Body (*see page 20*)

● **BIOCHEMICAL**
Body systems,
such as digestion

● **STRUCTURAL**
Muscles, bones,
joints, and nerves

● **PSYCHOSOCIAL**
Thoughts, feelings,
and relationships

Key: Evidence of Efficacy (*see page 182*)

❶ ❷ ❸ ❹ ❺

least evidence ◄─────────► most evidence

BIOCHEMICAL TREATMENT OPTIONS

CONVENTIONAL MEDICINE
Antiviral tablets such as acyclovir
(*see Drugs Glossary, page 179*), if taken
early on, can shorten attacks. Painkillers help ease mild discomfort, but
stronger analgesics may be necessary,
especially for postherpetic pain. If
sores become infected, doctors may
prescribe antibiotics.

COMPLEMENTARY THERAPIES
Western Herbalism ❸
(*see page 127*)
A practitioner may suggest
the immune-boosting

herb echinacea; licorice gel to ease
inflammation; lemon balm cream to
promote healing and prevent cold
sores; and ointment with capsaicin,
which can relieve the pain of postherpetic neuralgia.
Nutritional Therapies ❶
(*see pages 128–29*)
Therapists may advise you to eat lamb,
chicken, fish, potatoes, milk, beans,
and eggs, which contain the amino acid

Zinc-rich foods
may help control
the growth of the
HSV viruses.

lysine that may suppress HSV. Zinc supplements and ointments and zinc-rich
foods may inhibit the growth of HSV.
Some practitioners recommend garlic,
which is antiviral, and immunity-
enhancing supplements such as
bioflavonoids and vitamins C and E.
You may be advised to avoid chocolate,
peanuts, seeds, and cereals, which contain
arginine, which herpes viruses need.

SELF-HELP TECHNIQUES
• Avoid sugar, coffee, alcohol, and
tobacco, all of which can reduce
immune resistance.

STRUCTURAL TREATMENT OPTIONS

CONVENTIONAL MEDICINE
Doctors will prescribe ointments containing the antivirals idoxuridine or
acyclovir (*see Drugs Glossary, page 179*)
to apply to the affected area. Treatment
should begin as soon as the first symptoms occur. Atropine ointment may
ease shingles pain in the early stages
and transcutaneous nerve stimulation
(TENS – *see Glossary, pages 177–78*) may
help to reduce the pain
of postherpetic neuralgia.

COMPLEMENTARY THERAPIES
Acupuncture ❶ (*see page 125*)
A practitioner may needle local acupoints, which sometimes relieves postherpetic pain.

SELF-HELP TECHNIQUES
• As soon as a cold sore appears, hold
an ice cube wrapped in a dish towel to
it for at least 45 minutes, removing it
for 15 seconds every few minutes to
avoid "burning" • To ease the pain of

genital herpes, bathe the area in a solution of one teaspoon of salt dissolved
in 1 cup (250ml) of warm water • To
prevent infection from spreading, do
not squeeze or touch sores; wash your
hands frequently; keep your towels
and bed linen separate; avoid touching
or kissing (cold sores), oral sex, or sexual intercourse (genital herpes)
• Exercise regularly to help strengthen
the immune system.

PSYCHOSOCIAL TREATMENT OPTIONS

CONVENTIONAL MEDICINE
Because genital herpes is a highly
infectious sexually transmitted disease,
some people may feel ashamed and
anxious. A doctor may suggest counseling or couples therapy.

COMPLEMENTARY THERAPIES
Visualization ❸ (*see page 134*)
A practitioner might ask you to imagine postherpetic pain as something
such as a lump of ice

that melts or disappears to help alter
your perception of it and allow you to
feel more in control.
Biofeedback ❷ (*see page 136*)
This relaxation technique may help
with stress-related problems and persistent pain.

SELF-HELP TECHNIQUES
• Keep a stress diary (*see page 175*)
• Practice stress management and
breathing and relaxation techniques

(*see pages 168–71*)
to help you cope with
stressful events
• Get plenty of
rest during
periods of
overwork.

Breathing exer-
cises can help
relieve stress.

COLDS & FLU

Colds and flu are viral infections of the respiratory tract (the nose, throat, lungs, and bronchial tubes). New strains of the flu virus appear each year, and a cold may be the result of any one of 200 viruses. The symptoms they produce indicate that the immune system is fighting the virus. The flu virus produces symptoms similar to a cold, but worse, and, while a cold starts gradually, flu symptoms develop rapidly. A fever appears within 24 hours, along with loss of appetite, nausea, and aching muscles. The symptoms of colds and flu may be relieved and the duration possibly shortened, but the infection must run its course.

CASE STUDY

Elaine, an herbalist, was asked to help Diana, who was having difficulty recovering after a bout of the flu and needed to improve her resistance to infections. Diana said that she seemed to catch every virus going around and never fully recovered. She told Elaine that, for months, she had been overworked and was feeling tense. Elaine explained how stress affects the immune response and recommended that Diana review her work pattern and rejoin the yoga class she had once belonged to. She also prescribed echinacea tablets to boost Diana's immune system, and gave her a seven-day herbal remedy to use whenever she caught a cold. Diana was strongly advised not to return to work too soon. She quickly got over her bout of flu and had fewer respiratory infections that winter.

BIOCHEMICAL FACTORS

When the immune system is weak, a virus can overcome the body's primary defenses, which include the hairs and mucus in the nose and throat, and protective proteins, called immunoglobulins, in the mucous membranes. The virus infects cells lining the respiratory tract and rapidly multiplies. The infected cells secrete histamine, which causes inflammation, and toxins produced by the virus make the muscles ache. Yellow-green mucus results from the death of white blood cells summoned to fight infection.

BIOCHEMICAL TRIGGERS
• An immune system weakened by poor nutrition, stress, or exhaustion

PSYCHOSOCIAL FACTORS

Research shows that white blood cell activity, which helps fight infection, and antibodies are depleted by stress. Emotional stress has been linked to a greater susceptibility to colds and other viral infections.

PSYCHOSOCIAL TRIGGERS
• Loneliness • Depression • Overwork and lack of adequate sleep • Traumatic life events such as bereavement or divorce

STRUCTURAL FACTORS

A cold or flu virus is spread in tiny airborne droplets produced when an infected person breathes, coughs, or sneezes. Smoking and inhaling polluted air harm the body's defenses, increasing susceptibility to infection. Fighting the virus causes inflammation of the membranes that line the nose, sinuses, and throat, as well as a stuffy or runny nose, sneezing, a sore throat, and a cough.

STRUCTURAL TRIGGERS
• Close contact with an infected person

PRECAUTIONS

See a doctor if symptoms persist or worsen, or if you become short of breath or cough up blood or large amounts of yellow or green mucus. Consult a pharmacist about cold medications, which can interact with one another and affect preexisting conditions.

Realms of the Body (*see page 20*)

● BIOCHEMICAL
Body systems,
such as digestion

● STRUCTURAL
Muscles, bones,
joints, and nerves

○ PSYCHOSOCIAL
Thoughts, feelings,
and relationships

Key: Evidence of Efficacy (*see page 182*)

❶ ❷ ❸ ❹ ❺

least evidence ◄────────► most evidence

BIOCHEMICAL TREATMENT OPTIONS

CONVENTIONAL MEDICINE

Aspirin tablets

Flu immunization is useful for the elderly, people with respiratory problems, and those with weak immune systems. Over-the-counter drugs such as aspirin, acetaminophen, and ibuprofen ease symptoms; antibiotics are indicated only if there is a secondary bacterial infection. New nasal sprays may fight viruses.

COMPLEMENTARY THERAPIES

Naturopathy ❹ (*see page 126*)
For flu, a 48-hour fast will be advised to eliminate toxins, as well as plenty of fluids, rest, and warm baths. A naturopath will not suppress a fever unless it reaches 104°F (40°C).

Western Herbalism ❺ (*see page 127*)
Echinacea, which helps the immune system fight infection, may be recommended. Garlic has antibiotic, antiviral properties: Eat two crushed raw cloves when symptoms first appear, then one a day until they subside. Black elderberry extract may shorten the duration of the flu.

Homeopathy ❹ (*see page 130*)
Oscillococcinum (a remedy made from duck heart and liver), which reduced flu symptoms in one study, may be given.

SELF-HELP TECHNIQUES

• When symptoms appear, take a daily dose of both vitamin C (1000–1500 mg) and zinc gluconate (10–15 mg) or suck on 4–6 zinc lozenges daily.

STRUCTURAL TREATMENT OPTIONS

CONVENTIONAL MEDICINE

Pastilles or lozenges with local anesthetic soothe sore throats; decongestants and inhalants relieve runny or stuffy noses and blocked sinuses; cough suppressants ease dry, tickly coughs, and expectorants help moist chesty coughs.

COMPLEMENTARY THERAPIES

Aromatherapy ❸ (*see page 117*)
A steam inhalation using chamomile essential oil has been shown to reduce cold symptoms. Practitioners advise adding 4 drops of chamomile, eucalyptus, lavender, or tea tree oil to one quart of boiled water, and inhaling the steam for ten minutes, or instead, gargling with 1–2 drops in 1 cup (250 ml) of water.
Caution: Use steam inhalations with care if you have asthma.

Eucalyptus oil and plant

SELF-HELP TECHNIQUES

• Avoid close contact with people who have colds or flu • Avoid environmental pollutants and tobacco smoke, both of which irritate the mucous membranes • Rest, keep warm, and drink plenty of fluids, such as fruit juices, while symptoms persist
• For a sore throat, gargle several times a day with hot water, honey, lemon juice, and crushed garlic
• Use menthol products to help clear a stuffy nose and airways.

PSYCHOSOCIAL TREATMENT OPTIONS

CONVENTIONAL MEDICINE

If you often have colds, a doctor might suggest that you consider whether you are prone to stress. He or she may then suggest stress management techniques (*see pages 168–69*).

COMPLEMENTARY THERAPIES

Visualization ❷ (*see page 134*)
Imagining your white blood cells attacking and destroying the cold and flu viruses in your respiratory tract may boost the immune system. In one study, it raised levels of immuno-globulins (antibodies produced by the immune system) in the saliva.

Meditation ❷ (*see page 135*)
Regular meditation helps calm the mind and relax muscles. Long-term meditators seem to get fewer respiratory infections.

SELF-HELP TECHNIQUES

• A bad bout of flu is stressful and can leave you feeling tired and depressed for weeks afterward. Rest while the infection is acute, and allow yourself time to recover • Learn relaxation techniques (*see pages 170–71*).

Regular meditation may help ward off frequent colds.

PHLEGM & SINUSITIS

If the mucous membranes of the upper respiratory tract become inflamed, they produce excess mucus known as phlegm. This condition, which may be triggered by infections, allergies, or environmental irritants, may cause sneezing, a runny nose, and loss of smell and taste. Phlegm can also block the sinuses, which are cavities in the facial bones that form the nasal cavity. Blocked sinuses can lead to infection (*sinusitis*), which causes throbbing pain in the forehead, upper jaw, and cheek bones. The eustachian tube, linking the middle ear to the back of the nose, may also become blocked, leading to what is known as *glue ear*.

CASE STUDY

Christine, a homeopath, treated Marty, 35, a college lecturer with persistent sinusitis. His doctor referred him after medication had failed to help and the only alternative was a drainage operation, which Marty was anxious to avoid. Christine observed that Marty was quiet, reserved, and self-contained; he generally felt warm; and he had a craving for fish and salt. "I concluded his constitutional type was *Natrum mur.* and prescribed a single high-potency 200c dose of this remedy," she said. "I also suggested Marty avoid dairy products and sugar, take multivitamins, and use steam inhalations with tea tree oil every day." Over the next year the phlegm causing the sinusitis gradually cleared. Every 3–4 months Marty would have a slight relapse and need another dose of *Natrum mur. 200c.*

BIOCHEMICAL FACTORS

The immune system responds to invading viruses, bacteria, or allergens in the respiratory tract by sending infection-fighting white blood cells to the site. This reaction is accompanied by inflammation and excessive mucus secretion. Repeated ear infections in children can cause glue ear – constant production of sticky fluid in the middle ear – which can lead to a degree of deafness.

BIOCHEMICAL TRIGGERS

- Cold and flu viruses, or other infections
- Environmental and food allergies
- "Sick-building syndrome" *(see page 178)*
- Tooth abscess (for sinusitis)

STRUCTURAL FACTORS

If mucus in the upper respiratory tract is unable to drain away, bacterial infections can result. In the middle ear, the accumulation of sticky mucus interferes with the movement of delicate bones and affects hearing. Children are particularly susceptible to middle-ear infection because their eustachian tubes are shorter than those of adults.

STRUCTURAL TRIGGERS

- Irritation and inflammation of the linings of the nose, sinuses, and eustachian tubes caused, for example, by pressure, trauma, environmental particles, or chemicals
- Enlargement of the adenoids

PSYCHOSOCIAL FACTORS

Stress can result in a disturbed immune system and greater susceptibility to infections that lead to phlegm and sinusitis. Pain from blocked sinuses causes irritability and depression. In children, impaired hearing caused by glue ear may lead to behavioral and educational problems; the condition may be undetected until a routine hearing test is given.

PSYCHOSOCIAL TRIGGERS

- Anxiety • Overwork and lack of adequate sleep • Traumatic life events • Depression

Realms of the Body *(see page 20)*

● **BIOCHEMICAL**
Body systems,
such as digestion

● **STRUCTURAL**
Muscles, bones,
joints, and nerves

● **PSYCHOSOCIAL**
Thoughts, feelings,
and relationships

Key: Evidence of Efficacy *(see page 182)*

least evidence ◄————————► most evidence

BIOCHEMICAL TREATMENT OPTIONS

CONVENTIONAL MEDICINE
If phlegm is persistent, a doctor may
suggest decongestants. Antibiotics
are often prescribed for mucus in the
sinuses and middle ear, but can be
ineffective. There is concern that
over-prescribing antibiotics can lead
to antibiotic-resistant bacteria.

COMPLEMENTARY THERAPIES
Naturopathy ❷ *(see page 126)*
For sinusitis, holding hot packs or
menthol or eucalyptus packs over the

forehead and cheeks may be suggested.
Western Herbalism ❷ *(see page 127)*
Practitioners may suggest echinacea to
help boost the immune system and
eucalyptus to ease breathing.
Nutritional Therapies ❷
(see pages 128–29)
Therapists may suspect sensitivities to
foods such as milk, wheat, eggs, citrus
fruits, and sugar, and suggest that you
eliminate them from your diet.
Homeopathy ❷ *(see page 130)*
Various remedies may be recommended

for symptoms, including *Kali bich.*
for thick stringy discharge, *Sticta
pulmonaria* for chronic sinusitis,
and *Pulsatilla* for creamy discharge.

SELF-HELP TECHNIQUES
• Avoid dairy foods, which can increase
mucus • Drink lots of water and fruit
juice to expel toxins and eat a raw food
diet *(see page 129)*.

A diet rich in vitamin C
helps fight infection.

STRUCTURAL TREATMENT OPTIONS

CONVENTIONAL MEDICINE
If decongestants do not help glue ear,
a doctor can improve hearing by
inserting a tiny drainage tube (grommet)
through the eardrum. However, some
specialists believe the ear should clear
by itself. Surgery or washing out the
sinuses can help persistent sinusitis.

COMPLEMENTARY THERAPIES
Aromatherapy ❷ *(see page 117)*
To ease nasal congestion, you may be
advised to add lemon, eucalyptus, or
cedarwood essential oils to bathwater.
For sinusitis, a steam inhalation with
eucalyptus, lavender, or tea tree oil can
be very effective. **Caution:** Do not use
inhalations if you have asthma.

Osteopathy ❷ *(see page 119)*
Cranial osteopaths will gently
manipulate the skull of a child with
glue ear to improve fluid
drainage through the
middle ear.

Cranial osteopathy helps fluids
drain away from the head.

Hydrotherapy ❷ *(see page 126)*
A practitioner may suggest hot showers,
mustard baths, saunas, and steam
baths to help clear phlegm.

SELF-HELP TECHNIQUES
• Children who are breast-fed seem to
be less prone to glue ear (the shorter
nipples on bottles may not exercise
a muscle that opens the ear tubes,
allowing mucus to drain) • Ask your
doctor to perform a hearing test if you
or teachers at school suspect your child
has a mild hearing problem.

PSYCHOSOCIAL TREATMENT OPTIONS

CONVENTIONAL MEDICINE
Doctors support the use of stress
management methods *(see pages 168–69)*.

COMPLEMENTARY THERAPIES
Visualization ❷ *(see page 134)*
By helping you concentrate your mind
on positive images, visualization skills

can aid relaxation.
Relaxation & Breathing ❷
(see pages 170–71)
These techniques help you relax at
will, thus reducing the stress and
tension that can leave you susceptible
to viral and bacterial infections that
can lead to phlegm and sinusitis.

SELF-HELP TECHNIQUES
• Practice stress management
skills regularly *(see pages 168–69)*
• Be sure that you get plenty of restful
sleep • Make time to relax each day,
even if only for half an hour, and learn
relaxation and deep breathing
techniques *(see pages 170–71)*.

INDIGESTION

A blanket term for any discomfort in the upper abdomen, indigestion is also known as *dyspepsia* and *acid stomach*. Sometimes caused by overeating or rushed meals, its symptoms include belching, hiccups, heartburn (a burning acidic sensation behind the breastbone and at the same level in the mid-line of the back), nausea, and gas. Persistent indigestion may be a sign of a peptic ulcer, gallstones, or *esophagitis* – inflammation of the esophagus or gullet. Indigestion can cause severe chest pain similar to angina and is occasionally mistaken for heart disease. If this is the case, it may need to be investigated.

CASE STUDY

Hannah, a nutritionist, treated Barbara, 44, for indigestion, gas, and bloating. Medical tests had shown nothing wrong and Barbara was reluctant to continue her prescribed ranitidine (*see Drugs Glossary, page 179*), since it seemed to make no difference. "Acid production can go down or up if you are stressed," said Hannah. Tests confirmed that Barbara had low levels of stomach acid. "The enzymes that digest protein need an acid environment and poorly digested proteins in the lower bowel can create gas and bloating," Hannah explained. She advised a stomach acid supplement with each meal, a daily zinc supplement of 15 mg to help stomach acid production, and a diet rich in fruit and vegetables. Several weeks later, Barbara said her indigestion had begun to ease.

BIOCHEMICAL FACTORS

Chewed food passes down the esophagus into the stomach, where gastric acids and enzymes break it down further. Excessive gas and acid can flow back (reflux) into the esophagus. Since, unlike the stomach, the esophagus does not have a protective lining, when it is exposed to stomach acid it can become inflamed and painful.

BIOCHEMICAL TRIGGERS

• Eating too much rich, spicy, fatty, or fried food, especially near bedtime • Drinking excess alcohol • Rushing meals • Chewing food insufficiently • Swallowing air • Eating unripe fruit, which is high in indigestible pectin

STRUCTURAL FACTORS

Heartburn and reflux (*see right*) occur when the muscle at the bottom of the esophagus fails to keep gastric acid in the stomach. It is not clear why this happens but increased pressure on the digestive tract may be a factor. Smoking relaxes this muscle with the same effect. A hiatus hernia may cause frequent heartburn. This results when a small part of the stomach rises above the diaphragm (the muscle sheet that separates the stomach from the chest).

STRUCTURAL TRIGGERS

• Pregnancy • Being very overweight
• Hiatus hernia • Lying down after a meal
• Straining to lift • Constipation • Wearing tight clothing around the waist

PSYCHOSOCIAL FACTORS

Stress can lower or increase stomach acid production. It can also affect the secretion of enzymes, digestive juices, and hormones in the gut. Tension can make the gut irregular and reduce the flow of blood to the stomach and intestines (*see page 158*).

PSYCHOSOCIAL TRIGGERS

• Anxiety • Fear • Impatience

PRECAUTIONS

Consult a doctor if symptoms last more than a few days, if you are regularly taking antacids, or if you are over 40 and suddenly experience indigestion.

Realms of the Body (*see page 20*)

- BIOCHEMICAL
  Body systems,
  such as digestion
- STRUCTURAL
  Muscles, bones,
  joints, and nerves
- PSYCHOSOCIAL
  Thoughts, feelings,
  and relationships

Key: Evidence of Efficacy (*see page 182*)

❶ ❷ ❸ ❹ ❺
least evidence ◄————————► most evidence

BIOCHEMICAL TREATMENT OPTIONS

CONVENTIONAL MEDICINE
Antacids reduce the acidity of digestive juices. H_2 blockers (*see Drugs Glossary, page 179*) such as ranitidine limit the amount of acid released.

COMPLEMENTARY THERAPIES
Western Herbalism ❷ (*see page 127*)
Herbalists may suggest slippery elm to protect the digestive tract lining, peppermint and chamomile to settle the stomach, and dandelion and burdock before eating to enhance digestion and prevent indigestion.

Nutritional Therapies ❷
(*see pages 128–29*)
Hydrochloric acid deficiency is thought to cause indigestion, so a therapist may suggest a short course of betaine capsules. Food sensitivities and dysbiosis may also be suspected (*see pages 92–95*) and an exclusion diet recommended to identify offending foods. "Live" yogurt containing beneficial bacteria is thought to help. Food combining, or the Hay Diet (*see page 129*), in which proteins and carbohydrates are eaten separately, may be advised. Vitamin C, zinc, and beta carotene supplements may help repair the stomach lining.

Burdock and dandelion can help improve digestion.

SELF-HELP TECHNIQUES
• Eat regular small meals and follow a healthy, fiber-rich diet • Keep a food diary (*see page 147*) if you suspect a sensitivity • Avoid highly spiced, rich, or fatty foods • Steam, grill, or bake rather than fry • Avoid raw foods and acidic foods such as vinegar and pickles • Cut down on tobacco and alcohol, which increase stomach acidity; strong coffee, which irritates the stomach lining; and sodas, which cause gas.

STRUCTURAL TREATMENT OPTIONS

CONVENTIONAL MEDICINE
Swallowing antacid gels can help prevent reflux.

COMPLEMENTARY THERAPIES
Chiropractic ❷ (*see page 118*) and **Osteopathy ❷** (*see page 119*)
Practitioners may manipulate the area of the spine where nerve and blood supplies to the digestive organs arise.
Acupuncture ❷ (*see page 125*)
Some research suggests that acupuncturists can reduce high levels of acid production and relieve tension.

SELF-HELP TECHNIQUES
• Relax before and during meals and chew food thoroughly • If you get reflux or heartburn, avoid activities that involve bending from the waist or stooping just after meals • Eat at a table sitting upright rather than slumped in front of the TV • Get regular exercise to help circulation and induce relaxation • Raise the head of the bed by 6 in (15 cm) so gravity can help keep digestive acids in the stomach • Refrain from eating just before going to bed.

Take time to chew and to digest your food, and maintain an upright posture when eating.

PSYCHOSOCIAL TREATMENT OPTIONS

CONVENTIONAL MEDICINE
Stress management techniques may be suggested (*see pages 168–69*).

COMPLEMENTARY THERAPIES
Psychotherapy & Counseling ❷
(*see pages 132–33*)
Talking through problems may help identify areas of anxiety, and a practitioner will suggest ways of dealing with them.

Hypnotherapy & Meditation ❷
(*see pages 134–35*)
Learning techniques to focus the mind and induce relaxation may help to relieve underlying stress that can lead to "nervous" indigestion.

SELF-HELP TECHNIQUES
• Keep a symptom- and stress-trigger diary (*see pages 147 and 175*) • Practice relaxation and breathing techniques (*see pages 170–71*) to help deal with stress and anxiety.

IRRITABLE BOWEL SYNDROME

One of the most common gastrointestinal complaints, irritable bowel syndrome (IBS) may affect up to two people in ten. It is particularly prevalent among women 20 to 45 years old. IBS, also known as spastic colon, may come and go for years, with no infection or other apparent cause. The wavelike motion of the gut (peristalsis) becomes irregular, causing erratic bowel movements with possible constipation, diarrhea, or both, as well as gas and intermittent abdominal pain. Although IBS is not life-threatening, symptoms can cause distress and be difficult to control. Treatment can bring relief but does not always offer a cure.

CASE STUDY

Jane, an acupuncturist, treated Alison, 41, a divorcee with a teenage daughter. For two years, Alison had complained of insomnia, abdominal pains, diarrhea, and constipation, but medical tests found nothing wrong. Jane diagnosed her pattern of disharmony as Liver *qi* stagnation: "This is commonly associated with stress-related problems," she said. "I worked on acupuncture points between the knee and foot to release the blocked energy of the Liver. Meanwhile, Alison would relax deeply and often fall asleep." After six treatments, most of Alison's symptoms had gone.

BIOCHEMICAL FACTORS

Various nutritional factors can interfere with contractions of the colon, the release of digestive enzymes, and the absorption of food through the wall of the gut.

BIOCHEMICAL TRIGGERS

• Chemicals released by the body in response to stress • Intolerance of foods, especially dairy products, and grains such as wheat, barley, oats, rye, and millet • Dysbiosis (*see page 92*), when poorly digested food in the gut encourages the growth of unfriendly gut bacteria • "Leaky gut" (*see page 159*), which is especially likely after gastroenteritis or after a course of broad-spectrum antibiotics (*see Drugs Glossary, page 179*)

PSYCHOSOCIAL FACTORS

The stress response affects digestion and absorption by changing peristaltic rhythm, altering the secretion of juices and enzymes, and by affecting blood circulation. Over 50 percent of people with IBS report a history of emotional problems, and evidence indicates that people with anxiety or depression may be more likely to develop IBS after a gut infection. Poor sleep also seems to trigger IBS symptoms.

PSYCHOSOCIAL TRIGGERS

• Continual, low-level stress • Anxiety
• Inadequate sleep • Depression • Hostility

STRUCTURAL FACTORS

Peristalsis, the wavelike action of the gut that propels feces toward the rectum, becomes irregular with IBS. Symptoms can include mucus in the feces, an urgent need to have a bowel movement, and a feeling of incomplete evacuation.

STRUCTURAL TRIGGERS

• Muscles in the wall of the colon pushing its contents either too quickly, causing diarrhea, or too slowly, causing constipation • Muscular overactivity or spasm, causing cramps
• Bloating, rumbling, and gas caused by irregular peristalsis, excess gas produced by fermentation processes, or by swallowing air – a nervous habit sometimes linked with hyperventilation and eating too quickly

PRECAUTIONS

Consult a doctor if you are over 40 years old and your bowel habits have recently changed. Check with a doctor if there is blood in your stools. See a doctor if you are over 60 and have symptoms for the first time.

Realms of the Body (*see page 20*)

● **BIOCHEMICAL**
Body systems,
such as digestion

● **STRUCTURAL**
Muscles, bones,
joints, and nerves

● **PSYCHOSOCIAL**
Thoughts, feelings,
and relationships

Evidence of Efficacy (*see page 182*)

❶ ❷ ❸ ❹ ❺
least evidence ◄————————► most evidence

BIOCHEMICAL TREATMENT OPTIONS

CONVENTIONAL MEDICINE
A diet high in soluble fiber or bulking agents (psyllium or methylcellulose) may be advised to soften stools.

COMPLEMENTARY THERAPIES
Naturopathy ❹ (*see page 126*)
Exclusion and rotation diets (*see page 129*) may identify a food intolerance. Citrus fruits, tea,

Elimination diet has "neutral" foods.

coffee, and alcohol are often suspects, as are dairy products and wheat. A high-fiber diet may be advised if you have constipation. Live yogurt or supplements such as *lactobacillus* help normalize levels of bacteria in the gut.
Chinese Herbalism ❹ (*see page 124*)
A study reported in 1998 showed herbal formulas many herbalists prescribed could relieve symptoms.
Western Herbalism ❸ (*see page 127*)
Peppermint oil capsules sometimes help reduce muscular gut contractions.

SELF-HELP TECHNIQUES
• Keep a record of episodes of IBS. Do they coincide with certain foods or situations? • Check ingredients on food labels • Reduce fat intake • Avoid refined carbohydrates, which encourage muscle spasms • For constipation, increase water-soluble fiber (in leafy vegetables, fruit, and oat bran), which is easier to digest than insoluble fiber (in wheat bran and rice), which can irritate the gut • Drink at least 2 quarts of water a day.

STRUCTURAL TREATMENT OPTIONS

CONVENTIONAL MEDICINE
A doctor may prescribe antispasmodic drugs to relieve the pain of muscular spasms and cramps. A short course of antidiarrheal drugs may be suggested.

COMPLEMENTARY THERAPIES
Massage ❷ (*see page 116*)
Gentle massage of the lower abdomen is best demonstrated by a practitioner before you practice on yourself. It may relax muscular tension in the colon wall and help regulate the bowels.

Yoga ❷ (*see page 123*)
Postures such as the Half Shoulder Stand and the Cobra can stimulate digestion. Calming breathing exercises or *pranayama* help relieve stress.

Cobra pose aids digestion.

Acupuncture ❷ (*see page 125*)
An acupuncturist usually links IBS to one of the following: "stagnant Liver *qi*" (stress or hostility); "deficient Kidney or

Spleen" (poor digestion and food absorption); or "damp heat" (such as a disturbance in gut bacteria). Western acupuncturists believe that stimulating acupoints can positively affect the nerve system controlling the gut's contractions.

SELF-HELP TECHNIQUES
• At the first sign of pain, squeeze acupoints Colon 4 or Liver 3 (*see page 125*) • Get plenty of gentle exercise • Leave adequate time for meals • Make sure that you get enough sleep.

PSYCHOSOCIAL TREATMENT OPTIONS

CONVENTIONAL MEDICINE
Those with IBS are advised to learn stress management techniques (*see pages 168–69*).

COMPLEMENTARY THERAPIES
Psychotherapy & Counseling ❹ (*see pages 132–33*)
Cognitive behavioral therapy may help you change ways of thinking and behaving in response to stress. Counseling may help identify sources of stress and ways of coping.

Hypnotherapy ❹ (*see page 134*)
In a study by Dr. Peter Whorwell of the Withington Hospital, Manchester, England, reported in *The Lancet* (1989), hypnotherapy proved successful in relieving symptoms of IBS. Practitioners explain the gut's anatomy and function, then induce a state

Hypnotherapy may reduce symptoms.

of deep relaxation and a sensation of abdominal warmth before asking patients to imagine their gut working normally.

SELF-HELP TECHNIQUES
• Relaxation and breathing techniques (*see pages 170–71*) are important in reducing muscle tension and stress responses • Keep a diary of symptoms and possible stress triggers (*see page 147*) • Meditation (*see page 135*) may also help reduce stress symptoms.

INFLAMMATORY BOWEL DISEASE

The two main types of inflammatory bowel disease are Crohn's disease and ulcerative colitis. Both are becoming much more common in developed countries, particularly among people 15 to 35 years old. Crohn's disease affects any part of the digestive tract but especially the lower small intestine.

Common symptoms include pain, spasms, gas, diarrhea, fever, and weight loss. Ulcerative colitis inflames the colon and rectum, then ulcerates the gut lining. It can cause abdominal tenderness, diarrhea with cramps, mucus and blood in the feces, weight loss, a general feeling of being ill, and fever.

CASE STUDY

Tim, 42, an accountant, suffered from mild ulcerative colitis diagnosed by endoscopy (*see Glossary, pages 177–78*). Before going on anti-inflammatory drugs, Tim and his doctor agreed to try an alternative, and Tim consulted George, a naturopath. A challenge test and stool analysis pointed to a wheat intolerance with dysbiosis (*see page 93*) and yeast overgrowth. Tim's diet lacked vegetable fiber, so George advised him to eat grated apple or carrot before meals, as well as vegetable soups and brown rice. He also advised him not to include starch and protein in the same meal. Tim was given *lactobacillus* supplements to replace the abnormal gut flora, slippery elm porridge to soothe the gut, and licorice, wild yam, and barberry to help repair the intestinal lining. In three months, his condition had improved, but eating out could still cause a bout of diarrhea.

BIOCHEMICAL FACTORS

The exact cause of inflammatory bowel disease is unknown. In some cases it is part of an autoimmune disorder in which the immune system attacks the body's own tissues. Nutritional deficiencies occur if food is not properly absorbed by the gut.

BIOCHEMICAL TRIGGERS

• Family history • Food allergy or intolerance (*see pages 92–95*) • Bacterial or viral infection • Overusing antibiotics • A diet high in refined sugar and low in raw fruit, vegetables, fiber, and omega-3 fatty acids (found in oily fish) • Measles vaccination (?) (Crohn's disease) • Possibly ingesting the bacterium *Mycobacterium paratuberculosis*, found in milk (Crohn's disease) • Smoking (Crohn's disease)

PSYCHOSOCIAL FACTORS

Although there is little evidence that psychological factors can trigger either type of inflammatory bowel disease, emotional stress is thought to aggravate it. Symptoms of both conditions can often be a source of stress in themselves.

PSYCHOSOCIAL TRIGGERS

• Anxiety • Overwork and inadequate sleep • Traumatic life events

STRUCTURAL FACTORS

In Crohn's disease, chronic inflammation greatly thickens the intestinal wall and penetrating ulcers may form. The intestine can narrow so much that it becomes blocked. Complications of Crohn's disease include abscesses, fistulas (abnormal openings between loops of the intestines), and inflammation of the joints, spine, eyes, and skin. Complications of ulcerative colitis include a dangerously enlarged colon, rashes, mouth ulcers, anemia, arthritis, and conjunctivitis. Both conditions may go into remission for months or years, and so far there are no known structural triggers involved.

PRECAUTIONS

Consult a doctor if you have prolonged or unexplained diarrhea; any persistent change in bowel habits; blood or mucus in stools; or unexplained severe or persistent abdominal pain.

Realms of the Body (*see page 20*)

● BIOCHEMICAL
Body systems,
such as digestion

● STRUCTURAL
Muscles, bones,
joints, and nerves

● PSYCHOSOCIAL
Thoughts, feelings,
and relationships

Key: Evidence of Efficacy (*see page 182*)

❶ ❷ ❸ ❹ ❺
least evidence ◄─────► most evidence

BIOCHEMICAL TREATMENT OPTIONS

CONVENTIONAL MEDICINE
A doctor may prescribe sulfasalazine, corticosteroids, and mesalamine to ease inflammation (*see Drugs Glossary, page 179*), and a new antibody, infliximab, is being developed. A combination of antibiotics (rifabutin and clarithromycin) may be used to treat Crohn's disease.

COMPLEMENTARY THERAPIES
Nutritional Therapies ❹
(*see pages 128–29*)

Practitioners aim to improve digestion by resting the liver, and may suggest a bowel-cleansing juice fast. Supervised exclusion diets (*see page 129*) may help 50 percent of Crohn's disease patients – dairy products and wheat are often trigger foods. Oily fish and fish oil supplements may redress an imbalance of essential fatty acids. A practitioner may suggest "live" yogurt or *lactobacillus*

Live yogurt aids digestion.

supplements for dysbiosis and a "leaky" gut (*see page 159*). Vitamin and mineral supplements can aid nutrient absorption.

SELF-HELP TECHNIQUES
• Eat a diet high in complex carbohydrates, and take multivitamin and mineral supplements • For Crohn's disease, drink sterilized milk free of the *paratuberculosis* bacterium.

STRUCTURAL TREATMENT OPTIONS

CONVENTIONAL MEDICINE
A biopsy, barium X-ray, barium enema, colonoscopy, and sigmoidoscopy (*see Glossary, pages 177–78*) are used to make a diagnosis – similar symptoms can make it difficult to differentiate between the two conditions. In severe cases of either disease, damaged portions of intestine may be removed surgically. If the colon is removed, the patient is left with an ileostomy (*see Glossary, pages 177–78*). People with ulcerative colitis need regular checkups for bowel cancer.

COMPLEMENTARY THERAPIES
Massage ❸ (*see page 116*)
When combined with breathing exercises, massage may encourage sleep and the feeling of being in control of pain.
Acupuncture ❷ (*see page 125*)
A practitioner will aim to correct disturbances in the flow of *qi*. For ulcerative colitis, acupoints on the Gallbladder meridian may be stimulated with either needles or moxibustion.

SELF-HELP TECHNIQUES
• Practice yoga regularly. The breathing techniques, methods of mental focus, and body postures can all help relieve stress and improve circulation to the inner organs (*see page 123*).

Practicing the Half Shoulder Stand helps relieve stress.

PSYCHOSOCIAL TREATMENT OPTIONS

CONVENTIONAL MEDICINE
Your doctor may advise practicing one of the therapies listed below.

COMPLEMENTARY THERAPIES
Hypnotherapy ❷ (*see page 134*)
A practitioner will show you techniques that enable you to calm your mind at will to relieve stress. These may include visualization (*see page 134*), which can help you use your imagination to overcome stress and relax tense muscles.

Thinking about a restful scene can help reduce stress levels.

Biofeedback ❸ (*see page 136*)
By responding to signals on devices measuring body changes, you can learn to relax muscle tension.

SELF-HELP TECHNIQUES
• Keep a daily diary of diet, symptoms, and stress triggers (*see page 147*)
• Practice relaxation and breathing techniques (*see pages 170–71*) and learn stress management skills (*see pages 168–69*) to help you deal with the symptoms.

HIGH BLOOD PRESSURE

Blood pumped from the heart around the body exerts a constantly fluctuating pressure on the walls of arteries. Pressure levels are lowest early in the morning, and are highest during physical exercise. When blood pressure is consistently raised, it is known as high blood pressure, or hypertension.

This condition is estimated to affect up to 20 percent of adults in developed countries but, since there are usually no symptoms, it may go undetected until picked up during a medical checkup. Untreated, hypertension can damage blood vessels and increase the risk of stroke, heart and kidney disease, as well as other disorders.

CASE STUDY

James, a psychologist, saw Paul, a 35-year-old teacher with chest pains and borderline high blood pressure. Though Paul was eager to try drug treatment, the medicines had made him feel ill. James discovered that Paul's father-in-law had died recently and that a tree had crushed the greenhouse in which he used to unwind after work. James suggested that Paul buy another greenhouse and taught him autogenic techniques to help him relax.

"Paul's blood pressure came down ten points and a cardiogram showed his heart was fine. In fact the chest pains soon went away," said James. "So far Paul has no need for drugs, but his doctor checks his blood pressure twice a year just in case."

BIOCHEMICAL FACTORS

In 10 percent of cases, hypertension is attributed to disorders of the kidneys or adrenal glands, congenital abnormality of the aorta (the heart's main artery), pre-eclampsia in pregnancy, or to the use of certain drugs such as oral contraceptives. Estrogen seems to protect women until menopause begins, after which their risk equals and even exceeds that of men. A diet low in potassium and high in sodium is linked to high blood pressure in some people, and nicotine and epinephrine cause the arteries to constrict, resulting in a temporary rise in blood pressure.

BIOCHEMICAL TRIGGERS
- Excessive alcohol and caffeine consumption
- Being male or a postmenopausal female
- High salt intake • Smoking • Family history

STRUCTURAL FACTORS

In 90 percent of cases, hypertension is "essential" or "primary," meaning there is no specific cause. Untreated hypertension causes irreversible changes in the blood-vessel walls that increase the risk of fatty plaque deposits forming. These narrow the arteries and encourage blood clots, which can cause a heart attack or stroke (see Heart Disease, pages 48–51). Symptoms of hypertension, which occur only if blood pressure is very high, include dizziness, headaches, fatigue, and breathlessness.

STRUCTURAL TRIGGERS
- Race (black people suffer more from hypertension than other races) • Age • Obesity
- Inadequate physical activity • Environmental factors such as crowded living conditions

PSYCHOSOCIAL FACTORS

Under stress, the body undergoes a "fight or flight" response, which provokes a temporary rise in blood pressure. The heart beats faster, and extra reserves of the stress hormones epinephrine, nor-epinephrine, and cortisol flood the system. Arteries constrict so that less blood is lost in case wounds occur, and blood stickiness increases to form clots more easily. "Hostile" personality types react more strongly to stressful situations (see page 49).

PSYCHOSOCIAL TRIGGERS
- Hostility and aggression • Work or social stress • Anxiety

Realms of the Body (*see page 20*)

● **BIOCHEMICAL**
Body systems,
such as digestion

● **STRUCTURAL**
Muscles, bones,
joints, and nerves

● **PSYCHOSOCIAL**
Thoughts, feelings,
and relationships

Evidence of Efficacy (*see page 182*)

least evidence ◄————————————► most evidence

BIOCHEMICAL TREATMENT OPTIONS

CONVENTIONAL MEDICINE
For mild cases of hypertension, a doctor will suggest dietary and lifestyle changes (*see right*). Beta blockers, which reduce heartbeat force, and diuretics, which reduce blood volume, are usually prescribed first. (Tiredness and nightmares are fairly common side effects of beta blockers.) These may be followed by ACE inhibitors to dilate blood vessels, calcium channel blockers, and vasodilators (*see Drugs Glossary, page 179*).

COMPLEMENTARY THERAPIES
Nutritional Therapies ❸
(*see page 128*)
A practitioner may advise a vegetarian diet with plenty of potassium-rich fruit and vegetables, since studies suggest it lowers blood pressure and reduces the incidence of heart disease. Eating plenty of oat bran and psyllium seeds, garlic, and onion may be suggested, along with supplements such as omega-3 fatty acids (fish oils), magnesium to relax muscle tissue, vitamin C, and Coenzyme Q10.

SELF-HELP TECHNIQUES
• Reduce salt intake to no more than one teaspoon a day • Eat plenty of potassium-rich foods (bananas, celery, watercress, oranges)
• Cut back on processed foods, alcohol, and coffee
• Avoid foods high in saturated fats and cholesterol
• Stop smoking.

Watercress is an excellent source of potassium.

STRUCTURAL TREATMENT OPTIONS

CONVENTIONAL MEDICINE
Doctors recommend regular exercise, since it is known to help reduce mild hypertension.

COMPLEMENTARY THERAPIES
Massage ❷ (*see page 116*)
A practitioner may use long, slow strokes to help you unwind. Several studies show gentle, full-body massage temporarily lowers blood pressure and helps relaxation, but there is no evidence so far that it controls hypertension.

Aromatherapy ❷ (*see page 117*)
Many essential oils, including lavender and rose, are said to have sedative qualities. Aromatherapy can help if stress and tension are part of the problem, but it has not been shown to reduce hypertension in the long term.

Rose and essential oil

T'ai Chi ❸ (*see page 124*)
The combination of movement, breathing, and mental focus in t'ai chi has been shown to lower blood pressure raised by mental and emotional stress.

SELF-HELP TECHNIQUES
• Exercise regularly (consult your doctor first if you have moderate hypertension) • Lose any excess weight.

PSYCHOSOCIAL TREATMENT OPTIONS

CONVENTIONAL MEDICINE
A doctor may suggest cognitive behavioral therapy, which can help people with "hostile" personalities.

COMPLEMENTARY THERAPIES
Hypnotherapy ❸ (*see page 134*)
Recalling the memory of a hypnotically induced state of relaxation may enable you to reenter it when necessary.
Meditation ❸ (*see page 135*)
A practitioner will show you techniques that quiet and focus the

mind, which can help to generate deep alpha brain waves associated with relaxation.
Biofeedback ❸ (*see page 136*)
Monitoring devices can help you learn how to relax at will. Studies show that

Devices measure skin temperature.

Electrodes monitor brain wave activity.

biofeedback lowers mild hypertension so that medication can be reduced.
Relaxation & Breathing ❸
(*see pages 170–71*)
You will be taught how to breathe diaphragmatically to induce relaxation and combat the body's stress response.

SELF-HELP TECHNIQUES
• Keep a stress diary (*see page 147*) and practice stress management techniques (*see pages 168–69*) • Listening to music can temporarily lower hypertension.

HEART DISEASE

The heart is a hollow muscular organ at the center of the network of arteries and veins that circulates blood around the body. The blood supplies the tissues with oxygen and nutrients and removes waste products. Coronary arteries carry oxygenated blood from the lungs directly to the heart; any disease that damages or causes malfunction of these arteries affects the heart's ability to contract effectively. The conditions that result are known as *coronary artery disease* or *coronary heart disease*.

Coronary artery disease is one of the conditions caused by *atherosclerosis*, in which the insides of the coronary artery walls gradually become clogged with fatty plaque deposits called atheroma. This narrowing restricts blood flow to the heart muscle. Eventually, the arteries become so narrow that the heart muscle cramps when it has to work harder during exercise, causing pain known as *angina pectoris*. A *heart attack* (myocardial infarction) can be fatal. Part of the heart muscle dies because its blood supply is cut off by the narrowing of the arteries, or because a blood clot (thrombus) is blocking a coronary artery.

BIOCHEMICAL FACTORS

HIGH LEVELS OF BLOOD CHOLESTEROL contribute to atherosclerosis and angina (*see above*). Blood cholesterol is one of a group of fatlike substances known as lipids and is made by the liver. It is needed for digestion and to build cell membranes and hormones, but excess blood cholesterol is a health risk.

There are two types of cholesterol: high-density lipoprotein (HDL) and low-density lipoprotein (LDL). The latter makes up about two-thirds of cholesterol and is called "bad" cholesterol because its small molecules allow it to slip into the lining of damaged blood vessels and clog them up.

The higher your levels of LDL blood cholesterol, the greater your risk of heart disease. The arteries carry blood rich in oxygen and nutrients, which are vital for the growth, maintenance, and repair of cells and tissues. If LDL cholesterol builds up on artery walls, sticky blood-clotting cells (platelets) adhere so that plaque deposits form, impeding the flow of blood. When a coronary artery becomes blocked, the heart's blood supply is cut off, and the muscle may die (myocardial infarction or heart attack).

BIOCHEMICAL TRIGGERS

• Low levels of antioxidants, obtained from fruit and vegetables, which fight damaging free radicals that attack artery walls (*see page 161*) • A diet high in saturated fats and trans fatty acids (*see page 160*), which can raise levels of LDL blood cholesterol (*see left*)
• An inherited tendency toward high levels of blood cholesterol and a related blood fat, triglyceride
• High levels of fibrinogen, a blood-clotting agent that makes blood stickier and more likely to clot • Smoking, which quadruples the risk of heart attack: Toxic tobacco smoke chemicals in the bloodstream damage the arteries, increase blood cholesterol and fibrinogen levels, and raise blood pressure • Cortisol and epinephrine, chemicals produced under stress, which inhibit tissue repair and prevent artery walls from healing • Elevated levels of the amino acid homocysteine, a chemical "sandpaper" that damages the arteries and promotes atherosclerosis • The presence of *Chlamydia pneumoniae*, a common bacterium, in arterial walls, which may provoke a damaging immune system reaction

See page 50 for Biochemical Treatment Options

Realms of the Body (*see page 20*)

● BIOCHEMICAL
Body systems,
such as digestion

● STRUCTURAL
Muscles, bones,
joints, and nerves

● PSYCHOSOCIAL
Thoughts, feelings,
and relationships

STRUCTURAL FACTORS

DAMAGE TO ARTERY WALLS is exacerbated by high blood pressure, stress, and smoking, causing atherosclerosis (*see opposite*). This occurs when white blood cells cling to damaged areas of artery walls and attract fat, particularly cholesterol, which forms plaque deposits. The higher the cholesterol levels, the faster plaque narrows the arteries. High cholesterol also reduces levels of a muscle-relaxing substance in artery walls that encourages blood flow.

Damage and cracking of plaque deposits attracts platelet blood cells. These rapidly grow into a blood clot (thrombus) that further hinders blood flow through the artery and may completely block it. The clot may move into the bloodstream to cause harm elsewhere, particularly in the lung (pulmonary embolism) or brain (stroke, caused by a cerebroembolism).

STRUCTURAL TRIGGERS

● Stress, which raises blood pressure and triggers coronary artery spasms and abnormal heart rhythms. This in turn may lead to palpitations, hyperventilation, chest pain, and can even cause a heart attack
● Obesity, which puts the heart at risk; overweight, "apple-shaped" people, who carry fat around the middle rather than the hips, are at greater risk of coronary heart disease than others ● High blood pressure, placing a strain on the artery walls (*see page 46*) ● Lack of exercise, which reduces cardiac efficiency ● Smoking, which damages artery walls

See page 51 for Structural Treatment Options

PSYCHOSOCIAL FACTORS

IMPATIENT, AGGRESSIVE, WORKAHOLIC "Type A" personalities used to be considered more prone to heart disease. Now only one element of Type A behavior, "hostility" (*see right*), is considered a health risk. Hostility is a mixture of cynicism, self-involvement, and anger, and is often characteristic of people who feel they have little or no control over their lives.

When hostile, the mind and body are in "battle" mode. The heart works faster, the liver releases sugars and fats for fast energy, and blood clotting accelerates to seal injuries. If this condition is sustained, stress hormones, cholesterol, and fibrinogen (a clotting agent) rise to harmful levels. Hostile people also often tend to have poor health habits, such as overeating, smoking, and drinking alcohol to excess.

PSYCHOSOCIAL TRIGGERS

● Cumulative tiredness ● A life or work environment that is highly demanding and low in autonomy
● Poor ability to cope with situations ● Loneliness and lack of social support

See page 51 for Psychosocial Treatment Options

ARE YOU HOSTILE?

The more "yes" answers you give to these questions, devised by Dr. Redford Williams, the higher your risk of contracting heart disease. Use the Steps to a Trusting Heart exercise (see page 51) to help combat this risk.

● Do you always feel pressed for time?
● Do you hurry when you eat?
● At the end of the day, do you feel stretched to the limit?
● When angry, do you sulk or keep things bottled up inside?
● Do you always like to have the last word in an argument?
● If people ahead of you in the supermarket express line have too many items in their baskets, do you seethe but say nothing?
● If you see an able-bodied person park in a disabled driver's parking space, do you say nothing but fume inwardly?

HEART DISEASE

Key: Evidence of Efficacy (see page 182)

❶   ❷   ❸   ❹   ❺

least evidence ◀━━━━━━━━▶ most evidence

BIOCHEMICAL TREATMENT OPTIONS

CONVENTIONAL MEDICINE

Patients diagnosed with coronary artery disease may be recommended the following by their doctor: one aspirin (75 mg) twice a week to prevent blood clotting; vasodilator drugs to improve blood flow in narrowed arteries; drugs to improve the heart's pumping; beta blockers to treat high blood pressure, angina, and irregular heart rhythms; antiangina drugs such as nitrates and calcium channel blockers; cholesterol-lowering drugs such as statins; anticoagulant drugs (see Drugs Glossary, page 179). Postmenopausal women may be offered hormone replacement therapy (HRT),

Gentle exercise improves heart health.

which appears to reduce the risk of a heart attack by up to 50 percent, particularly if there is a family history of heart disease.

COMPLEMENTARY THERAPIES

Naturopathy ❹ (see page 126)

Changes in diet and lifestyle may help people with coronary heart disease. Cholestin, a nutritional supplement made from red rice, contains a statin shown to lower cholesterol. In the US, Dr. Dean Ornish's Ornish Lifestyle Program aims to reverse heart disease without surgery or drugs. It comprises a rigorous high-fiber vegetarian diet of which only 10 percent of calories come from fat (the usual recommendation for patients with coronary heart disease is 30 percent), 15–20 percent from protein, and 70–75 percent from complex carbohydrates. Patients must exercise one hour three times a week and attend group therapy sessions and yoga-derived daily stress management exercise classes. In one study, arterial blood flow improved and chest pain decreased in 82 percent of Dr. Ornish's patients, while symptoms worsened in 53 percent of a control group.

Western Herbalism ❸ (see page 127)

Practitioners may suggest the following herbs: the Chinese herb ginkgo to improve blood circulation in peripheral blood vessels and prevent a second heart attack or stroke; ginger to inhibit blood clotting; and garlic oil (allicin, in garlic) which lowers blood fats, lowers blood pressure, improves circulation to the skin, and thins the blood.

Ginkgo

Garlic bulb

The Ornish diet

Nutritional Therapies ❹

(see pages 128–29)

Diet has an important role in preventing and treating heart disease. Antioxidants may be advised to reduce damage from LDL cholesterol (see page 48). These include vitamin E (a UK study found this could reduce risk of a heart attack in patients with atherosclerosis by 77 percent), vitamin C, selenium, and Coenzyme Q10. Other supplements include omega-3 fatty acids such as fish oils and flaxseed oil, to lower blood fats and fibrinogen; omega-6 fatty acids, found in evening primrose and borage oil, to reduce cholesterol and improve heart function; vitamins B_6, B_{12}, and folic acid, to break down homocysteine.

SELF-HELP TECHNIQUES

Eating for a Healthy Heart

• Avoid saturated animal fats from red meats, hard cheese, cream, and butter• Avoid hydrogenated trans fatty acids, in some commercial baked goods, which may raise "bad" cholesterol levels

• Drink less coffee, especially if perked, drip, or made in a caffettiere; roasting releases cholesterol-raising substances.

Consume more

• Vegetable oils rich in mono-unsaturated fatty acids, such as olive and canola oil, to reduce cholesterol.

• Polyunsaturated spreads such as those from sunflower or canola oil

• Oily fish full of omega-3 fatty acids, such as salmon, herring, and sardines

• Antioxidant and flavonoid-rich fruit and vegetables (see page 162)

• Foods high in fiber, especially soluble fiber (oats, beans, and lentils)

• One or two glasses of flavonoid-rich red wine each day.

PRECAUTIONS

If you suspect a heart attack, call an ambulance immediately. Symptoms include intense chest pain possibly spreading down the left arm or up into the throat, or jaw. Sweating, breathlessness, nausea, and clammy skin may also occur.

STRUCTURAL TREATMENT OPTIONS

CONVENTIONAL MEDICINE
Surgery for severe cases may include angioplasty to widen arteries, or a coronary artery bypass to improve blood flow past damaged areas.

COMPLEMENTARY THERAPIES
Chiropractic ❸ (*see page 118*) and **Osteopathy ❸** (*see page 119*) Soft tissue manipulation may improve the circulation and nerve supply to the chest. **Yoga ❷** (*see page 123*) Exercise involving stretching movements and breathing helps relieve stress and encourages relaxation. **T'ai Chi and Qigong ❸** (*see page 124*) In a British study, heart

Qigong

attack patients who practiced t'ai chi had lower blood pressure and maintained their exercise program longer than others, speeding recovery and improving chances of survival. **Acupuncture ❸** (*see page 125*) There is evidence that electro-acupuncture may relieve angina.

SELF-HELP TECHNIQUES
• Exercise can reduce high blood pressure and cholesterol levels, and optimize the efficiency of the heart and circulation. It also provides a means of channeling hostility and burning off stress chemicals. Aim for 20 minutes of aerobic exercise three times a week. If you have a heart problem, consult your doctor first.

PSYCHOSOCIAL TREATMENT OPTIONS

CONVENTIONAL MEDICINE
Stress management techniques may be recommended by your doctor.

COMPLEMENTARY THERAPIES
Psychotherapy & Counseling ❹ (*see pages 132–33*) Cognitive behavioral therapy may help people with hostile personalities alter their behavior. The Trusting Heart program (Dr. Redford Williams of Duke University in North Carolina) includes meditation; monitoring cynical, hostile thoughts; learning to listen and forgive; and asserting yourself rather than bottling up anger.

Meditation can bring inner calm.

STEPS TO A TRUSTING HEART
• Avoid cynicism
• Be tolerant
• Keep things in proportion
• Practice trusting people
• Listen without interrupting
• Let go of resentful feelings

In a study at Duke University, results showed that having a spouse or close friend tripled a heart attack patient's chances of being alive five years later. Religious faith and involvement in a social group seemed to help patients survive and recover from open-heart surgery. Group therapy and self-help and support groups may sustain those lacking a social network.

Meditation ❸ (*see page 135*) Focusing on a particular object or activity to produce a state of "relaxed awareness" has been shown to induce relaxation and relieve stress (*see page 170*). Researchers into transcendental meditation claim it can reduce the major risk factors of heart disease.

Autogenic Training ❸ (*see page 136*) and **Biofeedback ❸** (*see page 136*) These show people how to induce relaxation at will. Autogenic classes teach a series of imagery techniques that most participants can follow and use in daily life.

SELF-HELP TECHNIQUES
• Use relaxation and breathing techniques (*see pages 170–71*) to reverse the heart-damaging effects of stress • Ask yourself if you are hostile (*see page 49*). If you feel you are at risk, try to follow the Steps to a Trusting Heart (*see left*), and let go of hostile feelings, aiming to be more trustful of yourself and others • Examine your lifestyle, and consider which activities and companions you find supportive and which tend to undermine you. Try spending more time with the former and less with the latter • Relax by listening to soothing music or taking part in music sessions; studies show that music can have a temporarily beneficial effect on blood pressure levels.

Listening to music can help lower blood pressure.

BACK & NECK PAIN

At least two-thirds of adults suffer from back and neck pain at some stage in their lives. In many cases, the cause of pain is unclear, and even severe pain often gets better with little treatment within four to six weeks. However, the problem commonly recurs and one-third of sufferers claim that these recurrences are long-term episodes. Those most likely to have back pain are physical laborers and office workers, athletes, tall or overweight people, and the elderly.

Simple back and neck pain is usually caused by injury to strained and tense muscles. Surprisingly, back problems seldom result from a prolapsed or "slipped" disk, in which the pad that separates two spinal vertebrae splits, putting pressure on a spinal nerve. This results in back stiffness and severe leg pain. Although serious spinal damage or disease is rare, correct diagnosis is nevertheless essential for everyone with acute, severe, or persistent back and neck pain to rule out the possibility of inflammatory arthritis, osteomyelitis, a bone fracture, or cancer.

BIOCHEMICAL FACTORS

A BONY ARCH on the back of each vertebra forms a protective canal through which runs the spinal cord, the main communication line between the brain and the body. Nerves from the spinal cord branch off between each vertebrae and spread throughout the body to control movement and regulate involuntary processes such as digestion and the immune response. Nerves feeding into the spinal column carry sensory impressions, including pain sensations, to the brain and hormonal system, which orchestrate all body functions.

When strains or injuries to joints, tissues, or muscles occur, they trigger a biochemical chain reaction. Injured body tissue releases histamine and other chemicals that cause inflammation and swelling; these chemicals also stimulate the nerves that transmit pain. Joints and muscles respond to pain and inflammation by tensing up to prevent further harm, which in turn restricts the circulation so that fewer of the nutrients needed for healing can reach the area. Waste products, including lactic acid (which irritates the muscles), tend to accumulate in the injured tissue, exacerbating the

problem. This vicious cycle of congested circulation and buildup of inflammatory chemicals and the toxic products of injury makes the muscles more irritable and prone to spasm.

Back and neck pain can be symptoms of more widespread disease, such as osteoporosis and other bone conditions, kidney disease, infections, and cancer. Also, some people's spinal disks are genetically predisposed to wear out too quickly. Usually, the onset of back and neck pain is gradual. If acute and sudden, the source of the problem is probably an injury (*see Structural Factors*). Acute infection or bone disease might be suspected only if other symptoms were present.

BIOCHEMICAL TRIGGERS
• Kidney infections and kidney stones
• Osteoporosis (brittle bone disease) • Infection or malignancy in the bone • Abdominal conditions such as peptic ulcers and pelvic infections indirectly causing pain in the back

See page 54 for Biochemical Treatment Options

Realms of the Body (*see page 20*)

● **BIOCHEMICAL**
Body systems,
such as digestion

● **STRUCTURAL**
Muscles, bones,
joints, and nerves

● **PSYCHOSOCIAL**
Thoughts, feelings,
and relationships

STRUCTURAL FACTORS

THE SPINE CONSISTS of 33 girdle-shaped bones, the vertebrae. There are 24 individual, movable bones; five fused sacral vertebrae; and, below them, four fused vertebrae in the coccyx ("tailbone"). The vertebrae are connected to each other by small facet joints, muscles, and ligaments that together enable the spine to bend and move in almost any direction. The most mobile areas, and therefore the most prone to problems, are the seven cervical (neck) vertebrae and the five lumbar (lower back) vertebrae that allow bending sideways, forward and backward, and rotation.

The vertebrae are separated by intervertebral disks, thick pads of cartilage that help the spine flex and bend and that act as shock absorbers to prevent the bones from rubbing together. The vertebrae are stabilized by interlocking facet joints. Poor posture, overloading, stiffness, and old age make problems with these joints and disks more likely. Body work and movement therapies counter this tendency, promoting better circulation of nutrient-rich blood and easier movement.

Back and neck pain may result after an injury, such as whiplash. If the pain does not start immediately after an injury, it is usually from strain on, or wear in, one of the small facet joints. Supporting

muscles and ligaments can become tense – even when there is no injury or inflammation. Then constant tension restricts blood circulation in the joints and muscles so that painful waste products accumulate, resulting in pain and stiffness. As the affected areas weaken, other muscles compensate and in turn come under strain, so that pain and stiffness build up in the large back, buttock, shoulder, and neck muscles. These areas can remain tense and irritated long after an acute backache seems to have gotten better, which may be why so many people find that backache becomes a recurring problem.

STRUCTURAL TRIGGERS
• Injuries, such as whiplash or bone fractures
• Lifting and carrying heavy objects • Poor posture: twisting while bending; sitting badly in one position for long periods of time • Using poorly designed chairs and sagging mattresses • Unaccustomed periods of physical labor • Pregnancy and excess weight, both of which put pressure on the back and abdominal muscles
• Osteoarthritis, which results in degenerating cartilage and stiffness • Minor skeletal abnormalities, such as legs of unequal length or exaggerated spinal curves; overflexible (hypermobile) joints; stretched ligaments

See page 55 for Structural Treatment Options

PSYCHOSOCIAL FACTORS

NEGATIVE FEELINGS AND ATTITUDES may contribute to back pain, which in itself is stressful and tiring. Personality and early negative experiences may result in habitual hunching, stooping, and other postural problems that encourage the very emotions that started them. Long-term, persistent back pain often has a psychological dimension and may be associated with anxiety and depression. Pain makes us tense, and the feeling of wanting to resist the pain may result in restricted breathing and tightening of muscles in the painful area. This response encourages a worsening cycle of pain and tension.

PSYCHOSOCIAL TRIGGERS
• Emotional upset, stress, and anxiety affecting posture and causing muscle tension, especially in the neck and shoulder muscles • Tense or rushed behavior resulting in sudden movements that risk back or neck strain and injury • Lack of the information, motivation, or support that could encourage those with back pain to exercise, which could relieve muscle tension and enhance mood
• Fear of worsening persistent pain leading to anxiety and inactivity, which increase existing muscle tension and soreness

See page 55 for Psychosocial Treatment Options

BACK & NECK PAIN

CASE STUDY

Andrew, an osteopath, treated Todd, 50, a bartender who had strained his back handling beer barrels three years ago and had suffered from pain, sexual problems, and insomnia ever since. Analgesic and anti-inflammatory drugs had not helped, and Paul had started to drink heavily. Andrew diagnosed areas of spasm and stiffness in Todd's back, and combined gentle manipulation with stretching techniques to restore normal function.

In discussing Todd's work, Andrew learned that the bar that Todd runs was understaffed, and suggested that he ask his employers for more physical help so he could concentrate on the managerial side of his job. Andrew also gave advice on posture, especially in handling heavy loads, and on sexual positions that could help lessen the strain on Todd's back. Three months later, Todd reported that his company had agreed to hire an extra person. "That has taken the pressure off me. I follow Andrew's instructions on lifting. The pain is mostly gone, sex with my wife has improved, I'm sleeping much better, and I'm less tempted to drown my sorrows in alcohol."

PRECAUTIONS

See a doctor immediately if back pain is accompanied by nausea, vomiting, fever, weakness, pain down one or both arms or legs, or loss of bladder or bowel control.

You should also consult a doctor if the pain worsens over a period of several weeks, does not get better when you lie down, or wakes you at night.

BIOCHEMICAL TREATMENT OPTIONS

CONVENTIONAL MEDICINE

A doctor may prescribe painkillers (such as ibuprofen or acetaminophen), muscle relaxants, and anti-inflammatories (*see Drugs Glossary, page 179*). Local injections of anti-inflammatory medication can help acute inflammatory back pain that results from facet joint disease and acute disk prolapse.

Acetaminophen relieves pain.

Arnica flowers used in the homeopathic remedy

COMPLEMENTARY THERAPIES

Western Herbalism ❷ (*see page 127*)
Herbal remedies may help alleviate pain and muscle tension. St. John's wort, valerian, and lavender are calming; crampbark and devil's claw have anti-inflammatory properties.
Caution: See page 21 before taking herbal remedies.

St. John's wort is relaxing.

Valerian has sedative properties.

Nutritional Therapies ❸
(*see pages 128–29*)
For acute back pain, a naturopath may prescribe bromelain enzymes to reduce joint inflammation. For persistent inflammatory joint pain, you may be put on a diet that is low in animal fat and high in fish oil, to reduce levels of arachidonic acid, which helps produce inflammatory chemicals. Glucosamine sulfate supplements may be given to help rebuild joint cartilage.

Homeopathy ❸
(*see page 130*)
Several homeopathic medicines are traditionally used to help relieve acute back pain. The principal injury remedy is *Arnica*, which should be taken every 30–60 minutes while acute symptoms persist. *Rhus tox* is frequently suggested for inflammatory pain, *Ruta* for muscle strains, and *Hypericum* for neuralgic pain that is referred (*see Glossary, pages 177–78*) into an arm or leg.

SELF-HELP TECHNIQUES
• For chronic back and neck pain, consider an anti-inflammatory diet (*see Nutritional Therapies, left*) • Eat oily fish such as sardines and salmon twice a week • Reduce your intake of animal fats by substituting low-fat dairy products, limiting red meat, and removing poultry skin.

Eating oily fish such as mackerel and sardines helps reduce joint inflammation.

STRUCTURAL TREATMENT OPTIONS

CONVENTIONAL MEDICINE

X-rays and scans may be used to determine the cause of persistent or severe back pain. Gentle exercise or physical therapy is recommended early

Protruding disk

A section view of the spine showing a prolapsed disk

on. Only in severe cases would traction, a collar or a corset be advised. Surgery is reserved for extreme cases of prolapsed disk, when a nerve is badly compressed.

COMPLEMENTARY THERAPIES

Massage ❸ *(see page 116)*
Practitioners use massage to reduce muscle tension and stiffness, and to promote better circulation.

Rolfing & Hellerwork ❸ *(see page 116)*
These therapies, which involve deep massage and stretching, are helpful in cases involving persistent, painful muscle tension.

Chiropractic ❹ *(see page 118)* and
Osteopathy ❹ *(see page 119)*
Manipulation of joints and vertebrae restores mobility. Studies show that chiropractic and osteopathy can be effective in relieving acute back pain.

Alexander Technique ❸
(see page 121)
An Alexander teacher will show you how to correct your posture to relieve strain on joints and muscles and to ease pressure on nerves in the back and neck. It is very helpful for recurring or persistent pain.

Hydrotherapy ❸
(see page 126)
"Compressing" can help ease pain that comes on suddenly. Hot and cold compresses are alternately held on the skin – the hot compress for three minutes, followed by the cold compress for one minute. This process, which is repeated every 20 minutes, helps to increase blood flow, relax the muscles, and reduce inflammation.

Acupuncture ❺ *(see page 25)*
To relieve pain, practitioners stimulate acupoints on the *yang* channels that flow down the back and legs. Studies suggest acupuncture is valuable for both acute and persistent back and neck pain.

Yoga ❺ *(see page 123)*
Gentle breathing exercises, or

The head and neck are aligned to relax the spine.

pranayama, relax back muscles in cases of acute pain. Gentle postures like the Child and the Corpse may relax and stretch the back. A full yoga program taught by a qualified teacher can help prevent persistent back pain and relapses.

SELF-HELP TECHNIQUES

• If pain is acute, try stimulating acupressure point Colon 4 *(see page 125)* • Use very gentle stretching movements to keep a spasm at bay • Wrap a hot-water bottle or a pack of frozen peas in a towel and hold it to the area • Use bed rest as little as possible if in severe pain, then begin gentle stretching exercises to get your back moving again *(see pages 154–55)* • Improving your overall level of fitness will reduce persistent pain • Pilates exercises *(see Glossary, pages 177–78)* may help prevent or diminish relapses • Invest in a well-designed chair and a mattress that supports the back • Make sure your computer and other equipment are at appropriate levels *(see page 151)* • Lift or carry heavy objects appropriately *(see page 150)* • Lose any excess weight.

PSYCHOSOCIAL TREATMENT OPTIONS

CONVENTIONAL MEDICINE

Your doctor may recommend stress management techniques if your pain is persistent, recurrent or is stress-related.

COMPLEMENTARY THERAPIES

Psychotherapy & Counseling ❷
(see page 132–33)
If you have persistent pain, cognitive behavioral therapy can help you understand how your thoughts and feelings may be involved. The therapy can offer strategies to help change your coping style and behavior.

Biofeedback ❸ *(see page 136)*
Training can make you aware of habitual muscle contractions that cause long-

term pain. You can then learn to relax the tense area.

Hypnotherapy ❷ *(see page 134)*
A hypnotherapist will help you recognize sources and signs of tension, and to relax.

Autogenic Training ❸ *(see page 136)*
Effective techniques can be learned to induce relaxation at will through autogenic training.

Autogenic exercises help relax the neck and shoulders.

SELF-HELP TECHNIQUES

• With acute pain, allow yourself time out. Rest completely for 2–3 days to recover. But don't be afraid to start gentle exercise as soon as possible; remember that remaining immobile means you will take longer to recover • Relaxation and breathing techniques *(see pages 170–71)* can help to ease tension • Long-term absence from work is associated with pain becoming persistent, so stay at work or return as quickly as possible.

Exercise eases tension and pain.

OSTEOARTHRITIS

The most common form of joint disease, osteoarthritis affects up to 80 percent of people over 50. Severe osteoarthrit is affects three times as many women as men. Symptoms range from mild pain, stiffness of one or more joints, and swelling and "creaking" to total loss of joint function, disrupting walking, dressing, and even sleep. Muscles may waste away around an arthritic joint, and the bones can change shape. Osteoarthritis tends to affect large weight-bearing joints, such as hips and knees, as well as small joints in the feet, hands, fingers, neck, and lower back. Symptoms may be more severe than actual physical damage.

CASE STUDY

Daniel, an osteopath, is treating Lucy, an active 65-year-old with osteoarthritis in her hip. Lucy's orthopedic surgeon has advised her to delay a hip replacement as long as possible. Daniel mobilizes Lucy's lower back and hips once a month, and uses acupuncture on trigger points (*see Glossary, pages 177–78*) to release tension in her hip and thigh muscles. On his advice, Lucy follows a low-sugar, low-fat vegetarian diet for a week each month, and takes glucosamine supplements and cod liver oil daily. She practices yoga regularly and has joined an aqua aerobics class to strengthen her hips and knees, which were beginning to stiffen. "The effort is worthwhile," says Lucy. "My arthritis feels manageable and my surgeon says X-rays show my hip is no worse than five years ago."

BIOCHEMICAL FACTORS

Faulty circulation may weaken cartilage, causing inflammation and swelling. Chemicals released when cartilage is damaged trigger the release of enzymes that destroy collagen, an important protein in connective tissue.

BIOCHEMICAL TRIGGERS

• Nutritional deficiencies • Food intolerances (in some forms of osteoarthritis, allergic-type reactions have been found in affected joints) • Family history

STRUCTURAL FACTORS

In osteoarthritis, the cartilage that protects the ends of bones at their points of contact gradually degenerates. Bony outgrowths can distort the joints and cause the misshapen appearance seen in badly arthritic hands. This leads to changes in joint use and posture. Surrounding muscles may become painfully stiff, tighten up, or waste away, and blood circulation around the area deteriorates.

STRUCTURAL TRIGGERS

• Aging • Overuse of joints • Injury • Obesity

PSYCHOSOCIAL FACTORS

Persistent pain is stressful and tiring. Feelings of anxiety, anger, denial, depression, and helplessness may make the pain feel worse and can affect family relationships.

PSYCHOSOCIAL TRIGGERS

• Loss of mobility and fitness • Problems in coping with disability • Pain

Realms of the Body (*see page 20*)

● **BIOCHEMICAL** Body systems, such as digestion

● **STRUCTURAL** Muscles, bones, joints, and nerves

● **PSYCHOSOCIAL** Thoughts, feelings, and relationships

Key: Evidence of Efficacy (*see page 182*)

❶ ❷ ❸ ❹ ❺
least evidence ◄———————► most evidence

BIOCHEMICAL TREATMENT OPTIONS

CONVENTIONAL MEDICINE
Aspirin and ibuprofen can relieve both pain and inflammation. Doctors may prescribe stronger nonsteroidal anti-inflammatory drugs (NSAIDS) and corticosteroid injections for severe cases (*see Drugs Glossary, page 179*).

COMPLEMENTARY THERAPIES
Western Herbalism ❸ (*see page 127*)
Ginger, bromelain and curcumin may reduce inflammation. Studies of an herbal remedy containing an avocado

and soybean compound, known as ASU, have shown promising results.
Nutritional Therapies ❸
(*see pages 128–29*)
Food avoidance and exclusion diets can identify food intolerances if these are suspected, and fish oil supplements may relieve pain and stiffness. Research supports the use of glucosamine sulfate (a major component of joint fluid) and green-lipped mussel extract to help relieve symptoms.

SELF-HELP TECHNIQUES
• Follow an anti-inflammatory diet low in sugar, salt, and saturated animal fats • Eat more whole-grain cereals, fresh fruit, vegetables, and fish.

An anti-inflammatory diet can help counter symptoms of osteoarthritis.

STRUCTURAL TREATMENT OPTIONS

CONVENTIONAL MEDICINE
Physical therapy, TENS (*see Glossary, page 178*), and heat treatment relieve symptoms. Disability aids may be given to help patients cope at home. Surgery for severe cases includes joint replacement and joint immobilization.

COMPLEMENTARY THERAPIES
Massage ❷ (*see page 116*) and **Osteopathy ❸** (*see page 119*)
Practitioners use massage and stretching to improve

joint mobility, increase circulation around joints, and relieve related muscle tension.
Yoga ❸ (*see page 123*)
Gentle stretching postures can release stiff joints. **Caution:** Practice exercises with care.
Hydrotherapy ❸ (*see page 126*)
Mineral and thermal baths relieve joint pain and enhance well-being.

Gentle twists aid flexibility.

Acupuncture ❸ (*see page 125*)
Practitioners stimulate acupoints with needles or moxibustion to relieve pain and reduce inflammation.

SELF-HELP TECHNIQUES
• Lose excess weight to relieve pressure on joints • Get gentle exercise such as walking or swimming to strengthen joint-supporting muscles (*see pages 154–55*) • Avoid activities that put pressure on the joints, such as walking over rough terrain or lifting.

PSYCHOSOCIAL TREATMENT OPTIONS

CONVENTIONAL MEDICINE
A doctor may recommend one of the following therapies to improve your morale and help you feel more in control of symptoms.

COMPLEMENTARY THERAPIES
Psychotherapy & Counseling ❸
(*see pages 132–33*)
Talking through problems and learning cognitive behavioral skills (*see page 133*) may help you cope with persistent pain.

Visualization ❸ (*see page 136*)
Training can enable you to feel in control of pain, and allow you to combat related stress.
Meditation ❸ (*see page 137*)
Relaxing through meditation can be an important coping skill, and some therapists believe meditation can harness the mind to relieve pain.

Meditating can bring both mental and physical benefits.

SELF-HELP TECHNIQUES
• Join a support group, or practice relaxation and breathing exercises (*see pages 170–71*) • Note pain attacks in a diary (*see page 147*) to identify possible triggers • Improve your self-esteem by staying as active as your physical condition permits and becoming involved with hobbies and events.

RHEUMATOID ARTHRITIS

Unlike osteoarthritis (*see pages 56–57*) rheumatoid arthritis is an autoimmune disease. The body produces antibodies that attack the membranes that line joints, which become painfully swollen and stiff. The smaller joints in the hands and toes are most susceptible, but the wrists, ankles, knees, hips, and neck may be affected. It usually strikes between the ages of 30 and 50, but can affect children and the elderly. Women are at three times greater risk than men. In severe cases the inflammation can spread to the cartilage and bone, destroying joints and causing deformity. Rheumatoid disease may affect other organs including the heart and eyes.

CASE STUDY

Linda, an acupuncturist, treated Susie, 34, a publicist, who had been diagnosed with early rheumatoid arthritis in her hands. Drugs could prevent the condition from worsening but, with her doctor's approval, Susie wanted to try acupuncture first. Linda found that Susie led a hectic life and had allowed herself to get run down. She told her, "Your immune system is impaired. Traditional Chinese Medicine (TCM) sees rheumatoid arthritis as an invasion of Wind, Cold, and Damp, which blocks Blood. In TCM, we say that Blood warms the sinews. If it stagnates, its quality becomes impaired." Linda stimulated various points with warming moxibustion to clear Damp and Phlegm, move *qi* in the Blood, and correct the underlying imbalance of Liver, Kidney, and Spleen. Weekly sessions for two months produced good results; follow-up treatment continued over the next year.

BIOCHEMICAL FACTORS

The blood and joint fluid of people with rheumatoid arthritis contains "rheumatoid factor" antibodies which are not found in other forms of inflammatory arthritis. As in all inflammatory joint diseases, rheumatoid arthritis involves abnormally high reactivity of the immune system (*see page 167*).

BIOCHEMICAL TRIGGERS

• Genetic predisposition • Food intolerances (*see pages 92–93*) • "Leaky" gut (*see page 159*)

STRUCTURAL FACTORS

Affected joints become warm, swollen, and stiff, and purple-red in color. Ligaments, tendons, and surrounding muscles may shorten, stiffen, and become weak and painful. Circulation in the area is congested and waste products accumulate. Episodes of pain and stiffness tend to come and go, with gradually worsening joint damage.

ASSOCIATED CONDITIONS

• Raynaud's syndrome (fingers turn white when exposed to cold) • Carpal tunnel syndrome (tingling and pain in the fingers caused by pressure on the median nerve in the wrist) • Tenosynovitis (inflamed tendon sheaths in the wrist)

PSYCHOSOCIAL FACTORS

Feelings of anxiety, anger, denial, depression, and helplessness may reduce pain tolerance, undermine the ability to cope (resulting in varying degrees of disability), and affect family relationships. High levels of stress appear to be associated with the onset of the condition and may provoke flare-ups.

PSYCHOSOCIAL TRIGGERS

• Loss of mobility and fitness • Problems in coping with disability • Pain

Realms of the Body (*see page 20*)

● **BIOCHEMICAL**
Body systems,
such as digestion

● **STRUCTURAL**
Muscles, bones,
joints, and nerves

PSYCHOSOCIAL
Thoughts, feelings,
and relationships

Key: Evidence of Efficacy (*see page 182*)

❶   ❷   ❸   ❹   ❺

least evidence ◄———————► most evidence

BIOCHEMICAL TREATMENT OPTIONS

CONVENTIONAL MEDICINE

Aspirin and nonsteroidal anti-inflammatories (NSAIDS) ease pain and reduce inflammation. Antirheumatic drugs may slow or halt the condition, but can have adverse side effects (*see Drugs Glossary, page 179*). New drugs are being developed to block the antibody responsible for inflammation.

Drugs can ease inflammation.

COMPLEMENTARY THERAPIES

Traditional Chinese Medicine ❷
(*see pages 124–25*)
An extract (T2) from the "thundergod vine" (*Tripterygium wilfordii*), an ancient arthritis remedy, may be given, since studies of its efficacy are promising.

Western Herbalism ❷ (*see page 127*)
Curcumin (turmeric), bromelain (a pineapple extract), and ginger are given for their anti-inflammatory effect.

Nutritional Therapies ❸
(*see pages 128–29*)
Food intolerance is an important factor in some cases of inflammatory arthritis. A therapist may recommend an exclusion diet, probably starting with cutting out wheat and dairy products. Several studies show that short-term supervised fasts and a vegetarian diet can benefit people with rheumatoid arthritis. Omega-3 fatty acids in flaxseed and fish oils can relieve pain and stiffness, and green-lipped mussel extract may also ease symptoms. Supplements of vitamins A, C, E, and B_6, as well as zinc, pantothenic acid, and selenium may also be suggested.

Homeopathy ❸ (*see page 130*)
Rhus tox has been found to be effective, and a practitioner will prescribe remedies according to your constitution.

SELF-HELP TECHNIQUES
• Follow a diet low in saturated animal fats (to reduce inflammatory arachidonic acid), sugar, and salt, and rich in whole-grain cereals, fresh fruit, vegetables, and cold-water fish
• Do not smoke and avoid drinking excess alcohol.

STRUCTURAL TREATMENT OPTIONS

CONVENTIONAL MEDICINE
Doctors recommend physical therapy to relieve muscle spasms and joint stiffness, and occupational therapy to help patients adapt their everyday activities. In severe cases, surgery can replace certain damaged joints.

COMPLEMENTARY THERAPIES
Massage ❸ (*see page 116*)
A therapist aims to stimulate circulation in and around the affected joint to aid flexibility and removal of waste products.

Yoga ❷ (*see page 123*)
Gentle stretching exercises with a yoga therapy teacher may ease stiff joints.

Acupuncture ❸ (*see pages 124–25*)
Therapists stimulate acupoints around the affected area to relieve pain. Traditional acupuncturists treat patients according to their constitution.

Hydrotherapy ❷ (*see page 126*)
Exercising in warm water helps maintain mobility. Therapy with mineral baths and mud packs can be effective in reducing inflammation and pain.

SELF-HELP TECHNIQUES
• Gentle exercise and stretching can maintain muscle strength, fitness, and flexibility.

Practice stretching exercises to ease stiff joints.

PSYCHOSOCIAL TREATMENT OPTIONS

CONVENTIONAL MEDICINE
If clinical depression becomes a problem antidepressants may be prescribed.

COMPLEMENTARY THERAPIES
Psychotherapy & Counseling ❸
(*see pages 132–33*)
Talking through problems may help, and learning cognitive behavioral therapy may be recommended.

SELF-HELP TECHNIQUES
• Self-management programs in which people take responsibility for their diet, exercise, and relaxation increase confidence and encourage a healthy coping style • Practice relaxation and breathing techniques (*see pages 170–71*) • Hobbies and interests may help maintain your activity level • Keep a pain diary to identify triggers (*see page 147*) • Being part of a support group may help you deal with psychosocial factors.

PERSISTENT MUSCLE PAIN

There are several causes of persistent muscle pain. When a joint is stiff, as in osteoarthritis, the muscles acting on that joint become inactive and tense. Even though a muscle heals after injury, strain, or postural misuse, painful and tender trigger points (TP) may persist (*see Glossary, pages*

177–78). More generalized muscle pain, with a characteristic pattern of tender spots around the neck and shoulders, lower back, hips, and buttocks, is known as *fibromyalgia syndrome* (FMS). Accompanied by fatigue, sleep disturbance, and poor concentration, FMS is linked with other conditions, including chronic fatigue syndrome.

CASE STUDY

Simon, a naturopath, treated Carol, a 39-year-old teacher, for muscle pain and stiffness with tender spots around her neck and lower back, and abdominal pain and bloating. Conventional medical tests were inconclusive, but Roger suspected "leaky" gut (*see page 159*). "This can trigger a release of inflammatory prostaglandins in muscle tissues, causing pain," said Simon. He prescribed slippery elm powder in water to soothe and heal the inflamed gut lining, and a soothing remedy of licorice, wild yam, and marshmallow. Simon also used body work (*see Naturopathy, page 126*) to stimulate digestion and lymph drainage processes and suggested a diet low in animal fat and a program of relaxation and exercise. Three months later Carol reported that all symptoms had abated considerably.

BIOCHEMICAL FACTORS

People with FMS tend to have other mind-body conditions, particularly hyperventilation and irritable bowel syndrome, dysmenorrhea, PMS, and chronic fatigue. These aspects of FMS may be linked to a deficiency of the brain chemical serotonin, which is also a cause of depression. Other factors that may be involved are a buildup of waste products in muscles caused by poor tissue circulation, food intolerances, infections, nutritional deficiencies, and hormone imbalances.

BIOCHEMICAL TRIGGERS
• Food intolerances • Low serotonin levels (*see Glossary, pages 177–78*)

STRUCTURAL FACTORS

Tense, aching muscles are a common sign of poor fitness and loss of well-being, and result in a self-perpetuating cycle of pain/muscle spasm/pain. Blood circulation around the area is poor so waste products tend to accumulate. Both FMS and trigger points can cause persistent tension and pain in muscles that are structurally normal.

STRUCTURAL TRIGGERS
• Stress and muscle tension • Poor posture
• Sleep disturbance • Hyperventilation syndrome (*see pages 170–71*) • Lack of exercise • Colds • Occupational strain from lifting and repetitive movements

PSYCHOSOCIAL FACTORS

Persistent unexplained pain is depressing, anxiety-provoking, and exhausting. It also perpetuates a cycle of inactivity, poor sleep, tension, and loss of physical fitness.

PSYCHOSOCIAL TRIGGERS
• Depression; the majority of people with clinical depression first see a doctor because of pain, often muscle pain • Sleep disturbance
• General anxiety • Low tolerance of pain

Realms of the Body *(see page 20)*

● **BIOCHEMICAL**
Body systems,
such as digestion

● **STRUCTURAL**
Muscles, bones,
joints, and nerves

● **PSYCHOSOCIAL**
Thoughts, feelings,
and relationships

Key: Evidence of Efficacy *(see page 182)*

❶ ❷ ❸ ❹ ❺

least evidence ◄——————► most evidence

BIOCHEMICAL TREATMENT OPTIONS

CONVENTIONAL MEDICINE
Painkillers such as acetaminophen and anti-inflammatories help in the short term, but they are of no benefit for persistent pain. Low-dose amitriptyline may be suggested for FMS (*see Persistent Pain, pages 106–09*).

COMPLEMENTARY THERAPIES
Western Herbalism ❷ *(see page 127)*
Valerian may be recommended if sleep is a problem for you.
Caution: Avoid if taking sleeping pills.

Nutritional Therapies ❸
(see pages 128–29)
A nutritionist may recommend an exclusion or rotation diet *(see page 129)* to identify any food intolerances. To help the body manufacture serotonin, the practitioner may recommend vitamins, magnesium, and the amino acid tryptophan. Calcium and zinc may help relieve disrupted sleep patterns.

Vitamin supplements remedy deficiencies.

Magnesium may be advised, since a mild deficiency can cause fatigue and muscle pain at rest.
Homeopathy ❸ *(see page 130)*
Practitioners claim constitutional homeopathy can help.

SELF-HELP TECHNIQUES
• Keep a food diary *(see page 147)* to figure out whether certain foods make the pain worse.

STRUCTURAL TREATMENT OPTIONS

CONVENTIONAL MEDICINE
A course of physical therapy exercises can improve mobility and circulation.

COMPLEMENTARY THERAPIES
Massage ❸ *(see page 116)*
A massage can stimulate the circulation and may ease pain by relaxing trigger points and areas of muscle stiffness.
Aromatherapy ❷ *(see page 117)*
Soothing essential oils such as lavender and rosemary can help relax muscles and promote a feeling of well-being.

Chiropractic ❷ *(see page 118)* and
Osteopathy ❷ *(see page 119)*
A practitioner will aim to relax and lengthen a muscle affected by TP, working around the spine and joints to improve flexibility. You will be advised about factors that cause muscle tension.
Yoga ❷ *(see page 123)*
Gentle stretching postures ease muscle stiffness and improve postural problems that could be causing pain.
Acupuncture ❸ *(see page 125)*
Research suggests that electro-

acupuncture may relieve FMS symptoms. Needle acupuncture also eased fibromyalgia in a 1998 study, in which results were ascribed to the stimulation of the body's natural painkillers.

SELF-HELP TECHNIQUES
• Knead tender areas to relax muscles
• Try acupressure *(see page 125)* on tender spots • Exercise for 20 minutes three times a week to release endorphins and enhance well-being.

PSYCHOSOCIAL TREATMENT OPTIONS

CONVENTIONAL MEDICINE
A doctor may suggest a cognitive behavioral approach if FMS causes a vicious cycle of pain and inactivity.

COMPLEMENTARY THERAPIES
Psychotherapy & Counseling ❷
(see pages 132–33)
A cognitive behavioral therapist helps those with FMS break cycles of depression and inactivity that reduce tolerance of pain. Short-term counseling may help if there are any

underlying psychological issues that are contributing to the pain.
Hypnotherapy ❸ *(see page 134)*
In a 1991 trial, people with FMS who had not responded to physical therapies reported less pain, fatigue, and stiffness and a greater sense of well-being after hypnotherapy.
Visualization ❷ *(see page 134)*,
Meditation ❸ *(see page 135)*,
Biofeedback ❷ *(see page 136)*
These techniques help relieve stress and release muscle tension.

SELF-HELP TECHNIQUES
• Learn relaxation and breathing techniques *(see pages 170–71)*
• Keep a stress diary *(see page 147)*.

Relaxation techniques relieve tension.

SPORTS INJURIES

From tennis elbow to swimmer's shoulder, there are many types of sports injuries, and a third are serious enough to need medical attention or to interfere with daily activities. Symptoms may include bruising, bleeding, swelling, and pain, and some can take longer to heal than broken bones. Practitioners advise the "RICE" response to hasten recovery; *rest* the injured part; apply *ice* in a towel for ten minutes every two hours for two days; *compress* the injury with a bandage; *elevate* it above the heart to reduce inflammatory fluids and swelling. Resume gentle movement when it is less painful, but stop if the pain returns.

CASE STUDY

Daniel, an osteopath, treated Graham, a 51-year-old teacher, who had pulled his shoulder during a vigorous game of tennis. Daniel diagnosed tendonitis: "Tennis was only a trigger," he said, "Graham's shoulder has been turning inward over a long period. The tendon inflammation would probably respond to a steroid shot, but his posture and the background tension in his neck and upper back make him prone to further injury." Daniel massaged and mobilized the shoulder to release strained, tight muscles and advised about posture and exercises to loosen the shoulders. Graham reported: "It took the best part of nine months before I felt ready for another match, but my upper body feels in much better shape now, and I don't get the tension headaches I used to."

BIOCHEMICAL FACTORS

A good training regime improves the muscles' capacity to process oxygen and to work harder, but frequent and intensive training can lower immunity and resistance to disease. There may be a connection between diet and the ability to recover.

BIOCHEMICAL TRIGGERS

• A diet high in saturated fats, which produces excess inflammatory chemicals
• Lack of essential fatty acids and antioxidants in the diet, which weakens the body's anti-inflammatory response

STRUCTURAL FACTORS

The most common sports injuries are sprains and strains to the lower limbs. Tendons most susceptible to injury are those in the shoulder, thumb, knee, and ankle and the Achilles' tendon on the heel. Half of all tennis players develop tennis elbow, a painful inflammation in the attachments of muscles around the elbow.

STRUCTURAL TRIGGERS

• Overuse of muscles • Lack of fitness
• Inadequate warming-up and cooling-down exercises • Ignoring warning aches and pains
• Cumulative wear and tear from a repetitive movement • Inappropriate style or technique
• Poor footwear

PSYCHOSOCIAL FACTORS

Too cavalier or too timid an attitude toward sports can lead to injury; for example, skiing on a run beyond your capability, or tensing up through fear. Lack of proper equipment and ignorance of correct techniques can also result in injury.

PSYCHOSOCIAL TRIGGERS

• Impatience • Desire to please • Timidity
• Stubbornness • Excessive competitiveness

PRECAUTIONS

Consult a doctor if the pain is severe, persistent, stabbing, radiating, or centered on a bone or a joint; if a joint is stiff or immobile; or if there is any numbness or tingling.

Realms of the Body (*see page 20*)

  BIOCHEMICAL
Body systems,
such as digestion

  STRUCTURAL
Muscles, bones,
joints, and nerves

  PSYCHOSOCIAL
Thoughts, feelings,
and relationships

Key: Evidence of Efficacy (*see page 182*)

❶ ❷ ❸ ❹ ❺

least evidence ◀——————▶ most evidence

BIOCHEMICAL TREATMENT OPTIONS

CONVENTIONAL MEDICINE
Painkillers and nonsteroidal anti-inflammatory drugs (*see Drugs Glossary, page 179*) help minor strains. Steroid injections relieve acute inflammation but can weaken joints if repeated.

COMPLEMENTARY THERAPIES
Western Herbalism ❸ (*see page 127*)
Arnica or St. John's wort, traditional herbs for muscle soreness, may be given.
Nutritional Therapies ❸ (*see page 128*)
Therapists may suggest supplements of

Pineapple speeds repair.

flavonoids, especially quercetin and citrus bioflavonoids, which can halve recovery times. Antioxidants beta carotene, vitamin C, vitamin E, zinc, and selenium may also speed healing, and bromelain, an enzyme in fresh pineapple, is thought to accelerate tissue repair. Essential fatty acids help produce anti-inflammatory prostaglandins.

Homeopathy ❶ (*see page 130*)
Remedies that a practitioner may advise include *Arnica* for bruising and for muscles aching from overuse in work or sports, or *Ruta* for sprains and strains of muscles, joints, and ligaments.

SELF-HELP TECHNIQUES
• Follow a balanced diet high in complex carbohydrates. (There is no evidence that high-protein diets build extra muscle.)

STRUCTURAL TREATMENT OPTIONS

CONVENTIONAL MEDICINE
X-rays can establish if any bones have been broken. A physical therapist may use ultrasound, which heats the area and improves circulation and drainage.

COMPLEMENTARY THERAPIES
Chiropractic ❹ (*see page 118*) and
Osteopathy ❹ (*see page 119*)
These therapies can help mobilize stiff joints, loosen tense muscles, rehabilitate muscle weaknesses, and prevent overuse injuries as well as muscular pain.

An ice pack can help reduce inflammation.

Massage ❸ (*see page 116*)
Many athletes use massage after injury to restore joint mobility and improve local circulation.
Acupuncture ❸ (*see page 125*)
A practitioner will stimulate acupoints and trigger points in the muscles to help relax a tense area prone to recurring injury.
Hydrotherapy ❷ (*see page 126*)
Practitioners recommend an ice pack or cold compress to reduce inflammation, and exercise in a warm pool to restore strength and flexibility. Jet showers, Jacuzzis, and whirlpool baths may ease pain. After swelling has subsided, dry heat from a heating pad or lamp can be used to ease stiffness.

SELF-HELP TECHNIQUES
• Warm up muscles by jogging in place, then stretching. Stretch again after exercise (*see pages 156–57*)
• Avoid sudden, vigorous, or repetitive movements • Get in shape before trying any new sport • Allow your body plenty of time to rest after injury.

Massage speeds recovery from sports injuries by improving circulation and relaxing muscles.

PSYCHOSOCIAL TREATMENT OPTIONS

CONVENTIONAL MEDICINE
Sports psychology is an expanding field that has been incorporated into conventional treatment. Cognitive behavioral therapy may help identify and change attitudes and behavior that increase the risk of injury. It can also improve athletic performance.

COMPLEMENTARY THERAPIES
Hypnotherapy ❸ (*see page 134*)
A practitioner may teach self-hypnosis techniques to foster a positive attitude and self-confidence. Hypnotherapy can be used as an adjunct to sports psychology to improve performance in ways that avoid risk of injury.

SELF-HELP TECHNIQUES
• Be patient and allow yourself time to recover from an injury • Make sure you are well prepared before starting any sport • Do not push your body beyond its limits and avoid over-competitiveness • Learn the correct techniques and practice them.

PREMENSTRUAL SYNDROME

A week or two before menstruation, women often suffer discomfort and distress. The symptoms of premenstrual syndrome (PMS) can be physical or emotional, and some experts categorize them into four types: anxiety (irritability, mood swings, and insomnia); craving (increased appetite, headache, palpitations, fatigue, and fainting); depression (forgetfulness, confusion, and lethargy) and fluid retention (weight gain, bloating, and breast tenderness). Symptoms are triggered by hormonal changes, but no single cause has been isolated and no consistent imbalance in progesterone and estrogen has been identified.

CASE STUDY

Tom, a Traditional Chinese Medicine (TCM) practitioner, was visited by Sara, who had left her job three years earlier to have a baby. Over the last two years her periods had gotten painful, and recently she found herself irritable and tearful during the week before menstruation. Tom explains: "In TCM, menstrual disorders and life events are closely connected, so I asked Sara how she was coping at home. Painful periods, along with PMS, indicate stagnation of Liver *qi*; and their starting after childbirth suggests deficiency of Blood. This, combined with the stress of change, may be causing discomfort."
Tom prescribed a traditional herbal remedy based on dong quai (angelica) taken over three months. Within a month, Sara's PMS symptoms were greatly reduced.

BIOCHEMICAL FACTORS

Hormones from glands all over the body help orchestrate the menstrual cycle; one hormone prompts an egg to develop, and another triggers ovulation. Various nutritional and hormonal imbalances may cause different symptoms.

BIOCHEMICAL TRIGGERS

• Low levels of vitamin B_6, vitamin E, magnesium, and essential fatty acids
• Disturbed levels of the hormone prolactin, which affects estrogen and progesterone levels • Excess estrogen, which may influence levels of the brain chemical serotonin, affecting mood • Rising levels of the hormone aldosterone, which may cause fluid retention
• Fluctuating levels of insulin-regulating hormones, leading to cravings

STRUCTURAL FACTORS

Excessive exercise can disrupt the hormonal cycle and exacerbate PMS symptoms. Poor circulation, fluid retention, and too much stress are often factors in PMS, and all can be reduced by moderate exercise, particularly in the two weeks before a period. Gentle exercise also eases aches and pains associated with PMS, because it stimulates the production of endorphins, the body's natural painkillers.

STRUCTURAL TRIGGERS

• Lack of exercise • Sustained, strenuous training

PSYCHOSOCIAL FACTORS

The hormonal cycle is controlled by those areas of the brain that are also affected by stress. Mild to moderate PMS symptoms may be exacerbated by psychological and lifestyle factors that reflect a general lack of well-being. Raised anxiety and muscle tension just before menstruation may be due to stress.

PSYCHOSOCIAL TRIGGERS

• Clinical depression • Relationship problems
• Stress from irregular or painful periods
• Perfectionistic personality with a tendency to take on too much • Stressful life events

Realms of the Body (*see page 20*)

● **BIOCHEMICAL**
Body systems,
such as digestion

● **STRUCTURAL**
Muscles, bones,
joints, and nerves

● **PSYCHOSOCIAL**
Thoughts, feelings,
and relationships

Key: Evidence of Efficacy (*see page 182*)

❶ ❷ ❸ ❹ ❺

least evidence ◄————————————► most evidence

BIOCHEMICAL TREATMENT OPTIONS

CONVENTIONAL MEDICINE
Prescribed drugs include progestogen, estrogen, and the contraceptive pill to regulate the normal menstrual cycle; bromocriptine, a hormone-suppressing drug; diuretics for fluid retention; lithium; tranquilizers; antidepressants; and painkillers (*see Drugs Glossary, page 179*).

COMPLEMENTARY THERAPIES
Western Herbalism ❸ (*see page 127*)
German studies show that *Agnus castus* may help adjust the hormone balance

by increasing the amount of progesterone available. If depression is a factor, St. John's wort, a traditional nerve tonic, may be suggested.
Nutritional Therapies ❹
(*see pages 128–29*)
Various studies suggest that for all PMS symptoms the following supplements are beneficial: vitamin B$_6$, vitamin E, magnesium, zinc, and evening primrose oil. Nutritionists recommend

Agnus castus

a diet low in fats, caffeine, and refined carbohydrates including sugar, and some practitioners consider food intolerances.

SELF-HELP TECHNIQUES
• To combat cravings, eat regularly
• Reduce your intake of salt, sugar, saturated fats, milk, and caffeine
• Taking 1200 mg of calcium carbonate daily may relieve symptoms • Eat plenty of phytoestrogenic foods – cereals, soy products, legumes, fruit, and vegetables – which help regulate hormones.

STRUCTURAL TREATMENT OPTIONS

CONVENTIONAL MEDICINE
Your doctor will recommend regular exercise to improve the circulation.

COMPLEMENTARY THERAPIES
Aromatherapy ❷
(*see page 117*)
Essential oils
of lavender,
clary sage,
and geranium,
especially if used

Lavender has
relaxing properties.

in massage (*see page 116*), appear to soothe, relieve tension, and reduce fluid retention.
Chiropractic ❷ (*see page 118*)
and **Osteopathy** ❷ (*see page 119*)
Practitioners may use soft tissue manipulation to aid relaxation and improve muscle tension and circulation in the pelvis.
Reflexology ❹ (*see page 120*)
A 1991 US study found stimulating certain acupoints in the feet to be effective in relieving PMS symptoms.

Yoga ❷ (*see page 123*)
The Triangle, Bow, Half Shoulder Stand, and Butterfly postures are recommended. **Caution:** Avoid upside-down postures during menstruation.
Acupuncture ❷ (*see page 125*)
Many women report that acupuncture brings relief from symptoms.

SELF-HELP TECHNIQUES
• Warm compresses or a hot-water bottle on the lower abdomen and back may help relieve discomfort.

PSYCHOSOCIAL TREATMENT OPTIONS

CONVENTIONAL MEDICINE
Some doctors may prescribe antidepressants. Stress management techniques may be suggested.

COMPLEMENTARY THERAPIES
Psychotherapy & Counseling ❷
(*see pages 132–33*)
Therapy may help those with severe PMS to resolve any emotional problems contributing to anxiety and tension. Relationship counseling may be useful. Cognitive behavioral therapy can help

women release negative attitudes and become more positive.
Autogenic Training ❸ (*see page 136*)
This structured approach to relaxation can induce a calm state of mind and help relieve stress-related symptoms.

SELF-HELP TECHNIQUES
• Keep a diary of daily events and moods to identify problem areas that need particular care before a period (*see page 147*) • Some experts suggest that you should try to regard the mood

swings of PMS not as an illness but as an opportunity to be assertive and creative • Relaxation and breathing techniques (*see page 170*) can relieve stress and reduce muscle tension.

Pinpoint factors
involved in PMS by
keeping a daily diary.

MENSTRUAL PAIN

At the beginning of a menstrual period, or just before, women commonly experience menstrual pain (dysmenorrhea), accompanied by dull aches in the lower back and headaches. "Primary" dysmenorrhea usually starts soon after puberty and tends to disappear between the ages of 25 and 30, or after childbirth. Pain begins shortly before the period and rarely lasts longer than 12 hours. "Secondary" dysmenorrhea, in which periods suddenly become painful after a number of years without problems, is usually caused by an underlying disorder. Pain starts several days before a period and continues throughout.

CASE STUDY

Rae, a homeopath, treated Pam, a 45-year-old executive, who had painful, flooding periods. Pam's doctor had diagnosed a fibroid, and suggested a hysterectomy if homeopathy didn't work. "Pam worked hard, but could be bad-tempered with her staff," said Rae, who concluded that Pam's constitutional type (*see page 130*) was *Lachesis*, a remedy derived from snake venom. Rae gave her a single dose in a dilution of *1m*.

"In three months, the pain and discomfort eased, and the flooding was less," said Pam. Now 50, she sees Rae 2–3 times a year and, so far, has avoided surgery. Pam's doctor expects the fibroids to shrink as she approaches menopause.

BIOCHEMICAL FACTORS

Primary dysmenorrhea may be caused by strong uterine contractions triggered when progesterone levels decline at the onset of a period. They are due to an excess of, or a sensitivity to, inflammatory prostaglandins, which are hormonelike fatty acids produced in the body (*see Glossary, pages 177–78*).

BIOCHEMICAL TRIGGERS
• Accumulating waste products in uterine and pelvic muscles • Inadequate nutrition

PSYCHOSOCIAL FACTORS

Stress, emotional upsets, and life events can lead to pelvic muscle tension and raise sensitivity to pain. Primary dysmenorrhea, along with premenstrual syndrome, tends to be associated with chronic fatigue syndrome, irritable bowel syndrome, and fibromyalgia syndrome (muscle pain). It can also indicate a general lack of well-being.

PSYCHOSOCIAL TRIGGERS
• Anxiety and/or depression • Poor posture and breathing • Work or emotional overload • Poor coping skills

STRUCTURAL FACTORS

Secondary dysmenorrhea is due to uterine congestion, a condition in which blood circulation in the pelvis is restricted and pelvic muscles become tense. It may be accompanied by heavy periods and should be checked by a doctor, since it is likely to be caused by an underlying condition. Poor fitness is a factor in both primary and secondary dysmenorrhea.

STRUCTURAL TRIGGERS
• Fibroids • Endometriosis • Pelvic inflammatory disease (infection of the uterus, fallopian tubes, and/or ovaries) • Sensitivity to an IUD (intrauterine device) • Lack of fitness

PRECAUTIONS

Consult your doctor if you suspect you have secondary dysmenorrhea.

Realms of the Body (*see page 20*)

● BIOCHEMICAL
Body systems,
such as digestion

● STRUCTURAL
Muscles, bones,
joints, and nerves

○ PSYCHOSOCIAL
Thoughts, feelings,
and relationships

Key: Evidence of Efficacy (*see page 182*)

❶ ❷ ❸ ❹ ❺

least evidence ◄———————► most evidence

BIOCHEMICAL TREATMENT OPTIONS

CONVENTIONAL MEDICINE
For primary dysmenorrhea a doctor will suggest acetaminophen, anti-inflammatories like ibuprofen, aspirin, or mefenamic acid, and/or muscle-relaxants (*see Drugs Glossary, page 179*). Severe pain is treated by suppressing ovulation with oral contraceptives or hormonal drugs such as danazol.

COMPLEMENTARY THERAPIES
Western Herbalism ❸ (*see page 127*)
Agnus castus may be recommended to regulate reproductive hormones.

Nutritional Therapies ❸
(*see pages 128–29*)
Supplements of magnesium, essential fatty acids, calcium, vitamins B_6 and B complex, and vitamin E may be advised. A high-fiber or vegan diet, containing 75 percent complex carbohydrates, 15 percent protein, and 10 percent fat, may be suggested.

Vegan diet

Homeopathy ❷ (*see page 130*)
Remedies include *Pulsatilla* for cramps with nausea, *Sepia* for pains with depression, *Nux vomica* for cramps and irritability, and *Magnesia phos.* for pain eased by warm pressure.

SELF-HELP TECHNIQUES
• Eat less animal fat and more essential fatty acids (*see pages 160–61*) • Balance hormones with natural phytoestrogens (*see Glossary, pages 177–78*) in celery, fennel, parsley, and soy products.

STRUCTURAL TREATMENT OPTIONS

CONVENTIONAL MEDICINE
Treatment of secondary dysmenorrhea will depend on the cause. A doctor may suggest exercise, which can help both types of dysmenorrhea by improving circulation and fitness.

COMPLEMENTARY THERAPIES
Chiropractic ❹ (*see page 118*) and **Osteopathy** ❹ (*see page 119*)
A practitioner will treat the spine, pelvis, and abdominal muscles, aiming to improve uterine circulation and relieve muscle tension. Trials show that chiropractic can relieve period pain.

Yoga ❷ (*see page 123*)
Postures that release tension in the lower abdomen, such as the Pelvic Lift, Triangle, Moon, Forward Stretch, and Corpse poses will be advised.
Caution: Experts warn against upside-down poses during periods.

Acupuncture ❹ (*see page 125*)
A practitioner will suspect "deficiency of *qi* or Blood" or "weakness of the Kidney and Liver" and treat accordingly. In one trial, 91 percent of patients improved with acupuncture.

SELF-HELP TECHNIQUES
• Lie on your back with knees bent and use the palm of your hand to massage the lower abdomen with circular motions. This relieves uterine muscle spasms and promotes blood flow • Heat, from sources such as a hot-water bottle, can boost circulation.

Hot-water bottle relieves pain.

PSYCHOSOCIAL TREATMENT OPTIONS

CONVENTIONAL MEDICINE
Your doctor may suggest that you practice one of the complementary therapies listed below.

COMPLEMENTARY THERAPIES
Hypnotherapy ❷ (*see page 134*)
You might be taught simple relaxation and imagery exercises to improve pelvic circulation and relieve pain.
Biofeedback ❸ (*see page 136*)
By responding to signals measuring minute body changes, you can learn to relieve muscle tension at will. You will be shown techniques to calm the mind and relax the muscles. Slow diaphragmatic breathing improves blood circulation to the pelvis.

SELF-HELP TECHNIQUES
• Try relaxation and breathing techniques (*see pages 170–71*) or meditation (*see page 135*), which can relieve muscle tension and improve circulation
• Regular exercise can improve circulation, tone muscles, and relieve tension (*see pages 150–52*)
• Keep a stress-trigger diary (*see page 147*) to learn what factors worsen symptoms of dysmenorrhea.

Regular meditation is excellent for relieving stress.

INFERTILITY IN WOMEN

Infertility is defined as the inability to conceive after a year or more of trying. In over 10 percent of cases no obvious reason can be found, but usually there is a specific problem in one or both partners (*see also Infertility In Men, pages 80–81*). Failure to ovulate and blocked fallopian tubes account for 60 percent of cases of female infertility. Complementary therapies may not trigger ovulation or clear tubes, but they do support conventional fertility techniques if they strengthen and regulate body systems. "Mind-body" techniques help in the same way and may counteract the stress that can affect biological factors involved in fertility.

CASE STUDY

James, a psychologist, saw Anne, 33, who had recently married for the second time. She had been trying to conceive for over a year and the medical investigations had found nothing wrong. "I discovered she had had an ectopic pregnancy at 28," said James. "Understandably she was anxious. She wanted a baby, but unconsciously feared disaster. I contacted her family doctor and eventually she saw a second gynecologist who said there was little chance of another ectopic pregnancy. I asked Anne to forget about trying to conceive and taught her self-hypnosis so she could relax and visualize becoming pregnant and carrying the baby to term." Anne started her "homework" right away and five months later became pregnant.

BIOCHEMICAL FACTORS

Absent or erratic menstrual periods usually indicate a failure to ovulate regularly. Problems with ovulation, the likely cause in a third of the cases of infertility, are often due to hormonal imbalances.

BIOCHEMICAL TRIGGERS

• Coming off the contraceptive pill
• Approaching menopause • Having inadequate levels of the hormone progesterone, which prepares the uterine lining for conception • Certain medications (ask your doctor) • Exercising excessively • An underactive thyroid gland • Inadequate nutrition • Environmental chemicals

PSYCHOSOCIAL FACTORS

Inability to conceive can be distressing, especially if there is no detectable reason. In animals, stress and underfeeding can cause temporary infertility and may have the same effect in humans. There is some evidence that reducing stress may reduce levels of the hormone prolactin (which in excess inhibits fertility). Striving to have a child and the burdens of infertility treatment can be enormously stressful. In one American study, infertile women were found to be as depressed as people with cancer or heart disease. Interestingly, couples with unexplained infertility who eventually reconcile themselves to childlessness or adoption often achieve a successful pregnancy.

PSYCHOSOCIAL TRIGGERS

• Stress and overwork • Subconscious feelings of fear or anger • Depression

STRUCTURAL FACTORS

Conception is impossible if the ovaries do not produce eggs; the eggs fail to reach the uterus because fallopian tubes are blocked; the uterus does not retain the fertilized egg; or the cervical mucus is hostile to sperm and prevents it from entering the uterus.

STRUCTURAL TRIGGERS

• Scarring or blocking of the fallopian tubes or ovaries caused by pelvic inflammatory disease (PID), sometimes caused by sexually transmitted diseases, for example, chlamydia • Multiple ovarian cysts • Endometriosis (growth of uterine lining in tubes and ovaries) • Fibroids • Extreme weight loss or gain • Genetic abnormalities • Cervical mucus that is too sticky, too acidic, or that contains spermicidal antibodies

Realms of the Body (*see page 20*)

● BIOCHEMICAL
Body systems,
such as digestion

● STRUCTURAL
Muscles, bones,
joints, and nerves

● PSYCHOSOCIAL
Thoughts, feelings,
and relationships

Key: Evidence of Efficacy (*see page 182*)

❶   ❷   ❸   ❹   ❺

least evidence ◀━━━━━▶ most evidence

BIOCHEMICAL TREATMENT OPTIONS

CONVENTIONAL MEDICINE

Investigation may include a blood test for progesterone and prolactin levels, and a sperm count. Antibiotics may be prescribed to clear up infections blocking the fallopian tubes. Other often-prescribed drugs include clomiphene, which helps trigger ovulation, and human chorionic gonadotropin (HCG), which stimulates the ovaries.

Wild yam has a progesterone-like effect.

COMPLEMENTARY THERAPIES

Western Herbalism ❷ (*see page 127*)
A practitioner will suggest herbs that regulate hormones and aid conception, such as agnus castus, false unicorn root, sarsaparilla, black cohosh, and wild yam.

Nutritional Therapies ❷
(*see pages 128–29*)
Vitamin and mineral deficiencies and exposure to chemical toxins are claimed to promote miscarriage. A therapist may suggest an organic diet and supplements such as essential fatty acids, folic acid and vitamins B_6 and B_{12}. A diet rich in vitamin E and alkaline foods is said to regulate acidity of cervical and vaginal secretions. Food intolerance tests and a detoxification regime may be advised.

SELF-HELP TECHNIQUES

• Have sex at the time of ovulation (urine dipsticks and daily waking temperature charts detect ovulation)
• Stop smoking • Try to maintain a healthy weight.

STRUCTURAL TREATMENT OPTIONS

CONVENTIONAL MEDICINE

Investigations include an ultrasound scan of the ovaries; special X-rays of the uterus; and an examination of the uterus, ovaries, and fallopian tubes with a laparoscope (an illuminated viewing tube). Blocked fallopian tubes may be cleared by surgery. Various kinds of "test-tube" or in vitro fertilization techniques (IVF) are available, but will only be suggested as a last resort.

COMPLEMENTARY THERAPIES

Yoga ❷ (*see page 123*)
Yoga or other body work therapies may be used with a detoxification program to improve circulation and reduce mucus in the case of tubal blockage or endometriosis.

Acupuncture ❷ (*see page 125*)
Chinese studies have suggested that acupuncture is helpful for PID or endometriosis.

SELF-HELP TECHNIQUES

• Use the "missionary position" during sex with the man on top and a folded pillow under your hips. Remain on your back with your knees raised for the 20–30 minutes the cervix needs to take in the semen • Do not use artificial lubricants because they can inhibit sperm movement • Do not douche after sex • Get regular, moderate exercise.

PSYCHOSOCIAL TREATMENT OPTIONS

CONVENTIONAL MEDICINE

If you are over 35, consult your doctor after trying to conceive for 6–9 months, or after two years if under 32. Sometimes seeking advice and feeling more in control may be sufficient to promote conception.

COMPLEMENTARY THERAPIES

Psychotherapy & Counseling ❷
(*see pages 132–33*)
The prospect of starting a family sometimes provokes unconscious fears. Discussing these issues may help put them in perspective. A program of cognitive therapy, relaxation techniques, and group support may aid conception.

Hypnotherapy ❸ (*see page 134*)
Hypnotherapy can reduce stress levels and help some women conceive. It may uncover fears about labor, motherhood, or the baby's potential threat to the relationship.

Discuss your feelings with your partner.

Meditation, Visualization, Autogenic Training ❷ (*see pages 135–36*)
Techniques that help you achieve deep relaxation will counter tension.

SELF-HELP TECHNIQUES

• Practice relaxation and breathing techniques (*see pages 170–171*)
• Talk openly about your feelings with your partner
• Focus on goals other than conception.

PREGNANCY

Pregnancy is a natural process, although modern medicine has, until quite recently, tended to treat it as a medical problem. Today there is a movement toward a less clinical approach and greater acceptance of the mother's involvement in monitoring her health and that of her unborn baby. As well as relieving ailments and enhancing well-being, complementary therapies can be useful in pregnancy if they encourage a woman's sense of control of her body. Therapies work well in tandem with conventional medical approaches and some midwives integrate aromatherapy and acupuncture as part of their care.

CASE STUDY

George, a doctor trained in homeopathy, saw Trisha early in her second pregnancy. Her first had ended in a difficult forceps delivery and this time she wanted to do everything possible to maintain well-being and avoid medical intervention. George recommended the homeopathic remedy *Sepia 6c* and elasticized acupressure wrist bands to relieve morning sickness. He encouraged her to follow a healthy diet and to join a natural childbirth class to learn relaxation, breathing techniques, and gentle prenatal yoga postures. To relieve low back pain in the last three months, George suggested McTimoney chiropractic, and two weeks before delivery he recommended the homeopathic remedy *Caullophylum*, which is derived from a Native American plant and is said to promote the normal onset of labor. The delivery of Trisha's son was easier and happier than the birth of her first baby and she breast-fed him immediately.

BIOCHEMICAL FACTORS

Women planning to conceive should take the opportunity to aim for optimum health. They should attempt to improve their diet and lifestyle, consult a doctor about any medical disorders, and avoid unnecessary medication. Adequate nutrition is vital at all stages of pregnancy since, increasingly, studies show that a mother's diet has long-term effects on her child's health. There is, for instance, a strong link between low birthweight and diabetes and heart disease in adult life.

PSYCHOSOCIAL FACTORS

Emotional highs and lows can result from hormonal changes and also from the expectation of a major life change. Our ancestors lived in groups, and frequently during pregnancy modern women become more aware of primitive instincts and feel in particular need of companionship.

PRECAUTIONS

Avoid anyone with German measles, or get vaccinated at least three months before trying to conceive. Do not take herbs in medicinal doses in the first three months of pregnancy and consult a trained herbalist thereafter. Do not take any essential oils internally and do not use thyme or chamomile essential oils externally. See a doctor immediately for prolonged nausea and inability to eat properly; frequent urination for more than two days, especially if accompanied by pain; prolonged flulike illness; fluid retention that has not decreased after three days; unusual headaches or unexplained pain; vaginal bleeding.

STRUCTURAL FACTORS

Many women feel easily exhausted and tired during pregnancy, especially if they are working or have other small children. All body systems are under strain, especially during mid- to late pregnancy, although they usually adapt. Strain on circulation is reflected in fluid retention, on the back in low back pain, and on digestion in acid reflux and indigestion.

Realms of the Body *(see page 20)*

● **BIOCHEMICAL**
Body systems,
such as digestion

● **STRUCTURAL**
Muscles, bones,
joints, and nerves

● **PSYCHOSOCIAL**
Thoughts, feelings,
and relationships

Key: Evidence of Efficacy *(see page 182)*

❶　❷　❸　❹　❺

least evidence ◄—————————► most evidence

BIOCHEMICAL TREATMENT OPTIONS

CONVENTIONAL MEDICINE
Consult a doctor or midwife as
soon as you suspect you are
pregnant. You will be told to take
folic acid (400 mcg daily) to prevent
defects in the baby's spinal cord and
nervous system. Iron, zinc, and
calcium supplements are sometimes
recommended. Small, regular meals
are advised for morning sickness.

COMPLEMENTARY THERAPIES
Western Herbalism ❸ *(see page 127)*
A practitioner may suggest chamomile

*Chamomile tea
is soothing.*

tea to induce sleep,
ginger capsules for
morning sickness,
and a compress
with witch hazel
for hemorrhoids.

Nutritional Therapies ❸
(see pages 128–29)
Suggested supplements may include
zinc for the baby's growth, vitamin B_6
and B_{12} for energy and to enhance the
working of folic acid in the body,
vitamin C and essential fatty acids for
brain growth. A therapist may suggest

bromelain (an enzyme in pineapple)
to reduce swelling after an episiotomy
(see Glossary, pages 177–78).

SELF-HELP TECHNIQUES
• Avoid large doses of multivitamins,
since too much vitamin A may cause
birth defects • Avoid foods that may
contain listeria: unpasteurized cheese,
raw undercooked meats, and food
with uncooked egg such as homemade
mayonnaise • Limit fatty foods, sugar,
and salt •Avoid alcohol in the first 12
weeks and give up smoking throughout.

STRUCTURAL TREATMENT OPTIONS

CONVENTIONAL MEDICINE
Regular tests are done to be sure you
are not suffering from problems such
as anemia, fluid retention, high blood
pressure, or poor placental growth.

COMPLEMENTARY THERAPIES
Chiropractic ❸ *(see page 118)* and
Osteopathy ❸ *(see page 119)*
Back pain is common in mid- to late

pregnancy. A practitioner will gently
stretch and manipulate the lower back
to ease symptoms.
Acupuncture ❹ *(see page 125)* and
Acupressure ❹ *(see page 125)*
A practitioner may stimulate the
Neiguan point, which is just below
the wrist on the Pericardium meridian,
since clinical trials have shown it can
relieve nausea in early pregnancy.

Acupuncture is useful for pain relief in
labor and moxibustion has been used
to avoid breech births.

SELF-HELP TECHNIQUES
• Get plenty of rest • Continue your
normal exercise program but replace
high-impact activities with walking,
yoga, or swimming • Practice pelvic
floor exercises before and after the birth.

PSYCHOSOCIAL TREATMENT OPTIONS

CONVENTIONAL MEDICINE
Prenatal classes help you prepare for
all aspects of birth and parenthood.
Postpartum support groups are
increasingly available.

COMPLEMENTARY THERAPIES
Visualization ❸ *(see page 134)*
You will be encouraged to focus on
positive feelings about your baby
during and after pregnancy. In one
study, mothers of premature babies
who listened to a guided imagery and
relaxation tape produced 63 percent
more breast milk than the control group.

Meditation ❷ *(see page 135)*
A practitioner will teach you
techniques that can provide effective
pain relief in labor.

SELF-HELP TECHNIQUES
• Get support from family, friends,
other mothers, and community
groups • Talk about your
feelings with your partner
and family and ask other
parents to share their
practical advice and
experiences
• Use relaxation

techniques *(see pages 170–71)* to
relieve tension • Your baby can hear
in the uterus as early as 20
weeks, so talk reassuringly to
your unborn baby and play
soothing music • Take
opportunities to enjoy
art and the beauty
of nature to enhance
your own well-being,
as well as that of
your baby.

*A hug is comforting
and reassuring.*

MENOPAUSE

The cessation of menstrual periods, which signals the end of childbearing years, is known as menopause. It occurs between 45 and 55, although it may take place as early as 35. The surgical removal of the uterus (hysterectomy) and ovaries results in immediate menopause. Hormonal changes take place over several years before and after periods stop. Known as perimenopause, this period may be accompanied by symptoms such as hot flashes, aches and pains, skin changes, and emotional upset. The severity of symptoms varies and it is thought that women with positive attitudes toward aging suffer less than others.

CASE STUDY

Tania, an acupuncturist, treated Clare, 51, for hot flashes, night sweats, insomnia, vaginal dryness, and anxiety. Clare's doctor had suggested HRT but recommended she try acupuncture first. Tania used methods of diagnosis from Traditional Chinese Medicine (TCM). "Clare's pulse was thin and rapid, and her tongue red – classic signs of *yin* deficiency. In TCM, Kidney *yin* energy is the body's cooling process and deficiency causes a slow, rumbling internal heat." She stimulated points on the Heart and Kidney meridians, chiefly Kidney 6 (*see page 124*).
"My night sweats disappeared after one treatment," reported Clare. "The other symptoms improved within six sessions."

BIOCHEMICAL FACTORS

A woman's estrogen levels decrease in her 40s, so eggs mature less regularly in the ovaries, producing less progesterone. This makes the uterus lining build up less, so periods become erratic and then cease. Many menopausal symptoms may result from the effect of less estrogen reaching the hypothalamus, which acts as a link between the hormonal and nervous systems. Adrenal glands and fat cells in the hips and thighs still manufacture small amounts of estrogen but are easily depleted by poor diet and stress. Falling estrogen levels also result in the following problems: disturbed blood circulation, loss of bone-building calcium and tissue-building collagen, anemia resulting from heavy periods in perimenopause, and increased likelihood of heart disease.

STRUCTURAL FACTORS

Although estrogen's primary role is in reproduction, it also helps preserve the health of the bones, heart and arteries, gut, skin, and even the brain. Common menopausal complaints include night sweats, hot flashes, headaches, palpitations, dizziness, weight gain, fatigue, itching and vaginal dryness, loss of skin elasticity and moisture, hair loss caused by thinning tissues, muscular aches and pains, increased urinary tract infections, osteoporosis, and increased risk of bone fractures. Menopausal problems are caused by declining estrogen levels, and most disappear when menopause is over; the exceptions are osteoporosis and complaints related to thinning tissues.

PSYCHOSOCIAL FACTORS

Common psychological menopause complaints are forgetfulness and difficulty in concentrating, loss of libido, depression, mood swings, and insomnia. Hormonal changes may disturb levels of endorphins, the body's natural painkillers and mood-enhancing chemicals. Menopause also often coincides with life changes, and some women may lose their sense of identity as children grow up and leave home. Women with a positive attitude toward aging and those who work seem to suffer less than others. Studies show women with premenstrual syndrome or dysmenorrhea (painful periods) are more likely to have menopausal complaints.

Realms of the Body (*see page 20*)

BIOCHEMICAL
Body systems,
such as digestion

STRUCTURAL
Muscles, bones,
joints, and nerves

PSYCHOSOCIAL
Thoughts, feelings,
and relationships

Key: Evidence of Efficacy (*see page 182*)

❶ ❷ ❸ ❹ ❺

least evidence ◀─────────────▶ most evidence

BIOCHEMICAL TREATMENT OPTIONS

CONVENTIONAL MEDICINE
Hormone replacement therapy (HRT), in the form of pills, skin implants, patches, and creams, is prescribed to replace estrogen. Treatment prevents many menopausal changes but may increase the risk of breast cancer if used long-term. Biphosphonates (*see Drugs Glossary, page 179*) and SERMs (Selective Estrogen Receptor Modulators) prevent bone loss.

HRT patches and creams

COMPLEMENTARY THERAPIES
Western Herbalism ❺ (*see page 127*)
A practitioner may prescribe agnus castus, licorice, and hops for hot flashes and night sweats; St. John's wort for mild depression; and valerian for insomnia.
Caution: Do not take licorice if you have high blood pressure, or valerian if you are taking sleeping pills.
Nutritional Therapies ❸
(*see pages 128–29*)
Suggested supplements may include

vitamin E for hot flashes, night sweats, and vaginal dryness; evening primrose oil for dry skin; calcium, magnesium, vitamin D, and boron for bone health; and vitamin B_6, B_{12}, and folic acid for heart and brain health.

SELF-HELP TECHNIQUES
• Follow a low-fat, high-fiber diet • Eat phytoestrogen-rich fruit and vegetables (*see Glossary, pages 177–78*) • Limit salt, red meat, and alcohol • Take 1500 mg of calcium daily (1000 mg if on HRT).

STRUCTURAL TREATMENT OPTIONS

CONVENTIONAL MEDICINE
Symptoms are treated individually (*see Headaches, pages 24–25; Persistent Muscle Pain, pages 60–61; Vaginitis, pages 74–75; and Cystitis, pages 76–77*).

COMPLEMENTARY THERAPIES
Massage ❷ (*see page 116*)
Visiting a practitioner for a regular massage can relieve tension and enhance feelings of well-being.
Aromatherapy ❷ (*see page 117*)
German chamomile, sandalwood,

or rose are among the essential oils recommended for hot flashes and mood swings.
Yoga ❷ (*see page 123*)
A teacher will demonstrate helpful poses. By focusing the mind on breathing, physical movement, and postures, yoga may relieve tension and improve body image.
Acupuncture ❷ (*see page 125*)
A practitioner will stimulate acupoints to regulate the hormonal system and relieve hot flashes.

SELF-HELP TECHNIQUES
• Exercise reduces the frequency and severity of hot flashes • Weight-bearing activities, such as walking and dancing, help maintain bone density
• Artificial lubricants such as KY Jelly can counteract vaginal dryness during sex.

Exercise helps menopause symptoms.

PSYCHOSOCIAL TREATMENT OPTIONS

CONVENTIONAL MEDICINE
A doctor may prescribe antidepressants if depression is severe. Stress management techniques may be advised (*see pages 168–69*).

COMPLEMENTARY THERAPIES
Psychotherapy & Counseling ❷
(*see pages 132–33*)
Talking through feelings can help resolve issues around the loss of fertility and self-esteem. Cognitive behavioral therapy may promote a

more positive approach toward aging. The period of psychological transition from fertility to postfertility can be an anxious time.

Focusing on a serene image can relieve anxiety.

SELF-HELP TECHNIQUES
• Stress can make symptoms worse. Practice relaxation, visualization, and breathing techniques (*see pages 170–71*) to relieve tension, promote relaxation, and improve coping skills
• Keeping a stress diary (*see page 147*) helps to pinpoint triggers • Share experiences with friends and make time for yourself and activities you enjoy • Stay as positive as possible. An optimistic outlook helps people cope successfully with life changes.

VAGINITIS

This infection, which is also known as vaginal thrush, yeast infection, or candidiasis, causes soreness and itching of the vulva, the skin around the opening of the vagina. A curdy, white discharge is a telltale sign. Vaginitis is common, particularly during pregnancy or after a course of antibiotics, but sometimes it can be difficult to keep at bay. Conventional treatment usually helps, but recurrences are frequent. Attention to all the contributing factors is important, especially if the condition is recurring. Since other infections can also cause vaginal soreness, it is important to confirm the diagnosis with medical tests.

CASE STUDY

Cathy, a nurse in her 30s, had recurrent vaginal infections. A laboratory culture had confirmed a diagnosis of vaginitis, and although antifungal medication had reduced her symptoms, it failed to prevent the infection from recurring. Susan, an herbalist, was asked to help. She gave Cathy vaginal suppositories, containing tea tree, marigold, and thyme extracts, to use each night for a week. A cream with the same ingredients was given for daytime use, and Cathy's partner was advised to use it too. Cathy found that the itching and discharge quickly cleared up. She also followed Susan's advice to eat a very low-sugar, high-fiber diet and increase her fresh fruit and vegetable intake to raise her levels of infection-fighting antioxidants.

BIOCHEMICAL FACTORS

"Friendly" bacteria in the vagina, mouth, and gut convert glucose into lactic acid, helping keep the area free of harmful microorganisms. Certain conditions, however, encourage the bacterium *Candida albicans* to overwhelm the friendly bacteria, resulting in vaginitis. Broad-spectrum antibiotics (*see Glossary, page 178*) kill friendly bacteria, so vaginitis is common after a course of antibiotics.

BIOCHEMICAL TRIGGERS

• Lowered immunity • Nutritional deficiencies
• Medication such as antibiotics, steroids, and immunosuppressants • Hormonal changes as a result of using oral contraceptives or being pregnant • Raised blood-sugar levels, as in diabetes • Allergies

STRUCTURAL FACTORS

Uncontrolled growth of *Candida albicans*, a common microorganism in the mouth, gut, and vagina, causes vaginitis. Many practitioners believe "candida overgrowth" in the gut contributes to problems from chronic fatigue syndrome and irritability to irregular periods and irritable bowel syndrome. They suspect that the microorganism damages the intestinal lining, allowing toxins to be absorbed into the bloodstream (*see page 159*). If the vagina is dry, its lining may be damaged during sex, increasing the likelihood of vaginitis.

STRUCTURAL TRIGGERS

• Sexual intercourse with an infected partner
• Overuse of douches, spermicides, and bath products that can disturb the acid/alkali balance in the vagina

PSYCHOSOCIAL FACTORS

Recurrent vaginitis may suggest that the immune system is impaired. Stress is known to increase susceptibility to infection in general.

PSYCHOSOCIAL TRIGGERS

• Overwork and lack of adequate sleep
• Anxiety • Depression • Traumatic life events

Realms of the Body (*see page 20*)

● **BIOCHEMICAL**
Body systems,
such as digestion

● **STRUCTURAL**
Muscles, bones,
joints, and nerves

● **PSYCHOSOCIAL**
Thoughts, feelings,
and relationships

Key: Evidence of Efficacy (*see page 182*)

❶ ❷ ❸ ❹ ❺

least evidence ◀ ──────────── ▶ most evidence

BIOCHEMICAL TREATMENT OPTIONS

CONVENTIONAL MEDICINE
If vaginitis recurs, a doctor will advise women on oral contraceptives to consider barrier methods.

COMPLEMENTARY THERAPIES
Naturopathy ❸ (*see page 126*)
A therapist sees vaginitis as possibly also indicating an overgrowth of *Candida* in the gut. Apple cider vinegar douches and *lactobacillus* yogurt may restore "friendly" bacteria and readjust the pH balance.

Nutritional Therapies ❸
(*see pages 128–29*)
A practitioner may advise you to exclude all dietary yeast, mold, and fungi (for example, yeast-based bread, blue cheese, or mushrooms), as well as starches and refined sugar on which yeast feeds. "Live" yogurt may be suggested to restore friendly bacteria in the gut, as well as natural antifungals, which include garlic, onions, aloe vera juice, and caprylic

Coconut extract has antifungal properties.

acid, an extract of coconut. Supplements to revive the immune system, such as vitamin B complex, beta carotene, and vitamins C and E, as well as zinc, selenium, magnesium, essential fatty acids, and folic acid, may be advised.

SELF-HELP TECHNIQUES
• Eat a healthy diet (*see pages 158–59*). • Avoid junk food and refined sugar.

STRUCTURAL TREATMENT OPTIONS

CONVENTIONAL MEDICINE
Examination of the vaginal discharge confirms diagnosis. A doctor will prescribe vaginal tablets of antifungal drugs, or nystatin or clotrimazole (*see Drugs Glossary, page 179*), or oral medication such as fluconazole. A vaginal swab tests for other infections, such as gardnerella or trichomonas, which cause soreness or discharge. A partner should be treated at the

Tea tree plant and oil

same time. Doctors believe candidiasis in the gut affects only people with impaired immune systems, such as those with AIDS.

COMPLEMENTARY THERAPIES
Aromatherapy ❸ (*see page 117*)
A practitioner may advise you to add antifungal or antiseptic essential oils, such as tea tree, to the bathwater.

Acupuncture ❷ (*see page 125*)
Where infection is recurrent, acupuncture may help boost an impaired immune system.

SELF-HELP TECHNIQUES
• Wear cotton underpants and avoid nylon panty hose and tight clothes that create a warm, moist environment
• Avoid vaginal deodorants and do not use scented soaps, bubble baths, and other products • Exercise regularly to enhance immunity.

PSYCHOSOCIAL TREATMENT OPTIONS

CONVENTIONAL MEDICINE
If vaginitis recurs, doctors will advise you to learn stress management techniques (*see pages 168–69*).

COMPLEMENTARY THERAPIES
Psychotherapy & Counseling ❷
(*see pages 132–33*)
Recurrent vaginitis may be part of an underlying sexual difficulty. It can also cause sexual problems and therefore relationships may suffer. Talking these through may help.

Visualizing pleasant images can help induce relaxation.

Visualization ❷ (*see page 134*)
You are encouraged to focus on calming scenes or use guided imagery to help you relax at will.

SELF-HELP TECHNIQUES
• Keep a stress-trigger and symptom diary (*see page 147*) • Try to get plenty of sleep • Practice stress management skills (*see pages 168–69*) • Learn relaxation and breathing techniques (*see pages 170–71*), which will help you deal with stressful events.

CYSTITIS

Over 20 percent of women have a cystitis attack once a year, and many cases result in a kidney infection. Cystitis is usually caused by a bacterial infection inflaming the lining of the bladder and urethra. Symptoms include burning or stinging when urinating, wanting to pass urine more often, abdominal pain, and unpleasant-smelling urine. Blood in the urine, chills, or fever may also be experienced. Recurrent cystitis indicates a low resistance to infection, which can be caused by a number of factors ranging from stress to oral contraceptives or a poor diet. If attacks persist, a doctor may advise seeing a gynecologist.

CASE STUDY

Abbey, a homeopath, saw Jill, 24, who had recurrent cystitis. Jill wanted to come off permanent low-dose antibiotics prescribed by her doctor because they seemed to give her indigestion. She said she felt depressed, and was uninterested in sex. She was better when busy but felt cold and craved sour tastes. All these characteristics were typical of the *Sepia* constitution. "Jill was well informed about the self-help treatments recommended for cystitis," said Abbey. "All I had to do was prescribe." With her doctor's agreement, Jill finished her course of antibiotics two weeks later and took a single dose of *Sepia 200c*. A month later, she was much happier and had had no further attacks. In the next six months she had two minor attacks, which were managed with the homeopathic remedies *Nux vomica 6c* and *Cantharis 6c*.

BIOCHEMICAL FACTORS

Recurrent attacks of cystitis suggest that the immune system is depleted, resulting in lowered resistance to infection. Poor diet can also reduce resistance to infection, as can hormone deficiency during and after menopause. Chemicals in foam baths, condoms, and spermicides can sometimes irritate the urethra.

BIOCHEMICAL TRIGGERS

• Spermicidal gels and contraceptive diaphragms • Oral contraceptives
• Sugar in the urine (caused by diabetes), which may encourage infection • Hormone deficiency during and after menopause
• Inadequate diet and food intolerances

STRUCTURAL FACTORS

Women are more susceptible to cystitis than men because their urethra is shorter and the opening is closer to the anus. Anything that prevents the bladder from emptying completely, for example during pregnancy, allows bacteria to multiply in stagnant urine. Bacteria can also find their way into the urethra from the anus after sex. Diaphragms can cause cystitis by putting pressure on the urethra and bladder.

STRUCTURAL TRIGGERS

• Prolapsed uterus, fibroids • Blockage in the bladder caused by a stone or tumor
• Bruising during intercourse ("honeymoon cystitis") • Enlarged prostate gland (in men)

PSYCHOSOCIAL FACTORS

Stress can put a strain on the immune system so that resistance to infection is low.

PSYCHOSOCIAL TRIGGERS

• Stress in the workplace • Problems with relationships • Anxiety and depression
• Emotionally traumatic events

Realms of the Body (*see page 20*)

BIOCHEMICAL
Body systems,
such as digestion

STRUCTURAL
Muscles, bones,
joints, and nerves

PSYCHOSOCIAL
Thoughts, feelings,
and relationships

Key: Evidence of Efficacy (*see page 182*)

❶ ❷ ❸ ❹ ❺
least evidence ◄———————————► most evidence

BIOCHEMICAL TREATMENT OPTIONS

CONVENTIONAL MEDICINE

If a urine test indicates a bacterial infection, antibiotics are given. These are effective, but may lead to a yeast infection. You will be told to drink plenty of fluids to flush out the bladder.

COMPLEMENTARY THERAPIES

Western Herbalism ❸ (*see page 127*)
A practitioner will suggest you drink unsweetened cranberry juice, which helps stop bacteria from sticking to the lining of the urinary tract. Dandelion

and chamomile are soothing, and echinacea boosts the immune system.
Nutritional Therapies ❷
(*see pages 128–29*)
If attacks recur, you may be tested for food intolerances, allergies, or *Candida albicans.* Supplements of vitamin C, zinc and bioflavonoids can help boost the immune system.
Homeopathy ❷ (*see page 130*)
Remedies include *Cantharis* if urination

Echinacea can improve immunity.

is painful; *Sarsaparilla* for burning after urination; *Staphysagria* for "honeymoon cystitis" (*see opposite*).

SELF-HELP TECHNIQUES

• Drink a teaspoon of bicarbonate of soda dissolved in 10 fl oz (300 ml) of water once an hour for the first three hours of an attack • Eat a whole-foods diet with garlic and onions • Avoid tea, coffee, alcohol, sugary and spicy foods, and acidic foods such as tomatoes, citrus fruits, and spinach.

STRUCTURAL TREATMENT OPTIONS

CONVENTIONAL MEDICINE

If a urine test finds no trace of bacterial infection, symptoms may be caused by an inflammation of the vagina or the urethra, the tube that carries urine from the bladder (urethritis). Bruising of the urethra during sex may also be a cause. In some cases a gynecological examination, X-ray of the kidneys, or cystoscopy (examination of the bladder with a viewing instrument) may be necessary for an accurate diagnosis.

COMPLEMENTARY THERAPIES

Acupuncture ❸ (*see page 125*)
A practitioner may stimulate the Bladder, Kidney, Spleen, Liver, and Conception Vessel acupoints. In a Norwegian study, when these points were stimulated twice a week for four weeks, 85 percent of women in the study were free of cystitis.

SELF-HELP TECHNIQUES

• To prevent cystitis, drink lots of water and urinate frequently

• Use lubrication during sex to avoid bruising, and urinate afterward
• Avoid foam baths, scented soaps, and vaginal deodorants
• Keep the genital area clean • Avoid tight-fitting or synthetic-fiber underwear • Hold a hot-water bottle to your lower back or between your legs to ease cystitis pain.

Water helps flush away cystitis bacteria.

PSYCHOSOCIAL TREATMENT OPTIONS

CONVENTIONAL MEDICINE

Doctors may suggest stress management techniques (*see pages 168–69*).

COMPLEMENTARY THERAPIES

Psychotherapy & Counseling ❷
(*see pages 132–33*)
Recurring cystitis may reflect or prompt sexual difficulties, so talking through relationship problems can help.
Relaxation & Breathing ❶
(*see pages 170–71*)
Relaxation and breathing techniques

can help you recognize tension in your body, and can teach you to calm your mind and relax your deep pelvic muscles.

Breathing through alternate nostrils has a calming effect.

SELF-HELP TECHNIQUES

• Keep a diary of cystitis attacks, noting any triggers that may be avoided
• Keep a symptom- and stress-trigger diary (*see page 147*) • Examine your lifestyle for persistent sources of stress and deal with them if possible
• Practice meditation techniques (*see page 135*) or stress management skills (*see pages 168–69*) • Mind-body techniques like yoga are useful for relaxing the muscles and calming the mind.

ENLARGED PROSTATE

The prostate is a small, walnut-shaped gland surrounding the urethra below the bladder, and secretes a fluid that contributes to semen. Enlargement of the prostate, known as *benign prostatic hyperplasia* (BPH), is increasingly common with age. More than 90 percent of men over 70 are affected. There may be no symptoms until the gland begins to press on the urethra and interfere with urine flow. Troublesome symptoms include frequent urination, incontinence, difficulty in urinating, urine and kidney infections, back pain, and pain between the legs. Symptoms of prostate cancer, the third most common cancer in men, are similar to those of BPH.

CASE STUDY

Carl, 66, consulted Jean, an herbalist, about a prostate problem. He complained of frequency and urgency in urination, and disturbed sleep because he had to get up at night to urinate. A urologist had recently diagnosed BPH and said that he would soon need surgery. Carl hoped for another approach; his doctor wanted to support him while he awaited surgery. Jean gave Carl saw palmetto and nettle root to protect the prostate from further enlargement, and couch grass and horsetail to heal irritated urinary membranes. She also advised taking 15 mg of zinc daily. Carl's symptoms lessened steadily. Within six months he had no discomfort or urgency when urinating and was getting up less often at night. His doctors were happy with his progress and no longer saw an immediate need to operate.

BIOCHEMICAL FACTORS

The cause of prostate enlargement is unclear, but hormonal changes related to aging may play a role. Falling levels of the male hormone testosterone, combined with rising levels of prolactin, encourage the conversion of testosterone to the powerful androgen dihydrotestosterone (DHT), which stimulates the growth of prostate tissue.

BIOCHEMICAL TRIGGERS

• Deficiencies of zinc and essential fatty acids encourage the conversion of testosterone to DHT • High alcohol intake (more than 4 units a day) is associated with BPH • High intake of saturated fat • Environmental pollution, which increases estrogen production in males

PSYCHOSOCIAL FACTORS

Embarrassment can prevent men from being examined soon enough for effective treatment. The symptoms of prostate enlargement can be humiliating and worrisome and may affect work, personal, and sexual relationships. Stress increases levels of the hormone prolactin, possibly leading to a buildup of DHT (*see above*).

PSYCHOSOCIAL TRIGGERS

• Overwork and anxiety • Fatigue caused by sleep that is disturbed by the need to urinate during the night • Shame and loss of self-esteem • Sexual difficulties • Stress

STRUCTURAL FACTORS

The bladder muscle may become over-developed from forcing urine through the compressed urethra. If the bladder is unable to expel all the urine, the tubes connecting it to the kidneys can become distended. Urine stagnating in the tubes may lead to a kidney infection and can leak around the obstruction, causing incontinence. The bladder may also become overactive, leading to a more frequent need to urinate.

STRUCTURAL TRIGGERS

• Aging • Lack of exercise • Poor posture or constipation, restricting circulation in the pelvis

PRECAUTIONS

Report any prostate problems to your doctor. Symptoms of BPH and prostate cancer are similar, so men over 60 should consider a yearly prostate examination and a prostate-specific antigen (PSA) test.

BIOCHEMICAL TREATMENT OPTIONS

CONVENTIONAL MEDICINE

Doctors screen for levels of PSA (prostate-specific antigen). High levels indicate prostate cancer, but slightly raised levels may not be significant. Alpha-adrenergic blockers (*see Drugs Glossary, page 179*), which help improve urine flow, may be prescribed, as well as the drug finasteride, which can shrink the prostate gland (although it occasionally causes impotence or loss of libido).

COMPLEMENTARY THERAPIES

Western Herbalism ❺ (*see page 127*)
Conventional doctors in Europe often prescribe herbal remedies. Several

Saw palmetto may shrink the prostate gland.

studies have shown that saw palmetto extract can improve symptoms as effectively as finasteride and with fewer side effects, but it may take 6–8 weeks for benefits to show. Other herbal remedies that may also be suggested include rye-grass pollen, extracts of flower pollen, pygeum bark extract, and stinging nettles.

Nutritional Therapies ❸
(*see pages 128–29*)
Zinc supplements may be given, since they seem to shrink the prostate, but

more studies are needed. Estrogens may interfere with zinc absorption, so older men may lack this mineral. Supplements of essential fatty acids, selenium, and vitamin A may help.

SELF-HELP TECHNIQUES

• Eat foods rich in zinc, essential fatty acids, and soy – natural sources of phytoestrogens that reduce BPH
• Avoid saturated fats and cholesterol
• Limit alcohol intake, especially beer.

Eat foods rich in zinc.

STRUCTURAL TREATMENT OPTIONS

CONVENTIONAL MEDICINE

A rectal examination will indicate whether the prostate is enlarged, a urine test will reveal any infection, and a blood test will assess kidney function. A physician may use ultrasound, a bladder X-ray, and a urine flow test to help diagnosis. If symptoms are mild, medical treatment may not be necessary. A procedure called transurethral resection (TURP) uses heat to destroy the enlarged prostate, and in more severe cases, the prostate gland may be removed

surgically (prostatectomy). Both procedures may cause sexual difficulties. Microwave treatment, laser surgery, and a new, high-frequency radio-wave procedure are alternative methods used to shrink the prostate.

COMPLEMENTARY THERAPIES

Alexander Technique ❷
(*see page 121*) Learning to improve posture can help

The Shoulder Stand posture

circulation of blood in the pelvis.
Yoga ❷ (*see page 123*)
The Triangle and Shoulder Stand are recommended to reduce prostatic swelling, and the Half Shoulder Stand and Supine Butterfly are suggested to improve pelvic circulation.

SELF-HELP TECHNIQUES

• Do not simply tolerate symptoms and hope they will improve. Seek advice and help • Take steps to improve general fitness.

PSYCHOSOCIAL TREATMENT OPTIONS

CONVENTIONAL MEDICINE

Doctors recognize the embarrassment and sexual difficulties associated with BPH and will advise counseling.

COMPLEMENTARY THERAPIES

Psychotherapy & Counseling ❷
(*see pages 132–33*)

Talking through feelings may help you to deal with symptom-related problems.

SELF-HELP TECHNIQUES

• Practice relaxation and breathing techniques (*see pages 170–71*) and stress management methods (*see pages 168–69*) • See a doctor when

symptoms first appear. Diagnosis is reassuring and natural treatments should begin early • Take practical steps to minimize embarrassment; for example, establish where toilets are in public places • Be honest about the problem; people are more understanding than you think.

INFERTILITY IN MEN

Infertility of some kind affects about 15 percent of couples, and male infertility may be the cause in 40 percent of cases. In normal circumstances, each ejaculation releases less than 1 teaspoon (3 milliliters) of semen, containing an average of 250 million sperm. A man's fertility is said to be impaired when there are fewer than 20 million sperm in a milliliter of ejaculate. Fertility can also be reduced by slow-moving, short-lived, or misshapen sperm. These conditions do not necessarily mean that a man will be unable to father a child, but they do indicate that he will need help and optimum conditions to do so.

CASE STUDY

Monica, an acupuncturist, was visited by Adam, 39. Adam and his wife wanted children but tests revealed a low sperm count and poor motility (slow-moving sperm). His doctor offered advice about diet and stress management, and referred him to Monica. "My diagnosis showed that Adam's Kidney *jing*, his vital essence, was depleted," said Monica. "Adam was working 60 hours a week as a sales manager and had become exhausted." Monica stimulated points on the Kidney meridian and the Governor vessel (*see page 124*) to warm and tonify the Kidneys and told Adam to rest, give up smoking, and eat "warming" foods. Adam's sperm motility slowly improved and, two years after taking a less stressful job, his son was conceived.

BIOCHEMICAL FACTORS

Falling sperm counts are reported in many countries, and the number of boys born with genital abnormalities is increasing. Both conditions may be due to a number of factors, possibly related to lifestyle and environment in developed countries, which can disrupt production of the male hormone testosterone.

BIOCHEMICAL TRIGGERS

• Smoking • X-rays • Various drugs, especially steroids • Alcohol • Caffeine
  • Drinking water contaminated with traces of pesticides, detergents, and other products containing forms of the female hormone estrogen, which may reduce sperm counts

STRUCTURAL FACTORS

The complex, partly external arrangement of the male genitals is vulnerable to a range of problems that can reduce fertility. Disorders of the testes, obstruction of the urethra, or problems that prevent erection or ejaculation can each be a factor. Illness may affect sperm production.

STRUCTURAL TRIGGERS

• Abnormal or undescended testes • Varicocele (varicose vein in scrotum) • Mumps or other infections that cause inflammation of the reproductive tract • High fevers
• Being over- or underweight • Too much or too little seminal fluid • Sperm duct blockage, from injury or a sexually transmitted disease • Ejaculation problems, such as retrograde ejaculation (semen forced back into bladder) • Erectile dysfunction (*see pages 82–83*) • Vasectomy

PSYCHOSOCIAL FACTORS

Constant production of stress hormones can interfere with the hormones regulating sperm production. In addition, anxiety and depression can contribute to problems in achieving and maintaining an erection that are not affected by low sperm counts. Anxiety about infertility can reduce libido and undermine the ability to enjoy lovemaking.

PSYCHOSOCIAL TRIGGERS

• Stress at work or in personal relationships
• Loss of confidence and self-esteem
• Depression

Realms of the Body (*see page 20*)

● **BIOCHEMICAL**
Body systems,
such as digestion

● **STRUCTURAL**
Muscles, bones,
joints, and nerves

PSYCHOSOCIAL
Thoughts, feelings,
and relationships

Key: Evidence of Efficacy (*see page 182*)

least evidence ◄———— ❶ ❷ ❸ ❹ ❺ ————► most evidence

BIOCHEMICAL TREATMENT OPTIONS

CONVENTIONAL MEDICINE
A doctor will investigate underlying hormonal problems, which can occasionally cause male infertility. If low sperm counts are due to hormonal imbalance, testosterone injections or drugs such as clomiphene or gonadotropin may be prescribed (*see Drugs Glossary, page 179*).

COMPLEMENTARY THERAPIES
Traditional Chinese Medicine ❶
(*see page 124*)
Practitioners treat infertility with acupuncture and herbal remedies, but there is little supporting research.

Western Herbalism ❷
(*see page 127*)
A practitioner may suggest ginseng and and saw palmetto, which are traditionally used to improve male reproductive function.
Caution: Do not take ginseng if you have high blood pressure.

Dried ginseng

Ginseng capsules

Nutritional Therapies ❸
(*see pages 128–29*)
A nutritionist may recommend foods or supplements with the following nutrients that are potentially beneficial

for healthy sperm function: zinc, selenium, folate, vitamins C and E, arginine, and essential fatty acids. In one study in 1993, folinic acid, a type of folate, treated a type of male infertility called round cell idiopathic syndrome, and a 1995 study at Sheffield University in the UK showed that a three-month course of vitamin E may help sperm bind to the egg.

SELF-HELP TECHNIQUES
• Eat a balanced, whole-grain diet of organic produce, free of pesticides
• Avoid smoking, caffeine, and alcohol
• Maintain a healthy weight.

STRUCTURAL TREATMENT OPTIONS

CONVENTIONAL MEDICINE
A sperm analysis is usually performed early in the investigation of a couple's fertility. If the sperm count is found to be low and the woman is fertile, artificial insemination may be an option to consider. Surgery can correct a varicocele (varicose vein in the scrotum) and possibly reverse a vasectomy.

COMPLEMENTARY THERAPIES
Massage ❷ (*see page 116*)
Massage by your partner can be introduced as a useful aid for stress management and may act as a welcome boost to libido and lovemaking.

Sensual massage can encourage relaxation and boost lovemaking.

SELF-HELP TECHNIQUES
• Avoid tight clothing, hot baths, and saunas, since overheating the testicles can slow sperm production
• If necessary, during sex use a nonartificial lubricant (such as cocoa butter) that will not interfere with sperm quality • Do not overexercise
• Immersing the testicles in cool water for ten minutes three times daily is said to improve the circulation and raise sperm count.

PSYCHOSOCIAL TREATMENT OPTIONS

CONVENTIONAL MEDICINE
As long as the sperm count is not very low, a small but effective increase may be achieved with an integrative approach that uses both conventional and complementary methods. If there is no structural or biochemical cause, a doctor may suggest making lifestyle changes to improve general health and practicing relaxation and stress management techniques (*see pages 168–69*).

COMPLEMENTARY THERAPIES
Psychotherapy & Counseling ❷
(*see pages 132–33*)
If sperm production problems are not treatable, talking through feelings about fatherhood with a counselor may help you come terms with the situation.
Autogenic Training & Biofeedback ❸ (*see page 136*)
It is possible that cognitive behavioral approaches, including autogenic training

and biofeedback, may make a difference if sperm production is borderline.

SELF-HELP TECHNIQUES
• Practice relaxation and breathing techniques (*see pages 170–71*) and stress management skills to relieve tension and reduce the effects of stress
• Consider changing your job if you work with lead, radiation, pesticides, solvents, or in a hot environment.

MALE SEXUAL DYSFUNCTION

Most men, particularly as they grow older, have problems in achieving or maintaining an erection at some time. When this is short-term or occasional, the problem is usually psychological. One in ten men experience *persistent erectile failure* – often, though incorrectly, known as impotence – which is likely to have a structural or biochemical cause, although there is often an accompanying psychological element. Many men are reluctant to seek help, although 90 percent of sufferers could be successfully treated. Any persistent problem may be the first symptom of a disease and should always be referred to a doctor.

BIOCHEMICAL FACTORS

Prescribed and other drugs are a frequent reason for difficulties in achieving and maintaining an erection. Hormonal imbalances are a less common cause.

BIOCHEMICAL TRIGGERS

• Alcohol and medication, especially antidepressants, antihypertensives, and diuretics *(see Drugs Glossary, page 179)*• Low levels of the male hormone testosterone• High levels of the female hormone prolactin (all men produce small amounts of female hormones) • High blood cholesterol levels, resulting in atherosclerosis *(see pages 48–51)*

STRUCTURAL FACTORS

When there is a physical cause, erectile dysfunction usually begins gradually and occurs in all sexual situations. Structural causes of persistent erectile failure include disorders of the nervous system, and circulation problems that affect the flow of blood into the penis.

STRUCTURAL TRIGGERS

• Deficient blood flow into the penis because of atherosclerosis • Excessive drainage of blood from the penis ("leaking veins") • Damage of the nerves going to and from the penis as a result of injury, surgery, or disease • Diabetes, alcohol, smoking, and drug abuse, which can cause nerve or circulatory problems • Conditions that damage the central nervous system, such as stroke and spinal cord injury • Pelvic surgery, for example, removal of the prostate gland

CASE STUDY

Aisha, a psychologist, was visited by Jerry, 32, who had enjoyed a normal sex life until his current relationship. Now he was unable to maintain an erection. "I can't understand it when I love her more than anyone else," he said. Aisha suspected a problem with emotional intimacy and discovered that Jerry had suffered a broken love affair when he was 20. She encouraged Jerry to grieve for this lost love and to acknowledge that, as a result, subconsciously he believed being close to somebody meant getting hurt. Aisha suggested that the couple explore intimacy without intercourse for a period. Six months later, Jerry reported that he felt sexually confident and enjoyed lovemaking again.

PSYCHOSOCIAL FACTORS

If erectile dysfunction begins suddenly and occurs in some circumstances and not in others, then there is usually a psychological cause. In competitive macho societies, size of the penis and sexual prowess are given disproportionate importance. Erectile dysfunction and other genitourinary conditions may influence a man's attitude toward sex and affect relationships. In one study, 21 percent of patients' relationships broke up as a result of sexual dysfunction.

PSYCHOSOCIAL TRIGGERS

• Fear of failure and worry about poor sexual performance • Stress and anxiety • Marital conflicts and dissatisfaction • Sexual boredom • Unresolved sexual orientation • Loss of libido because of prostate problems, depression, or chronic illness

Realms of the Body *(see page 20)*

● **BIOCHEMICAL**
Body systems,
such as digestion

● **STRUCTURAL**
Muscles, bones,
joints, and nerves

● **PSYCHOSOCIAL**
Thoughts, feelings,
and relationships

Key: Evidence of Efficacy *(see page 182)*

❶ ❷ ❸ ❹ ❺
least evidence ◄──────► most evidence

BIOCHEMICAL TREATMENT OPTIONS

CONVENTIONAL MEDICINE
A doctor may prescribe sildenafil
(Viagra – *see Drugs Glossary, page
179*), which helps relax blood vessels
in the penis, allowing blood to flow
in and cause an erection. It should be
taken an hour before sexual activity
and requires sexual desire and
stimulation to be effective. However,
there are side effects and it is not
suitable if you have heart or liver
problems. Testosterone replacement
may be prescribed, if laboratory
tests indicate a deficiency.

COMPLEMENTARY THERAPIES
Tradional Chinese Medicine ❷
(see pages 124–25)
Erectile failure is associated with Kidney
weakness and Liver *qi* stagnation. A
practitioner may suggest ginseng to
enhance blood flow and potency.
  Acupuncture points on the
Conception, Spleen, and Bladder
meridians may be stimulated to
increase the flow of *qi* to sexual
organs. **Caution:** Avoid ginseng if
you have high blood pressure.
Needles are used to stimulate acupoints.

Western Herbalism ❹ *(see page 127)*
A practitioner may recommend saw
palmetto, a traditional tonic
for the male reproductive
system, and ginkgo. In one
study ginkgo helped 50
percent of men with
erectile problems
caused by poor blood
flow in the arteries.

Ginkgo
leaves

SELF-HELP TECHNIQUES
• Follow a healthy whole-foods diet
to optimize well-being.

STRUCTURAL TREATMENT OPTIONS

CONVENTIONAL MEDICINE
If there is a mild vascular problem, a
doctor may offer a constriction device.
This uses a pump to create a vacuum
around the penis to draw blood into
it. Penile implants can be inserted
to stiffen the penis. Several drugs
including sildenafil can be injected
into the penis to produce an erection,
while alprostadil is inserted into the
urethra *(see Drugs Glossary, page 179)*.

COMPLEMENTARY THERAPIES
Massage ❷ *(see page 116)*
Partners may help arouse one another
by massaging areas of the other's body
in ways they find mutually relaxing
and erotic.

SELF-HELP TECHNIQUES
• If erectile dysfunction is due to
leaking veins, try Kegel exercises,
which can be as effective as surgery.

Stop midflow when urinating and note
which muscle is used. Hold for four
seconds, then continue. Contract this
muscle for four seconds, then relax
and repeat four times, at least twice
a day. After a week, try holding the
contraction for eight seconds, then ten.
You should see some improvement in
4–12 weeks • Exercise regularly to
improve cardiovascular fitness
• Reduce alcohol intake.

PSYCHOSOCIAL TREATMENT OPTIONS

CONVENTIONAL MEDICINE
Depression is a major cause of sexual
difficulty. Erectile problems often
respond well to placebo medication.
A doctor may also suggest stress
management *(see pages 168–69)*,
psychotherapy, hypnotherapy, marital
counseling, and sex therapy.

COMPLEMENTARY THERAPIES
Psychotherapy & Counseling ❷
(see pages 132–33)
A therapist might explore underlying
subconscious reasons for the condition;

for example, sexual difficulties are
often a result of unacknowledged
relationship problems. Sexual
counseling encourages activities that
do not depend on an erection, such
as affectionate cuddling and caressing.
Men are asked to concentrate on
communication and the enjoyment
of sensual touch rather than on
penetration and are told to avoid
intercourse for an agreed-upon
period of time. Erection often follows
spontaneously, if the expectation to
perform is removed.

SELF-HELP TECHNIQUES
• Practice relaxation
and breathing *(see pages
170–71)* and other stress
management techniques
to relieve anxiety
and tension.

Meditation
relieves
underlying
anxieties.

STRESS

We experience psychological and physical stress in situations that tax our resources or endanger our well-being. We need some stress to prompt us into action, however, since too little leaves us bored and inert. Stress becomes a problem if body and mind remain in "emergency" mode because of continuing external stresses or internal conflicts. Persistent stress can lead to lifestyles that harm individuals and their relationships. People vary in their response to stress, depending on their ability to cope with it psychologically, structurally, and biologically. This capability can be boosted in all three areas.

CASE STUDY

Claudia, a nutritionist, helped Steve, a middle manager in his 30s, deal with stress more effectively. Steve's energy levels had recently plummeted, he had mood swings, and lost sleep over impending deadlines. He used coffee as an "upper" and drank 10–12 cups a day, but still could not pick himself up. "The caffeine in coffee is a stimulant," explained Claudia. "Combined with other repetitive stressors over time, it can exhaust the adrenal glands and cause extreme fatigue." Steve gave up coffee and suffered from caffeine-withdrawal headaches for four days. He switched to natural coffee substitutes and herbal teas, started a regular exercise routine, and used a relaxation tape. "After seeing you I had to reevaluate my lifestyle and work habits," he told Claudia a few months later. "I have more energy and I'm less moody now."

BIOCHEMICAL FACTORS

The body's reaction to an emergency is called the "fight or flight" response (*see pages 168–69*). It causes the stress hormones epinephrine, norepinephrine, and cortisol to enter the system. In response, the digestion slows down as blood is diverted to the muscles, the liver releases sugar and fats for immediate energy, saliva dries up, and perspiration increases. Persistent stress reactions can weaken the immune system and lead to recurring infections.

BIOCHEMICAL TRIGGERS
• Poor nutrition • Alcohol • Caffeine
• Nicotine • Additives • Recreational drugs
• Environmental chemicals

PSYCHOSOCIAL FACTORS

In modern life, the causes of stress are more often emotional than physical. People most vulnerable to stress are obsessive, silent worriers and impatient, hostile, "type A" personalities (*see page 49*). Psychological symptoms of persistent stress include lack of concentration, irritability, tearfulness, anxiety and panic attacks, sexual difficulties, insomnia, compulsive eating, obsessive behavior, addictions, and depression.

PSYCHOSOCIAL TRIGGERS
• Stress-prone personality • Repressed strong emotions, such as fear, anger, or grief • Unresolved conflicts • Loneliness, bereavement, or major loss of any kind • Traumatic events or shock • Inability to relax and feel calm • A challenge, exam, or competition • Time pressure or long or irregular working hours • Monotony and boredom • Feelings of hopelessness and helplessness

STRUCTURAL FACTORS

The "fight or flight" response (*see pages 168–69*) anticipates physical action. The heart pumps faster, blood pressure rises, and muscles tense. If the body does not discharge this tension, the effects accumulate. Persistent stress can cause muscle tension in the back, neck, and shoulders. Tension in the gut, heart, and diaphragm can lead to poor digestion, irritable bowel syndrome, constipation or diarrhea, nausea, hyperventilation, and palpitations. Skin irritation and nervous system problems, like fatigue or dizziness, may also occur.

STRUCTURAL TRIGGERS
• Injury • Poor posture • Noise • Lack of exercise and physical relaxation

Realms of the Body (*see page 20*)

● **BIOCHEMICAL**
Body systems,
such as digestion

● **STRUCTURAL**
Muscles, bones,
joints, and nerves

● **PSYCHOSOCIAL**
Thoughts, feelings,
and relationships

Key: Evidence of Efficacy (*see page 182*)

❶ ❷ ❸ ❹ ❺
least evidence ◄————————► most evidence

BIOCHEMICAL TREATMENT OPTIONS

CONVENTIONAL MEDICINE
Tranquilizers and sedatives (*see Drugs Glossary, page 179*) are now seldom prescribed, except if circumstances are causing severe problems.

COMPLEMENTARY THERAPIES
Western Herbalism ❸
(*see page 127*)
Traditional remedies include Siberian ginseng, to help

Valerian can induce calm.

the body withstand stress, valerian to calm the mind and induce sleep, and kava kava to relieve anxiety and muscle tension. A practitioner will suggest a combination of herbs based on individual symptoms. **Caution:** Do not take ginseng if you have high blood pressure or are pregnant. Do not take valerian if you already take sleep-inducing drugs.
Nutritional Therapies ❷
(*see pages 128–29*)
Certain nutrients are used up more

rapidly during stressful periods. To support the nervous system, a practitioner may recommend B-complex supplements, as well as a diet rich in this vitamin, and vitamin C and zinc, which increase resistance to infection.

SELF-HELP TECHNIQUES
• Eat a whole-grain diet with plenty of antioxidant-rich vegetables and fruit (*see pages 158–59*) • Limit caffeine, alcohol, and smoking, and avoid other nonprescription stimulants.

STRUCTURAL TREATMENT OPTIONS

CONVENTIONAL MEDICINE
A doctor may advise regular exercise, since it discharges tension and releases endorphins (mood-enhancing chemicals) into the bloodstream.

COMPLEMENTARY THERAPIES
Massage ❸ (*see page 116*)
All forms of touch can release endorphins (*see above*). Massage can relieve muscle tension and induce the relaxation response (*see page 170*).
Aromatherapy ❸ (*see page 117*)
Lavender, rose, ylang ylang, neroli,

or geranium essential oils may reduce tension and induce relaxation.
Yoga ❸ (*see page 123*)
A teacher will recommend stretching and breathing exercises to promote the relaxation response, relieve tension, and calm the mind. The Corpse posture and alternate nostril breathing can be particularly useful.
Traditional Chinese Medicine ❸
(*see pages 124–25*)
Acupuncture can promote deep calm, and the mental focus induced during t'ai chi and qigong encourages the

relaxation response. Research shows t'ai chi can lower stress hormone levels.

SELF-HELP TECHNIQUES
• Exercise regularly to release endorphins, break down accumulated stress chemicals, and discharge tension.

The flowing movements of t'ai chi relieve stress.

PSYCHOSOCIAL TREATMENT OPTIONS

CONVENTIONAL MEDICINE
As many as 80 percent of visits to a family doctor are for stress-related complaints. Your doctor will suggest that you try to identify causes of persistent stress and will help you find ways of dealing with them.

COMPLEMENTARY THERAPIES
Psychotherapy & Counseling ❹
(*see pages 132–33*)
Cognitive behavioral therapy can help

you change the way you perceive and respond to pressure.
Visualization ❸ (*see page 134*)
This is one of the many established techniques that induce the relaxation response.
Meditation ❹ (*see page 135*)
Studies in the US show that regular meditation can reverse the "fight or flight" response to stress. Meditation can also induce a state of deep physical relaxation and mental alertness.

Autogenic Training ❸ (*see page 136*)
A practitioner will teach you a series of exercises that involves elements of relaxation, self-hypnosis, and meditation. Once taught you will be able to treat yourself.

SELF-HELP TECHNIQUES
• Practice relaxation and breathing techniques (*see pages 170–71*) • Keep a stress diary (*see page 147*) • Discover your own healthy coping strategies.

ANXIETY & PANIC ATTACKS

Anxiety is a normal reaction to threatening situations – part of the "fight or flight" response to stress (*see pages 168–69*), when the mind and body go on alert. Prolonged stress can lead to a variety of physical ailments, including headaches, raised blood pressure, and palpitations. Panic attacks – sudden surges of intense anxiety – may occur at random. They are usually accompanied by disturbing bodily sensations and are often so intense that they interfere with daily activities. About one in ten people suffers from intense anxiety, irrational fears, phobias, and obsessive-compulsive behavior at some point in life.

CASE STUDY

Andrew, a psychologist, treated Jane, a 21-year-old student who had started to get panic attacks. She told Andrew, "I start to feel frightened. My heart pounds, I get breathless, and then my hands sweat and my lips and fingers tingle. I was sure I had a bad heart, but medical tests showed I had nothing to worry about." Apparently her grandmother had had a stroke just before Jane's exams, when she was unable to visit, and had died soon after. "At the time she had to put it out of her mind," explained Andrew. Her tingling and numbness were due to hyperventilation, but made her feel like she was going to have a stroke. Andrew taught her diaphragmatic breathing, and arranged for bereavement counseling. Once she began to accept the link between her panic attacks and her grief, she began to feel in control again.

BIOCHEMICAL FACTORS

Stress triggers the "fight or flight" response; when stress-hormone levels rise, the heart pumps faster and muscles tense. Breathing becomes rapid, shallow, and irregular, coming from the upper chest instead of the diaphragm. This causes hyperventilation because too much carbon dioxide leaves the body, affecting blood chemistry, circulation, and nerves. People who are hyperventilating can feel breathless or faint, with tingling or numbness, muscle pain or spasms; they may feel as if they are dying, which accentuates panic.

BIOCHEMICAL TRIGGERS
• Low blood sugar (hypoglycemia)
• Stimulants, such as caffeine or alcohol
• Inadequate nutrients in the diet
• Food intolerance • Body chemistry changes due to overbreathing • Persistent high levels of adrenaline

STRUCTURAL FACTORS

Physical effects from the strain of being constantly on alert can be mistaken for symptoms of serious illness, which further increases anxiety. In the long term, anxiety may undermine the immune system and contribute to disorders such as high blood pressure or irritable bowel syndrome. Structural symptoms include sweating, chest pains and palpitations, digestive disturbances, headaches, and back and neck pain.

STRUCTURAL TRIGGERS
• Muscle tension • Lack of exercise
• Overbreathing

PSYCHOSOCIAL FACTORS

The causes of anxiety are not always clear. Anxious tendencies may partly be genetic, or may be rooted in past events. Pessimistic, perfectionist, impatient people are more likely to suffer from stress. Many anxious people "over-breathe," or hyperventilate, which increases anxiety and causes physical symptoms.

PSYCHOSOCIAL TRIGGERS
• Overawareness of small changes in the body, such as minor pain, heart rhythm, and gut movements • A conviction that symptoms are dangerous • Family behavior patterns
• Overload from a combination of generalized stresses • Bad experiences in the past

Realms of the Body (*see page 20*)

● **BIOCHEMICAL**
Body systems,
such as digestion

● **STRUCTURAL**
Muscles, bones,
joints, and nerves

● **PSYCHOSOCIAL**
Thoughts, feelings,
and relationships

Key: Evidence of Efficacy (*see page 182*)

❶ ❷ ❸ ❹ ❺
least evidence ◀━━━━━━▶ most evidence

BIOCHEMICAL TREATMENT OPTIONS

CONVENTIONAL MEDICINE
Short-term minor tranquilizers (benzo-diazepines) or beta blockers (*see Drugs Glossary, page 179*) reduce symptoms of acute anxiety. Anti-depressants may be prescribed to help panic.

COMPLEMENTARY THERAPIES
Western Herbalism ❸
(*see page 127*)
At least one study has shown that the traditional Polynesian

Passion flower

herb kava kava can reduce anxiety. A practitioner may prescribe valerian to stop the mind from racing, passionflower for long-term anxiety, and St. John's wort for associated depression.
Caution: Do not take St. John's wort if you have been given conventional antidepressants, or valerian with sleeping pills.
Nutritional Therapies ❸
(*see pages 128–29*)
An exclusion diet may reveal an intolerance for a mood-

affecting food. Some nutritionists link magnesium and calcium deficiencies to anxiety and prescribe supplements of these minerals; others suggest vitamin B-complex supplements to support the nervous system.

SELF-HELP TECHNIQUES
• Eat regular meals high in protein and complex carbohydrates • Avoid caffeine and alcohol • In an acute panic attack, breathe into a bag to increase levels of carbon dioxide in the blood.

STRUCTURAL TREATMENT OPTIONS

CONVENTIONAL MEDICINE
Your doctor may suggest one of the complementary therapies below.

COMPLEMENTARY THERAPIES
Massage ❸ (*see page 116*)
Regular massage can relieve muscle tension, and reduce stress and anxiety.
Aromatherapy ❸ (*see page 117*)
Many people find massage with calming essential oils such as lavender, neroli, and clary sage helpful. In hospital studies, patient anxiety decreased after

massage with Roman chamomile oil and neroli oil.
Caution: Do not use chamomile essential oil during pregnancy.
Therapeutic Touch ❸
(*see page 122*)
A practitioner will use touch to balance your "energy flow." Therapeutic touch has reduced anxiety in hospital patients more efficiently than casual touch or conversation.

Theraputic touch reduces anxiety.

Acupressure ❷ (*see page 125*)
Acupressure points Liver 3, Lung 14, Heart 7, Pericardium 6, and yintang may be stimulated to relieve anxiety.

SELF-HELP TECHNIQUES
• Practice yoga and t'ai chi (*see pages 123 and 25*) to ease physical tension • Get regular aerobic exercise, which boosts mood-enhancing brain chemicals and encourages the relaxation response.

PSYCHOSOCIAL TREATMENT OPTIONS

CONVENTIONAL MEDICINE
If symptoms are severe, a doctor will refer you to a psychiatrist. Counseling can be especially important if anxiety attacks follow a traumatic event (Posttraumatic Stress Disorder). Obsessive-compulsive disorders and phobias that interfere with daily life need expert help.

Counseling can restore perspective.

COMPLEMENTARY THERAPIES
Psychotherapy & Counseling ❹
(*see pages 132–33*) Psychotherapy can help sufferers to recognize, understand, and come to terms with the reasons for their anxiety. Cognitive behavioral therapy changes patterns of thinking and behavior that reinforce anxiety.

Hypnotherapy ❷ (*see page 134*)
During treatment you will be taught techniques that may be helpful in undoing conditioned responses such as test anxiety.
Meditation ❸ (*see page 135*)
Studies show that "mindfulness" techniques can relieve panic disorders.

SELF-HELP TECHNIQUES
• Relaxation and breathing techniques (*see pages 170–71*) help • Remember symptoms are harmless and will pass.

DEPRESSION

The term "depression" is used to describe a range of negative feelings, from feeling unhappy or low occasionally to being so crippled by despair that life does not seem worth living. The incidence of clinical depression is rising, affecting one-third of all people during their lives and five percent of the population at any one time. Two-thirds of diagnosed depression sufferers are women, with an equal number of men likely to develop manic depression, a genetic disorder in which moods swing between extremes. Complementary therapies can help mild cases, but clinical and manic depression always require conventional medical help.

WARNING SIGNS

See a doctor if at least four of the following symptoms have applied to you for more than two weeks with no obvious cause:
- Loss of interest and enjoyment in life
- Lack of drive and motivation that makes even simple tasks seem impossible
- Overwhelming fatigue and loss of energy
- Unexplained aches and pains
- Agitation, irritability, and restlessness
- Loss or gain in appetite and weight
- Sleeplessness, early-morning waking, or excessive sleeping
- Loss of affection for those close to you
- Loss of interest in sex
- Loss of self-confidence
- Feelings of uselessness, guilt, inadequacy, shame, helplessness, and hopelessness
- Mood swings
- Thoughts of suicide – a certain sign that help is needed

BIOCHEMICAL FACTORS

A reduction in neurotransmitters (brain chemicals), is thought to be a factor in depression. Many drugs and supplements seek to treat depression by raising levels of serotonin and other neurotransmitters, which affect mood by stimulating certain brain cells. Physical illness or hormonal changes can affect mental state and cause depression, and there is also a family tendency toward depression, which could be partly genetic.

BIOCHEMICAL TRIGGERS
- Genetic predisposition • Hormonal changes caused by pregnancy (postpartum depression), premenstrual syndrome, oral contraceptives, and menopause • Alcohol • Certain drugs • Viral illnesses such as flu, hepatitis, or Epstein-Barr disease (glandular fever) • Some types of disease including cancer and endocrinal, neurological, and autoimmune conditions (see Glossary, pages 177–78) • Food intolerances

STRUCTURAL FACTORS

Most depressed people first see a doctor with symptoms such as extreme fatigue or pain. Depression manifests itself in other physical ways: Depressed people are more prone to heart disease and osteoporosis. Research shows that recurrent depression disrupts nerve cell connections that generate positive feelings. Environmental triggers may be important. Seasonal affective disorder is a type of depression related to low levels of daylight during the winter months.

STRUCTURAL TRIGGERS
- Physical illness • Chronic pain
- Infections • Inadequate sleep

PSYCHOSOCIAL FACTORS

Stress-related events are thought to trigger 50 percent of all cases of depression, and stress encountered in early life could predispose people to depression at a later stage. Those with certain personality types, for example, people who are pessimistic, introverted, and anxious, are more vulnerable to depression.

PSYCHOSOCIAL TRIGGERS
- Stressful events in childhood and adolescence • Family traits • Personality type, such as anxious, pessimistic, perfectionist, or introverted • Loss or bereavement • Anxiety • Unemployment • Overwork • Loneliness • Relationship problems

Realms of the Body (*see page 20*)

- **BIOCHEMICAL**
  Body systems,
  such as digestion
- **STRUCTURAL**
  Muscles, bones,
  joints, and nerves
- **PSYCHOSOCIAL**
  Thoughts, feelings,
  and relationships

Key: Evidence of Efficacy (*see page 182*)

❶ ❷ ❸ ❹ ❺

least evidence ← → most evidence

BIOCHEMICAL TREATMENT OPTIONS

CONVENTIONAL MEDICINE
A course of antidepressants (*see Drugs Glossary, page 179*) can be lifesaving for a depressed person. Three main types of antidepressants are commonly prescribed: selective serotonin reuptake inhibitors (SSRIs), such as Prozac; tricyclics; and monamine oxidase inhibitors (MAOIs). Norepinephrine reuptake inhibitors, which are relatively new, may also be given. Lithium is useful for recurrent depression and manic-depressive illness.

COMPLEMENTARY THERAPIES
Western Herbalism ❹

St. John's wort

(*see page 127*)
St. John's wort may be recommended. It has been shown to be as effective as antidepressants in treating cases of mild depression, but produces far fewer side effects.
Caution: Taking St. John's wort with antidepressant medication may increase the drugs' side effects.

Nutritional Therapies ❸
(*see pages 128–29*)
Vitamin B_6 and magnesium may help premenstrual depression. A therapist may suspect deficiencies affecting brain chemistry, including lack of folic acid and B vitamins, or test for food intolerances. Supplements 5-HTP and SAM-e need more research.

SELF-HELP TECHNIQUES
• Eat a healthy, balanced diet • Avoid alcohol and recreational drugs.

STRUCTURAL TREATMENT OPTIONS

CONVENTIONAL MEDICINE
Regular exercise can help relieve moderate depression by triggering natural mood-enhancing chemicals. Aerobic exercise has proved as effective as psychotherapy and relaxation techniques with mild depression. Studies show that it can help prevent depression, and that working on physical inertia and negative body image can be highly therapeutic. In the future, people with depression may be offered treatment in which high-powered magnetic pulses are directed at specific brain areas; in experiments it temporarily relieved severe depression.

COMPLEMENTARY THERAPIES
Massage ❷ (*see page 116*)
Massage aids relaxation, enhances mood, and relieves depression.
Aromatherapy ❷ (*see page 117*)
Aromatherapists use various essential oils, including bergamot, rose, neroli, ylang ylang, and lavender, to promote relaxation and elevate mood.

Acupuncture ❸
(*see page 125*)
Acupuncture, especially electro-acupuncture, can help.

SELF-HELP TECHNIQUES
• Yoga classes may improve posture and provide a supportive environment.

Regular aerobic exercise is an excellent way to elevate mood.

PSYCHOSOCIAL TREATMENT OPTIONS

CONVENTIONAL MEDICINE
Depression may be associated with bottled-up feelings, particularly those of rage and loss. Mild depression might not require any medication, since counseling and help with practical difficulties may be sufficient. A doctor may recommend cognitive behavioral therapy – studies show it can be as effective as antidepressants in relieving mild to moderate depression. Medication and psychosocial approaches work well together.

COMPLEMENTARY THERAPIES
Psychotherapy & Counseling ❹
(*see pages 132–33*)
A cognitive behavioral therapist may suggest the following: more involvement in pleasant activities; identifying negative behavior and pessimistic thought patterns, and improving social skills to relate to other people more easily.

SELF-HELP TECHNIQUES
• Practice any stress-reduction method that appeals to you (*see pages 168–69*)
• Learn relaxation and breathing techniques (*see pages 170–71*) to reduce tension and relieve anxiety
• Listen to favorite pieces of music
• Do not bottle things up; learn to talk through problems with others • Break larger problems down into smaller, achievable tasks so that the problems can be tackled a little at a time • Try not to brood over problems • Take care of your appearance to boost your self-esteem • Remind yourself that negative feelings will eventually pass.

INSOMNIA

Adequate sleep can help the body repair and regenerate tissue, build bone and muscle, and strengthen the immune system. The inability to get enough of the right kind of sleep can lead to fatigue and irritability. Insomnia is common when people are over-stressed or depressed, particularly as they get older. Sleeplessness falls into three categories: being unable to go to sleep, which is linked to anxiety; falling asleep but waking frequently; and waking early in the morning, then being unable to go back to sleep. Difficulty in remaining asleep may be linked to depression, illness, persistent pain, or changes in daily body-clock rhythms.

CASE STUDY

Jane, an herbalist, treated Joe for long-term insomnia. After many years of shiftwork he found it difficult to drift off and his sleep was often disturbed by dreams. Sometimes he got no more than five hours' sleep a night. Jane prescribed an herbal mix to take as a tea in the evening. It included valerian and passionflower to promote relaxation and peaceful sleep, and kava kava to relax the body and relieve the anxiety that may have been causing his restless dreaming. Jane told him where he could get a good relaxation tape and suggested he exercise for half an hour a day. Joe gradually found he went to sleep more quickly and woke refreshed, without the "hangover" sleeping pills had produced.

BIOCHEMICAL FACTORS

During deep, nondreaming (NREM) sleep, human growth hormone (HGH) is secreted, which stimulates tissue and liver regeneration, maintains the immune system, and helps convert fat to muscle. The pineal gland responds to darkness by producing melatonin, a chemical that helps make us feel sleepy, while other chemicals promote wakefulness. The overall balance of brain chemicals influences when we feel tired or wakeful. For as yet unexplained reasons, deep sleep decreases with age and at least half of those between 40 and 55 have occasional problems sleeping.

BIOCHEMICAL TRIGGERS

• Changes in daily body-clock rhythms, due to jet lag or shiftwork • Caffeine • Alcohol • Nicotine • Drugs such as beta blockers or thyroid preparations • Balance of brain activity

STRUCTURAL FACTORS

Sleep entails alternating periods of rapid eye movement (REM) sleep, when most dreaming occurs, and deep slow-wave sleep (SWS), also known as non-REM (NREM) sleep. The body needs to be comfortable enough to relax during sleep. Opinions vary, but seven to eight hours' sleep is generally considered the optimum amount of sleep for adults, and most people seem to need six hours to function without feeling tired.

STRUCTURAL TRIGGERS

• Lack of exercise • Illness or chronic pain • An inadequate sleeping environment, caused by heat, cold, noise, or an uncomfortable mattress

PSYCHOSOCIAL FACTORS

Dreaming (REM) sleep is thought to be important in helping people process the day's events and emotional issues. Stress and anxiety, work deadlines, concern over family, health, and personal crises probably account for at least 50 percent of sleep disturbance; these factors are most commonly the cause if the insomnia began suddenly. In the absence of such factors, depression or an anxiety disorder should be considered. Psychological strategies can be most effective in helping people sleep.

PSYCHOSOCIAL TRIGGERS

• Worry (associated with trouble falling asleep) • Depression (linked to difficulty in remaining asleep)

Realms of the Body (*see page 20*)

● **BIOCHEMICAL**
Body systems,
such as digestion

● **STRUCTURAL**
Muscles, bones,
joints, and nerves

PSYCHOSOCIAL
Thoughts, feelings,
and relationships

Key: Evidence of Efficacy (*see page 182*)

❶ ❷ ❸ ❹ ❺

least evidence ◀━━━━━━▶ most evidence

BIOCHEMICAL TREATMENT OPTIONS

CONVENTIONAL MEDICINE
Your doctor will advise sleeping pills or tranquilizers (*see Drugs Glossary, page 179*) only as a short-term solution or last resort. Waking early because of depression is usually relieved by a course of antidepressants.

COMPLEMENTARY THERAPIES
Western Herbalism ❹ (*see page 127*)
St. John's wort can help, especially if moderate depression is the cause. Valerian, passionflower, and hops are traditional remedies and studies support the use of valerian.
Caution: Do not take valerian with other sleep-inducing drugs. Taking St. John's wort with antidepressants may make side effects more likely.
Nutritional Therapies ❸
(*see pages 128–29*)
You may be prescribed supplements of the hormone melatonin,

Passionflower infusion

which can help revive a body clock disturbed by jet lag or shift work.

SELF-HELP TECHNIQUES
• Avoid stimulants such as caffeine, alcohol, and nicotine before bedtime
• Do not eat a meal within two hours of bedtime; digestion interferes with sleep • Snack on carbohydrate foods high in natural tryptophan, which makes melatonin (bananas, milk, or whole-grain crackers) • Go to bed at a regular time; late nights disrupt the body clock.

STRUCTURAL TREATMENT OPTIONS

CONVENTIONAL MEDICINE
Light therapy can help synchronize the body clock. Bright light in the morning helps those who go to bed progressively later and cannot wake up; light in the evening helps those who go to bed progressively earlier.

COMPLEMENTARY THERAPIES
Massage ❷ (*see page 116*)
Massage can relieve muscle tension, reduce anxiety, and promote sleep-enhancing brain chemicals.
Aromatherapy ❸ (*see page 117*)
Lavender essential oil, inhaled, added to a bath, or used in massage, may enhance sleep. In one study, the constant odor of essential oil of bitter orange was sedative and improved sleep even for those under mental stress.
Hydrotherapy ❷ (*see page 126*)
A warm bath can improve circulation, relax muscles, and may encourage deep sleep just as well as exercise.

SELF-HELP TECHNIQUES
• Exercise regularly to reduce stress hormones and increase secretion of HGH (*see opposite*) • Avoid strenuous activity (excluding sex) within three hours before bedtime • Be sure your bedroom is well-ventilated; 75°F (24°C) is the optimum room temperature
• Choose a firm mattress • Avoid drinking before bedtime • If early daylight wakes you, use an eye mask or invest in heavy curtains.

PSYCHOSOCIAL TREATMENT OPTIONS

CONVENTIONAL MEDICINE
A doctor may suggest "sleep hygiene" (learning habits to help you sleep) and sleep-restriction therapy, which allows only six hours in bed. Stimulus control therapy restricts bed for sleep or sex only, breaking the association between bed and sleeplessness.

COMPLEMENTARY THERAPIES
Hypnotherapy ❹ (*see page 134*)
Self-hypnosis can induce and enhance sleep. Intrusive thoughts are calmed by focusing on relaxation and breathing.

Meditation ❸ (*see page 135*)
Meditation, either on its own or combined with another relaxing therapy, can aid sleep by releasing tension and helping relaxation.
Biofeedback ❸ (*see page 136*)
This technique can allow you to calm the body by monitoring your stress levels on sensitive instruments.

SELF-HELP TECHNIQUES
• Stop any work an hour before bedtime to calm mental activity, and keep work materials out of the bedroom

• Practice relaxation and breathing techniques (*see pages 170–71*) in bed.

Getting up and reading a book is a useful distraction for those who are unable to sleep.

FOOD SENSITIVITY

Any kind of abnormal reaction to a food or food additive is known as a *food sensitivity*. An acute *food allergy* is relatively rare but can be very dangerous. The body's immune system reacts immediately to a particular food protein or carbohydrate as if it were harmful, forming immunoglobulin E (IgE) antibodies that cause acute inflammation of the skin and mucous membranes, a sudden fall in blood pressure, and shock (known as anaphylaxis). In severe cases, this type of acute allergic reaction can be fatal.

The far more common type of food sensitivity is *food intolerance*. Symptoms occur after eating certain foods, but reactions are not acute or severe. They generally either appear one or two days after eating the trigger food, or build up gradually with regular intake. The immune system does not react in the same way as it does to a food allergy. Tests show no trace of IgE antibodies, although other types may be detected. The sensitivity may go unrecognized for years because continued intake appears to be tolerated. However, problems eventually develop and only improve if treatment for food sensitivity begins. The trigger food should then be avoided for at least six months, after which it can usually be eaten again in moderation.

Although some conventional doctors are skeptical, food intolerance can sometimes be a factor in certain long-term illnesses. These include chronic fatigue syndrome; hypoglycemia (low blood sugar); arrhythmia (abnormal heartbeat); persistently swollen glands; skin disorders; digestive conditions such as irritable bowel syndrome; urinary problems; frequent infections; musculoskeletal disorders such as muscle pain, migraine, arthritis, and back pain; and psychological problems such as depression, hyperactivity, and anxiety disorders.

BIOCHEMICAL FACTORS

IN CASES OF FOOD ALLERGY, it is the production of immunoglobulin E antibodies (*see above*) that triggers the acute allergic response. A substance called histamine is released, which in turn causes inflammation in various body tissues. Food allergies often occur in people who also suffer from other allergic conditions, such as eczema or hay fever. In cases of food intolerance, there is recent scientific evidence suggesting that faulty non-IgE antibodies (known as IgA and IgG) may allow incompletely digested food molecules to cross the lining of the intestinal tract and enter the bloodstream.

BIOCHEMICAL TRIGGERS
Food allergies: Early exposure to inappropriate food proteins, such as cows' milk • Allergic tendency in family • Peanuts and other nuts • Shellfish • Eggs • Strawberries
Food intolerances: Lack of specific digestive enzymes (for example, lactase, responsible for the digestion of cows' milk) • Dairy products • Gluten – a protein in wheat (celiac disease) • Preservatives (especially benzoic acid) • Colorings (especially Yellow Dye No. 5) and other additives • Pesticides • Antibiotics and other drugs

See page 94 for Biochemical Treatment Options

Realms of the Body (*see page 20*)

BIOCHEMICAL
Body systems,
such as digestion

STRUCTURAL
Muscles, bones,
joints, and nerves

PSYCHOSOCIAL
Thoughts, feelings,
and relationships

STRUCTURAL FACTORS

IN AN ACUTE ALLERGIC REACTION to a food (*see left*), the release of histamine and other chemicals causes blood vessels to widen and blood pressure to fall dramatically. Other reactions may include an itchy raised rash, constriction of the airways in the lungs so that breathing is difficult, swelling of the tongue and throat, pain in the abdomen, and diarrhea. Practitioners of nutritional therapies believe many cases of long-term food intolerance are due to "dysbiosis" (the overgrowth of "unfriendly" gut bacteria) and a "leaky gut," which lets partly digested substances be absorbed into the bloodstream, affecting all body systems (*see page 159*). Overconsumption of certain foods, particularly wheat, dairy products, and refined sugar (for which the gut is poorly adapted), may also be responsible.

STRUCTURAL TRIGGERS

Food intolerance: Poor blood circulation in the intestines • Irritated gut lining • "Leaky gut lining," allowing absorption of partly digested food proteins into the bloodstream (*see below*)

See page 95 for Structural Treatment Options

PSYCHOSOCIAL FACTORS

STRESS AFFECTS DIGESTION and is a common factor in food intolerances (*see below*). People with food intolerances may also have difficulties in coping with stress because they feel under par. Those with allergies of all kinds tend to find their condition is worse when they are stressed.

PSYCHOSOCIAL TRIGGERS

• Stress • Poor health • Lack of coping skills • Anxiety
• Depression • Overwork; lack of sleep • Traumatic events

See page 95 for Psychosocial Treatment Options

Stress leads to biochemical imbalances.

Toxin-induced ailments lead to pain and general poor health, which is stressful.

Effect on gut:
• Fewer digestive enzymes
• Poor intestinal circulation
• Iregular peristalsis (*see Glossary, pages 177–78*)

Various biochemical waste products can act as irritating "toxins."

Toxins overload the liver and kidneys and irritate other organs.

Food is not properly broken down or absorbed.

May lead to:
Dysbiosis: Poorly digested food in the gut encourages overgrowth of "unfriendly" bacteria, resulting in candidiasis, for example.
Leaky gut: Toxins from poorly digested food "leak" from the gut into the blood.

FOOD SENSITIVITY

BIOCHEMICAL TREATMENT OPTIONS

CONVENTIONAL MEDICINE

If you have an acute allergic reaction, a doctor will suggest a RAST (Radio Allergo Sorbent Test), which is a very reliable method of detecting food allergies. Antibodies are extracted from a blood sample and added to the suspect allergen. Radioactive or colored markers indicate an allergic reaction. A food allergy is lifelong, so you will be advised to avoid the food responsible permanently. Acute food allergies are treated with epinephrine injections and antihistamine and corticosteroid drugs (*see Drugs Glossary, page 179*), which can be lifesaving.

COMPLEMENTARY THERAPIES

Nutritional Therapies ❹
(*see page 128–29*)

The skin reacts to foods causing sensitivity.

A practitioner is likely to recommend diagnostic tests such as a skin-prick test (*see page 131*) or a RAST (*see above*), but only if they suspect a true food allergy. For food intolerance they will suggest an elimination or exclusion diet (*see page 128*) to identify the culprit food. Compared with the plant-rich, raw, and unrefined diet for

which our bodies evolved, the modern Western diet is unsuitable for many people, containing too much protein, refined sugar, and wheat, as well as excess fat and additives. Short fasts and "detox" diets give the body a rest from irritant foods and allow the digestion and elimination to recover. A practitioner will suggest supplements to suit your needs, since people with food sensitivities are sometimes deficient in various vitamins and minerals. If dysbiosis (*see page 159*) is suspected, live yogurt and *lactobacillus* supplements will be given to promote healthy gut bacteria.

Environmental Medicine ❸
(*see page 131*)
Clinical ecologists believe that the Western diet, combined with exposure to synthetic chemicals, encourages food intolerances. These intolerances are, they claim, the cause of chronic illnesses. Controversial diagnostic methods include cytotoxic tests, pulse-testing, hair analysis, Vega-testing, and applied kinesiology (*see Glossary, pages 177–78*), but most conventional doctors doubt their accuracy. Some doctors and nutritionists test for immunoglobulin G (IgG) abnormalities, but this is a relatively new procedure. Also recommended may be Enzyme Potentiated Desensitization (EPD), in which an enzyme is used to make the skin absorb a safe dilution of common allergens.

Placing desensitization drops under the tongue.

Some complementary practitioners prepare highly diluted "desensitization drops," taken by mouth and believed to work by "turning off" the intolerance. This is a controversial form of treatment.

SELF-HELP TECHNIQUES

• Keep a food-trigger diary (*see page 147*) to help identify those foods that may be the cause of sensitivities
• Consider a "Stone Age" diet (*see page 129*) if you have any chronic illness
• Remember that excluding food triggers from your diet may initially make your symptoms worse, as will the reintroduction of any food to which you have a sensitivity.

A detox diet includes raw fruit and vegetables, as well as whole-grain cereals and plenty of filtered or pure mineral water.

Maria, a nutritionist, saw Sarah, 34, whose lifelong mild asthma was starting to get significantly worse. Medical tests had found nothing wrong. "Dust was mainly responsible for Sarah's condition," said Maria, "but I find that removing irritating foods often helps alleviate respiratory allergies because it reduces the total demand on the body.

"Sarah was eating wheat at almost every meal," Maria continued. "She had muesli for breakfast, whole-grain bread for lunch, frequent pizzas and pasta, and snacks of plain cookies and wheat crackers." Wheat is a common food intolerance, so Maria suggested Sarah avoid it for a month to see if it helped reduce her bouts of wheezing, which it did. When wheat was reintroduced, her wheezing became worse again.

Maria advised Sarah to replace wheat with rye bread, to eat buckwheat pasta, and to make muesli from flakes of rice, millet, rye, barley, and oats. "I thought my diet was varied," said Sarah, "but it was in fact based around one food. I now eat more fruit and vegetables, and my symptoms are under control."

PRECAUTIONS

Call an ambulance immediately if you suspect an anaphylactic reaction.

Those at risk of an acute allergic reaction should avoid the food responsible, carry a syringe that has been preloaded with epinephrine, and wear a medical alert tag.

The following symptoms are all associated with acute allergic reactions to food. Consult a doctor if any of them develop within an hour or two of eating: itching or swelling in the mouth or on the skin on any part of the body, breathlessness, severe diarrhea, and abdominal cramps.

Practicing yoga postures and breathing exercises can reduce the severity of symptoms.

STRUCTURAL TREATMENT OPTIONS

CONVENTIONAL MEDICINE
Doctors see allergies as biochemical problems with no structural component. However, some doctors believe that food intolerance can be a significant underlying factor in certain long-term diseases.

COMPLEMENTARY THERAPIES
Yoga ❷ (see page 123)
In common with other movement therapies, yoga may be of help in alleviating mild food intolerance. Any exercise that improves circulation to the gut, lungs, and kidneys helps body systems function efficiently and can be beneficial. Yoga practitioners are likely to recommend postures and practices that support digestion and elimination, including Half Shoulder Stands, the Relaxation pose, spinal twists, and breathing exercises (pranayama).

SELF-HELP TECHNIQUES
• Exercise regularly to improve the circulation, aid digestion, and relieve tension (see page 152).

Aerobic exercise such as jogging can help body systems function efficiently.

PSYCHOSOCIAL TREATMENT OPTIONS

CONVENTIONAL MEDICINE
Doctors believe that no psychological treatment should be offered for a condition as dangerous as an acute food allergy. However, in the case of long-term intolerances, the severity of the reaction will often vary according to the patient's stress levels. Psychotherapy may be of use in helping patients cope with stress and to identify the times when they are most likely to suffer a reaction.

COMPLEMENTARY THERAPIES
Psychotherapy & Counseling ❷
(see pages 132–33)
Sometimes food intolerances are blamed inappropriately for ill health and psychological problems. In addition, some people become over-concerned about food sensitivity and condition themselves to expect symptoms. Talking through problems with a trained counselor can help identify unacknowledged areas of psychological difficulty.
Relaxation & Breathing ❷
(see pages 170–71)
Hyperventilation (rapid breathing) stimulates the release of histamine, involved in the allergic response. A practitioner will demonstrate techniques to regulate breathing in order to reduce the severity of the stress response. Relaxation techniques also help relieve muscle tension and stress.

SELF-HELP TECHNIQUES
• Keep a stress diary (see page 147) and choose a stress management technique (see page 168–69). Food sensitivity is often a matter of high reactivity to the trigger food, and personal unhappiness can drastically undermine normal immune responses.

HAY FEVER & RHINITIS

Harmless airborne substances trigger allergic reactions in some people. Membranes lining the nose, throat, sinuses, and eyes become inflamed, increasing mucus production. Symptoms can include itchy, watery eyes, a blocked or runny nose, sneezing, a heavy head, drowsiness, fatigue, and a sore throat. Some allergens, notably pollen, cause *seasonal rhinitis*, or hay fever. This affects one in five people; half also suffer from asthma and many people have eczema as well. Nonseasonal allergens, such as house dust, can cause year-round *perennial rhinitis*, although food intolerances can contribute. Allergies often ease with age.

CASE STUDY

Andrew, 36, dreaded the summer, when his hay fever led to a stuffy nose and very itchy, sore, and swollen eyes. Antihistamines helped, but made him rather drowsy. Jill, an herbalist, prescribed an herbal remedy containing ephedra to reduce allergic reaction, and eyebright, elderflower, goldenseal, and plantain to reduce mucus production and soothe the membranes of his eyes and nasal passages.

Within a few hours of taking his first dose, Andrew found his symptoms much relieved, and he was able to go outside and enjoy the summer weather. He continues to take his herbal remedy when the pollen count is high, and feels he is becoming less susceptible to pollen allergies after several seasons.
Caution: Take ephedra only with professional supervision.

BIOCHEMICAL FACTORS

Hay fever and rhinitis are more likely to occur in "atopic" individuals (those with a family history of asthma, eczema, and hay fever). For unknown reasons, their immune system overreacts to proteins in airborne pollens and dust, and produces immunoglobulin E (IgE) antibodies, which stimulate an excessive release of histamine. This normally helps protect the body from infection by dilating blood vessels so they are more permeable and white blood cells can fight invading organisms. However, the result is inflammation with pain and swelling.

BIOCHEMICAL TRIGGERS
• Genetic tendency for allergies • Grass and tree pollen • Fungal spores • House-dust mites • Animal dander (particles of skin, fur, and feathers) • Food intolerances

STRUCTURAL FACTORS

Once inflamed, the mucous lining of the nose, throat, and sinuses becomes increasingly sensitive. It then takes fewer allergens to trigger an attack, and nonseasonal irritants such as perfume, environmental chemicals, dust, or cigarette smoke can exacerbate symptoms. Swollen mucous membranes may lead to blocked sinuses, sinusitis, and headaches.

STRUCTURAL TRIGGERS
• Cigarette smoke • Environmental chemicals, such as pesticides • Perfumes • Airborne particles, such as traffic fumes

PSYCHOSOCIAL FACTORS

Allergy symptoms are stressful in themselves but, according to complementary practitioners, stress from other sources can exacerbate the immune system's reaction. Other allergies, such as eczema and asthma, are known to be made worse by psychological stress. A study of 128 patients with perennial rhinitis or hay fever concluded that psychological factors are of more significance in perennial rhinitis than in hay fever.

PSYCHOSOCIAL TRIGGERS
• Anxiety • Overwork • Lack of adequate sleep • Traumatic life events

Realms of the Body (*see page 20*)

● BIOCHEMICAL
Body systems,
such as digestion

● STRUCTURAL
Muscles, bones,
joints, and nerves

PSYCHOSOCIAL
Thoughts, feelings,
and relationships

Key: Evidence of Efficacy (*see page 182*)

❶ ❷ ❸ ❹ ❺

least evidence ◄————————► most evidence

BIOCHEMICAL TREATMENT OPTIONS

CONVENTIONAL MEDICINE
Antihistamine tablets, eyedrops, nasal inhalers, and sprays (*see Drugs Glossary, page 179*) may be prescribed to reduce inflammation. Decongestant sprays and drops are effective but may damage nasal membranes if overused. Sodium cromoglycate eyedrops, ointments, inhalers, and nasal sprays inhibit allergies, and anti-inflammatory corticosteroids can ease severe cases. Immunotherapy is a specialized treatment that involves injecting increasing

Eyedrops can be soothing.

amounts of an allergen under the skin monthly for up to two years.
Caution: Some remedies interreact; always consult a pharmacist first.

COMPLEMENTARY THERAPIES
Western Herbalism ❸ (*see page 127*)
Herbalists may suggest a course of echinacea or licorice to boost the immune system before the pollen season. **Caution:** Avoid licorice when pregnant.
Nutritional Therapies ❷
(*see pages 128–29*)
Practitioners may recommend a 48-hour detoxifying fast, followed by a raw-food, cleansing diet to relieve an overloaded

coping system. Vitamin C is said to support the mucous membranes. You might be advised to avoid wheat, dairy products, and food additives.
Homeopathy ❹ (*see page 130*)
Taking homeopathically potentized pollens (*see page 130*) before the pollen season begins may help prevent symptoms. Several studies have found *Galphimia glauca* effective. Other popular remedies are available in pharmacies and health-food stores.

SELF-HELP TECHNIQUES
• Eating garlic and onions may help boost the immune system.

STRUCTURAL TREATMENT OPTIONS

CONVENTIONAL MEDICINE
Masks or caps that cover the mouth or nose help sufferers by filtering air.

COMPLEMENTARY THERAPIES
Aromatherapy ❷ (*see page 117*)
A steam inhalation can ease congestion. Adding 3–4 drops of menthol or eucalyptus essential oils may help. **Caution:** If you have asthma, use steam inhalations with care.
Acupuncture ❸ (*see page 125*)
Traditional Chinese Medicine regards hay fever as "Wind invasion" occurring

Eucalyptus

because the body's defenses (*wei chi*) are weak. Medical acupuncturists in the West claim that acupuncture can affect nerves controlling mucus production and swelling of nasal blood vessels.

SELF-HELP TECHNIQUES
• Try to stay inside and keep windows closed, especially mid-morning and early evening, when the pollen count is highest •Vacuum regularly and dust surfaces with a

damp cloth • Keep any pets out of bedrooms • Splash your face with water to flush away pollen and dust • Shower and wash your hair to remove pollen each evening
• Cover your bed during the day
• Wash bedding and pillows at over 140°F (60°C) to kill dust mites.

Wash your hair to remove allergens.

PSYCHOSOCIAL TREATMENT OPTIONS

CONVENTIONAL MEDICINE
Your doctor may recommend that you reduce stress levels with one of the therapies listed below.

COMPLEMENTARY THERAPIES
Hypnotherapy ❸ (*see page 134*)
A practitioner may demonstrate breathing techniques that can help

alleviate symptoms.
Visualization ❷ (*see page 134*)
You will be shown techniques to relieve physical and mental tension which may reduce stress.
Biofeedback ❷ (*see page 136*)
This technique allows you to monitor your reactions to stress. Used with methods of relaxation and meditation,

it may help to relieve the swelling of perennial rhinitis.

SELF-HELP TECHNIQUES
• Keep a symptom diary (*see page 147*) to identify possible allergic triggers, including foods • Practice stress management techniques (*see pages 168–69*).

ASTHMA

The episodes of breathlessness and wheezing that are characteristic of asthma result when the membranes lining the small airways of the lungs (the bronchioles) become constricted and inflamed, and airflow is restricted. Production of phlegm then increases and worsens the obstruction.

Asthma is becoming very common, especially in industrialized countries, and affects over 200 million people worldwide, including one child in seven. About a quarter of sufferers have severe attacks with sweating and a racing pulse, which can be frightening and dangerous and must be treated with conventional medicine.

CASE STUDY

Louise, a homeopathic doctor, treated Rebecca, 10, for worsening asthma attacks. She advised continuing with the steroid inhalers and performed skin tests for common allergens. Louise decided that Rebecca had the typical characteristics of a *Phosphorus* constitution and prescribed *Phosphorus 30c* daily for a week. Ten days later she added a daily homeopathic dilution of house-dust mite, the allergen to which Rebecca had reacted most strongly. Louise continues to see Rebecca. "The steroid dose she was on has been slowly reduced and she has had no further severe attacks."

PRECAUTIONS

Always keep emergency medicines on hand. If an attack does not respond quickly to self-administered bronchodilator drugs, call a doctor or go to the hospital immediately.

STRUCTURAL FACTORS

A combination of tense bronchial tube muscles and inflamed, swollen membranes narrows the airways so that airflow is restricted. Production of white sticky phlegm increases, making the blockage worse, and breathing becomes a struggle. The chest feels tight, and attempts to clear the airways may produce a dry cough, especially at night.

STRUCTURAL TRIGGERS

• Vigorous physical exertion, especially in cold, dry air • Cold, damp, dry, or stormy weather • Fluctuations in body rhythm make attacks more likely between midnight and 3 A.M.

BIOCHEMICAL FACTORS

When an asthmatic person inhales airborne allergens or irritants, the immune system overreacts, producing immunoglobulin E antibodies. These stimulate histamine release in the lining of the bronchial tubes, causing inflammation. Dietary factors or even viral infections can also trigger the immune response in susceptible individuals.

BIOCHEMICAL TRIGGERS

• House-dust mites, cockroaches, mold, or pollen from grasses, trees, and other plants • Animal dander (particles of fur, skin, and feathers) • Environmental pollutants such as tobacco smoke, exhaust fumes, and industrial fumes • Allergy to foods such as dairy products, seafood, yeast, nuts, and wheat, and of food additives and alcohol (see page 92) • Food intolerances may increase susceptibility to inhaled allergens • Monosodium glutamate; preservatives • Deficiency of nutrients such as vitamin C, magnesium, or essential fatty acids • Viral infections

PSYCHOSOCIAL FACTORS

An asthma attack can be triggered by any kind of psychological stress, be it anxiety, overwork, relationship and family problems, depression, or even apprehension about the next attack. Anxiety constricts the bronchial tubes, and the severity of an attack is often related to the degree of anxiety felt.

PSYCHOSOCIAL TRIGGERS

• Stress and anxiety • Strong emotions • Fear of the next asthma attack • Repressed feelings

BIOCHEMICAL TREATMENT OPTIONS

CONVENTIONAL MEDICINE
Your doctor will discuss a treatment plan with you and might perform skin or blood tests to identify allergens. Sodium cromoglycate or inhaled cortiocosteroid sprays, which reduce inflammation and mucus, are prescribed for daily use to prevent attacks (*see Drugs Glossary, page 179*).

COMPLEMENTARY THERAPIES
Western Herbalism ❷ (*see page 127*)
A practitioner may prescribe coleus,

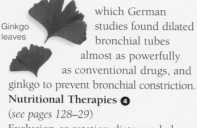
Ginkgo leaves

which German studies found dilated bronchial tubes almost as powerfully as conventional drugs, and ginkgo to prevent bronchial constriction.
Nutritional Therapies ❹
(*see pages 128–29*)
Exclusion or rotation diets can help identify food intolerance. Supplements of vitamin C and B_6 may be suggested.
Homeopathy ❹ (*see page 130*)
In a study published in *The Lancet* in

1994, asthmatics taking homeopathic remedies showed an improvement.

SELF-HELP TECHNIQUES
• Eat oily fish and whole-grain cereals, rich in omega-3 fatty acids and magnesium, and avoid salt
• Protect against house-dust mites with synthetic bedding and carpets, and a powerful vacuum cleaner
• Avoid animals, tobacco smoke, and polluted air • Consider a new job if you are exposed to allergens at work.

STRUCTURAL TREATMENT OPTIONS

CONVENTIONAL MEDICINE
Bronchodilators such as albuterol, cromolyn sodium, or inhaled steroids (*see Drugs Glossary, page 179*) may be given. During an attack, they are taken via nebulizers or inhalers to open the airways.

Asthma inhaler

COMPLEMENTARY THERAPIES
Osteopathy ❸ (*see page 118*) and
Chiropractic ❸ (*see page 119*)

Practitioners use manipulation to relax and stretch the chest muscles and diaphragm, so breathing is easier.
Yoga ❹ (*see page 123*)
Breathing and stretching postures help chest muscles work better, expand the lungs, and calm the mind and body.
Acupuncture ❸ (*see page 125*)
Studies suggest that stimulating acupoints may relieve symptoms.

SELF-HELP TECHNIQUES
• Regular exercise increases lung

capacity and strengthens the heart (*see pages 152–53*) • If an attack is brought on by exercise, use a bronchodilator inhaler beforehand • Diaphragmatic breathing and progressive muscle relaxation (*see pages 170–71*) can help • In the controversial Buteyko method, asthma is attributed to hyperventilation (rapid breathing). Patients are taught how to shallow-breathe and hold their breath, but there is still very little evidence for this method's effectiveness.

PSYCHOSOCIAL TREATMENT OPTIONS

CONVENTIONAL MEDICINE
Discuss any family, social, or psychological problems with your doctor, who may suggest counseling (*see below*). There is evidence that repressed feelings make people more susceptible to asthma attacks.

COMPLEMENTARY THERAPIES
Psychotherapy & Counseling ❸
(*see pages 132–33*)
Cognitive behavioral therapy can reduce the frequency of attacks by

reducing the expectation of panic and giving a greater sense of control.
Hypnotherapy ❸ (*see page 134*)
By teaching you to relax and cope with unpleasant sensations, hypnosis can relieve symptoms and reduce the need for medication.

SELF-HELP TECHNIQUES
• The unpredictability of an attack is wearing; keep a diary (*see page 147*) to identify stresses, environmental factors, dietary factors, and even

emotions that trigger attacks • Join a support group • Learn coping skills (*see pages 172–73*).

Making notes in a diary helps pinpoint factors involved in attacks.

CANCER

The second biggest killer after heart disease, cancer affects about a third of people who live in developed countries. It occurs when cells in certain tissues multiply uncontrollably and most commonly affects the breasts, lungs, bowel, skin, stomach, ovaries, pancreas, prostate, bladder, and lymph glands. Cancer is not a single disease and its severity depends, among other things, on the kind of tissue affected. Some forms are relatively mild and, if caught in time, have a 100 percent cure rate. The incidence of certain cancers varies considerably, from country to country, and differences in diet and lifestyle are significant. It seems as many as 70 percent of cancer cases could be prevented if people avoided known trigger factors, such as tobacco, ultraviolet light, and certain foods.

In the past, complementary medicine sometimes claimed "miracle" cures for cancer that were later proved to be ineffectual or even fraudulent. Now a combination of conventional and complementary therapies offers a promising way forward, and many leading cancer treatment centers, hospices, and self-help groups have adopted the integrative approach, using gentle therapies such as massage, relaxation, and healing to help relieve symptoms. Complementary therapists aim to ease pain and anxiety, alleviate the side effects of conventional medicine, help patients come to terms with their situation, and, where the outlook is poor, to enjoy whatever time is left. There is some evidence that the resulting enhancement of emotional and spiritual well-being prolongs life.

BIOCHEMICAL FACTORS

THERE ARE MORE THAN 200 FORMS OF CANCER, but all have one thing in common: abnormal cells whose growth is out of control. All cells multiply by splitting in two, a process stimulated by genes called oncogenes, and slowed by others known as tumor suppressors. Genetic mutations can throw this process out of balance, so that cells divide at breakneck speed, faster than the tumor suppressors can restrain them. As the tumor grows, it eventually invades neighboring tissues, and tumor cells metastasize (spread) through the bloodstream and lymph system to distant parts of the body where they form "secondary" tumors.

A tendency for cells to mutate can be inherited. Certain types of cancer – like colon and breast cancer – run in some families. Other types may be triggered by viral infections and lifestyle factors. Diet is estimated to account for up to 80 percent of cancers of the bowel, breast, and prostate.

BIOCHEMICAL TRIGGERS

• Genetic disposition • Infection with hepatitis B and C, or HIV viruses, and *Helicobacter pylori* • Smoking (lung, mouth, throat, esophagus, pancreas, bladder, and cervix) • Heavy drinking (mouth, esophagus, pharynx, larynx, and liver) • Obesity (breast, uterus, and gallbladder) • Chemicals and food additives
• Processed and smoked foods, charred food • Diet high in red meat and other foods containing saturated animal fats • Diet low in selenium and other antioxidants

See page 102 for Biochemical Treatment Options

Realms of the Body (*see page 20*)

⬤ BIOCHEMICAL
Body systems,
such as digestion

⬤ STRUCTURAL
Muscles, bones,
joints, and nerves

⬤ PSYCHOSOCIAL
Thoughts, feelings,
and relationships

STRUCTURAL FACTORS

EXTERNAL FACTORS SUCH AS POLLUTION, industrial chemicals, and radiation may trigger cell mutation and abnormal cell growth. Cultural differences seem to make certain cancers more prevalent in some countries. Breast cancer rates, for example, are higher in the affluent US, where early onset of menstruation and the postponement of childbearing are common, than in poorer countries like Poland, where slower growth rates delay menstruation. There are more cases of stomach cancer in Japan than in other countries, possibly caused by high salt intake and greater rates of infection with the stomach bacteria *Helicobacter pylori*, which some experts believe might trigger cancer of the stomach.

STRUCTURAL TRIGGERS

• Ultraviolet radiation (skin cancer) • Environmental and chemical irritants • Pesticides, traffic fumes • Ionizing radiation (for example, excessive X-rays) • Inactivity (studies show inactive men are twice as likely to develop cancer as active men) • Unprotected sex (cervical and anal cancer are linked to a sexually transmitted virus)

See page 103 for Structural Treatment Options

PSYCHOSOCIAL FACTORS

A PERSON'S SUSCEPTIBILITY TO CANCER has been attributed to stress, personality and emotional events. Some books have even implied that cancer is caused by repressed emotions or a lack of "spiritual development." These theories and the related idea that recovery depends on the amount of mental effort put into it should be treated with skepticism. There is no firm evidence that stress, personality, emotional states, thoughts, or feelings in themselves can *cause* cancer, nor that negative feelings will make tumors grow faster.

On the other hand, most experts now believe that the onset of the disease is complex. It requires a number of predisposing factors, from genes to lifestyle, which all need to be involved before one acts as a trigger. A stressful situation, such as bereavement or loneliness, may undermine normal immune processes, but this might only trigger tumor formation if the person is already suffering from poor nutrition, adverse environmental factors, or has a genetic tendency to develop cancer.

POSITIVE ATTITUDE

How we cope with cancer may be important. One study of women with early breast cancer found that those who had a positive "fighting spirit" fared better than those who felt negative or helpless. There is also evidence that supportive social environments and psychological factors may increase chances of recovery or lengthen the survival time of patients.

See page 103 for Psychosocial Treatment Options

WARNING SIGNS

Cancer can cause a variety of symptoms. Consult a doctor as soon as possible if you have any of the following:

• Unexplained, persistent weight loss
• A mole that changes shape, gets bigger, itches, or bleeds
• Sores, scabs, or ulcers on the skin that do not heal
• A lump in the breast; discharge or bleeding from the nipple or flattening of the nipple; change in the shape or size of the breast; dimpling or puckering of the skin
• Change in the shape or size of the testicles

• Unexplained severe headaches
• Constant hoarseness; persistent sore throat; nagging cough; difficulty in swallowing; repeatedly coughing up blood
• Persistent abdominal pain or indigestion
• Blood – either red or black – in the stools or urine
• Change in bowel habits, for example, persistent constipation (especially in those over 40)
• Vaginal bleeding between menstrual periods, after sex, or after menopause

CANCER

Key: Evidence of Efficacy (*see page 182*)

1 **2** **3** **4** **5**

least evidence ◄————► most evidence

BIOCHEMICAL TREATMENT OPTIONS

CONVENTIONAL MEDICINE

Radiation therapy (*see Glossary, pages 177–78*) to mop up cancer cells left after surgery, or chemotherapy to destroy cells that have traveled to other parts of the body, may be given. The success of these methods varies with the type of cancer. Retinoids, carotenoids, aspirin, and hormones such as tamoxifen are being investigated as treatments, and new approaches include biological therapies and gene therapy. Vaccine therapy may eventually help the immune system fight specific cancers, notably skin and prostate cancer.

COMPLEMENTARY THERAPIES
Traditional Chinese Medicine 3

(*see pages 124–25*)
You may be given remedies to alleviate the side effects of chemotherapy and radiation therapy. *Fu zheng* therapy, which relies on an herbal formula with ginseng and astragalus, is claimed to improve life expectancy. Many studies show ginseng to have protective qualities.

Lycopene in tomatoes and peppers helps protect against cancer.

Western Herbalism 2

(*see page 127*)
Practitioners aim to boost the body's defenses. A cleansing program with herbs such as burdock may be followed by restorative remedies for the liver, digestion, circulation, and nervous system. Canadian herbalists have developed a remedy known as Essiac, based on a Native American formula, but their claims of its effectiveness require more research.
Caution: Take herbal remedies only under professional supervision and with the consent of your doctor.

Nutritional Therapies 3

(*see pages 128–29*)
Some foods seem to have protective qualities, and the natural combination of nutrients, especially in fruit and vegetables, may be more powerful than taking isolated supplements. Many doctors and nutritionists recommend fiber – to improve elimination and mop up potentially carcinogenic substances – and foods rich in antioxidants (*see page 162*), which work together to protect against "free radicals" that can stimulate cancer cell growth. Important antioxidants include vitamins A and E to improve immune function; vitamin C to prevent carcinogenic nitrosamines (*see Glossary, pages 177–78*) from forming; selenium to protect the cell membranes; and bioflavonoids to strengthen the capillaries. B-complex vitamins neutralize certain carcinogens.

Healing foods A nutritionist might recommend eating garlic and onions, which contain allicin, said to help prevent gastrointestinal and bladder cancer; tomatoes and red peppers, which are rich in lycopene, shown to lower the risk of prostate and cervical cancer; oily fish, which seems to have an antitumor effect; cabbage,

Shiitake mushrooms may be protective.

broccoli, and soy, which protect against prostate, ovarian, and breast cancer; and shiitake and maitake mushrooms, which may inhibit cancer cell development.

Cancer-fighting diets There are a number of dietary therapies, such as the Gerson raw foods diet, the Hippocrates wheatgrass diet, and the Kelley-Gonzalez and Livington-Wheeler programs that claim to *treat* cancer. However no single program has been scientifically proven to cure cancer or stop its spread, and these extreme regimens can cause weight loss and psychological strain in people who may already be stressed and underweight. The Bristol Diet devised in the late 1980s at the Bristol Cancer Help Centre in the UK is a less rigorous regimen, with an emphasis on natural, unprocessed foods.

Homeopathy 3 (*see page 130*)
Iscador, an extract of mistletoe, may be suggested. Tests show it can inhibit the growth of tumors, but there is no conclusive evidence for its effectiveness.

SELF-HELP TECHNIQUES

• Eat more organic vegetables, fruit, and whole grains • Cut down on fat; red meat; salt-cured, salt-pickled, and smoked foods • Drink alcohol only in moderation • Throw away moldy food, since some molds are carcinogenic.

Protect against cancer with oily fish, vegetables, and grains.

PRECAUTIONS

If you have cancer, consult a doctor before undertaking any complementary therapy and do not stop taking conventional medication.

STRUCTURAL TREATMENT OPTIONS

CONVENTIONAL MEDICINE
Diagnosing cancer may require a biopsy (*see Glossary, pages 177–78*) to determine if a tumor is malignant. A CT or MRI scan may be arranged; nuclear medicine imaging allows three-dimensional views of tumors. Surgery aims to remove the cancer, possibly along with the local lymph nodes.

COMPLEMENTARY THERAPIES
Massage ❹ (*see page 116*)
Therapeutic massage, now available in many cancer centers and hospices, can relieve muscle pain and tension, reduce anxiety, and encourage relaxation. After a mastectomy, you may be offered a very gentle form of massage called lymphatic drainage to help reduce the swelling. Massaging someone with cancer demands knowledge and skill, but family and friends can also learn techniques that bring comfort and reassurance through physical touch.

Reflexology is relaxing and may help relieve cancer symptoms.

Reflexology ❷
(*see page 120*)
Reflexology is increasingly available in US cancer centers and hospices, where it is often given by nurses. It is relaxing, and practitioners claim it can help relieve symptoms, including pain, constipation, and nausea.

Healing ❸ (*see page 122*)
Healers are available in some cancer centers, and many patients and their families report that healing, or "laying on of hands," provides support, strength, symptom relief, and spiritual solace.

Therapeutic Touch ❸ (*see page 122*)
A growing number of nurses, particularly in the US, use therapeutic touch, and studies report that it can help pain management.

Acupuncture ❺ (*see page 125*)
A practitioner will show you how to stimulate acupoints, especially Pericardium 6, to relieve nausea caused by chemotherapy. Acupuncture can encourage the release of endorphins, natural painkillers that increase feelings of well-being.

SELF-HELP TECHNIQUES
• Exercise regularly to improve digestion and circulation
• Examine your skin, breasts, or testicles regularly • If you already have cancer, get as fit as your age and condition allow.·

Gentle qigong is excellent exercise (*see pages 124–25*).

PSYCHOSOCIAL TREATMENT OPTIONS

CONVENTIONAL MEDICINE
A doctor may suggest one of the therapies below. Once considered unconventional, they are now widely recommended to cancer patients and their families.

COMPLEMENTARY THERAPIES
Psychotherapy & Counseling ❹
(*see pages 132–33*)
Therapy aims to promote a relaxed, optimistic outlook, which, studies show, seems to increase the activity of natural killer cells that destroy cancerous cells. One US study found that weekly support groups, coupled with relaxation and self-hypnosis, doubled the length of survival of women with advanced breast cancer.

Visualization ❷ (*see page 134*)
Visual imagery can be used to alleviate symptoms and promote healing, although there is no definite evidence that it affects the outcome. While in a state of relaxation, you will be asked to

focus on feeling stronger or better, or to picture the destruction of tumor cells. One technique, in which patients visualize remaining calm and relaxed at each step during various treatment procedures, can help control nausea before chemotherapy.

Hypnotherapy ❸ (*see page 134*)
Hypnosis can help people cope with pain and other symptoms of cancer, and with nausea and vomiting, which are side effects of chemotherapy.

Art Therapy ❸ (*see page 137*)
Drawing, painting, and sculpture, available in many cancer centers, can enable people to find a nonverbal way of expressing strong feelings and encourage pleasure in creativity.

Art therapy can help people with cancer express emotions.

SELF-HELP TECHNIQUES
• Practice relaxation, breathing, and stress management techniques (*see pages 170–71 and 168–69*)
• Encourage a sense of connectedness by developing a supportive network of friends and becoming involved in community life • Enjoy pleasurable and creative activities as much as possible (*see page 173*).

CHRONIC FATIGUE SYNDROME

Characterized by extreme physical and mental exhaustion, chronic fatigue syndrome (CFS) can last for years. Symptoms may begin suddenly, sometimes after a viral infection, and can be wide-ranging. They include muscle aches, joint pains, headaches, depression, swollen glands, memory loss, inability to concentrate, recurring minor infections, digestive disorders, and food intolerances. CFS is now accepted by doctors as a diagnosable disease, and experts believe it may be caused by a complex interaction of factors such as stress, viral infections, brain chemistry, psychological problems, and social factors.

CASE STUDY

Alice, 31, had suffered from CFS for three years following a flulike viral infection. Medical tests had found nothing wrong so her doctor suggested she try complementary therapies. Adam, a naturopath, advised a calcium and magnesium bedtime drink to ensure a good night's sleep, and breathing techniques, massage, and autogenic training to help her relax. Alice cut back on milk and cheese after an exclusion diet suggested a mild dairy intolerance, and took *lactobacillus acidophilus* and *Bifidobacteria* supplements to normalize gut bacteria. She also took echinacea, goldenseal, and barberry to boost immunity. Adam suggested Alice visit a counselor. She found herself expressing intense grief over her mother's death three years previously. Alice slowly improved and 12 months later was able to return to full-time work.

BIOCHEMICAL FACTORS

It is uncertain how viral infections are involved in CFS although they can clearly trigger it. However, high levels of antibodies to certain viruses, for example, to the Epstein-Barr virus, which causes glandular fever are sometimes found in CFS patients. These viruses can possibly interfere with the body's normal homeostatic processes (*see Glossary, pages 177–78*). Hormone imbalances, genetic susceptibility, vaccinations, environmental chemicals, and other toxins have all been implicated, but not conclusively.

BIOCHEMICAL TRIGGERS

• Epstein-Barr virus (glandular fever) • Viral hepatitis, viral meningitis • Any viral infections if already run down

STRUCTURAL FACTORS

Inactivity can lead to muscle cell abnormalities. There is little evidence that CFS is caused by a muscle disorder, but muscle pain (*see page 60*) is often associated with it. Some sufferers have a form of low blood pressure in which the nervous system mistakenly tells the body to lower blood pressure when standing. Since CFS often makes people feel anxious, sufferers may overbreathe (hyperventilate). If persistent, this could intensify CFS symptoms.

STRUCTURAL TRIGGERS

• A form of low blood pressure (neurally mediated hypotension) • Excessive bed rest, lack of exercise, and loss of fitness

PSYCHOSOCIAL FACTORS

CFS was thought to be more prevalent among educated, professional people, but research suggests it affects all social classes and cultures. A particular personality profile appears most susceptible: perfectionist, conscientious people who feel obliged to take on too much, come under a lot of stress, find it hard to relax and are inclined to become depressed and introverted. Many people with CFS rightly resist the idea that it is "all in the mind". Nevertheless, psychological elements seem to be involved, whether as causes or effects.

PSYCHOSOCIAL TRIGGERS

• Stress and overwork • Anxiety • Depression • Perfectionism, inability to delegate and excessive conscientiousness • Pessimistic expectations about illness

Realms of the Body (see page 20)

- **BIOCHEMICAL** Body systems, such as digestion
- **STRUCTURAL** Muscles, bones, joints, and nerves
- **PSYCHOSOCIAL** Thoughts, feelings, and relationships

Key: Evidence of Efficacy (see page 182)

❶ ❷ ❸ ❹ ❺
least evidence ◄━━━━━━━━► most evidence

BIOCHEMICAL TREATMENT OPTIONS

CONVENTIONAL MEDICINE

Prolonged fatigue is a symptom of other diseases, including anemia, chronic infection, diabetes, cancer, and autoimmune or thyroid disorders. Only when these have been ruled out will CFS be diagnosed; then a healthy diet and vitamin and mineral supplements will be suggested.

COMPLEMENTARY THERAPIES

Western Herbalism ❷ (see page 127)
An herbalist may advise echinacea and astragalus to improve immunity,

Siberian ginseng to increase resistance to stress, St. John's wort to improve mood, and ginkgo to boost circulation. **Caution:** Avoid ginseng in pregnancy or if you have high blood pressure. Do not take St. John's wort with conventional antidepressants.

Nutritional Therapies ❸ (see pages 128–29)
A practitioner will test for

Siberian ginseng combats stress.

dysbiosis (see page 93) and food sensitivities. Exclusion diets, detoxification programs, and high-energy diets may be recommended. Suggested supplements might include evening primrose oil, coenzyme Q10, and vitamins A (as beta carotene), C, E, and B-complex. Injections of magnesium or vitamin B_{12} help some people.

SELF-HELP TECHNIQUES

- Eat a healthy balanced diet with fruit, vegetables, and whole grains
- Limit caffeine and alcohol.

STRUCTURAL TREATMENT OPTIONS

CONVENTIONAL MEDICINE

Doctors will advise gentle but gradually increasing levels of exercise. Avoiding all activity may be tempting but it can make CFS worse, since underused muscles lose power, and bulk or tense up, causing even more aches and pains.

Gentle exercise can relieve debility and pain.

COMPLEMENTARY THERAPIES

Massage ❷ (see page 116)
Massage can help combat CFS by relieving muscular discomfort and tension and encouraging relaxation.

Yoga, T'ai chi, and Qigong ❷ (see pages 123 and 125)
All three therapies make use of gentle stretching movements and breathing techniques that focus the mind and may increase energy levels.

Acupuncture ❷ (see pages 125)
Practitioners associate CFS with deficiencies of Kidney and Liver

energy, defined by exhaustion and a low ability to cope with stress. Combining acupuncture with Chinese herbal remedies and *tuina* (Chinese massage therapy) may be even more effective than acupuncture alone.

SELF-HELP TECHNIQUES

- Get regular daily exercise • Pace yourself, avoiding sudden exertion that might set you back • Allow time to relax, particularly after an infection. Remember that any improvement could take several months.

PSYCHOSOCIAL TREATMENT OPTIONS

CONVENTIONAL MEDICINE

Antidepressants might not relieve CFS as such, but they can be highly effective at alleviating associated symptoms such as anxiety, depression, or disturbed sleep.

COMPLEMENTARY THERAPIES

Psychotherapy & Counseling ❹ (see pages 132–33)
Counseling can help with CFS.

Patients need someone to acknowledge how frustrated and anxious the illness makes them feel. It can also help them reevaluate lifestyle and career goals and manage stress more effectively. Several studies have found that cognitive behavioral therapy helps people with CFS. People who reframe their beliefs about illness improve more quickly than those who do not.

Relaxation & Breathing ❸ (see pages 170–71)
Diaphragmatic breathing improves circulation and helps relieve a tight chest caused by hyperventilation, which affects some people with CFS.

SELF-HELP TECHNIQUES

- Learn to pace yourself and allow time to relax during the day • Practice stress management (see pages 168–69).

PERSISTENT PAIN

Short-term, acute pain, which ranges from nagging discomfort to excruciating agony, is the body's warning signal that something specific is wrong, whether it is a cut finger or acute appendicitis. Chronic, or persistent, pain is defined as pain lasting for six months or longer. It may have a clear source, such as chronic inflammation (a symptom of some types of arthritis), nerve damage from a herpes infection, or tumor growth. Very often, however, there is no clear explanation, even after extensive examination and testing. This kind of persistent, incapacitating pain can affect work and relationships, and is viewed by doctors not so much as a symptom, but as a disorder in itself.

About 75 percent of people who visit complementary practitioners do so because of various sorts of painful conditions, and usually because they have found conventional treatments inadequate. Often the cause of pain is clear and, as in migraine, it comes and goes. Persistent pain, however, usually involves physical *and* psychological factors and so holistic approaches that take account of a person's lifestyle and attitudes may ultimately increase the chances of relief.

Certain manipulative therapies and acupuncture can stimulate the production of endorphins, the body's natural painkillers. Other techniques, such as hypnosis and relaxation, aim to help people improve their tolerance of pain. Increasingly these approaches are employed alongside conventional treatments in hospital pain clinics. Practitioners have found that a combination of methods within an overall pain management program often achieves good results.

BIOCHEMICAL FACTORS

SENSORY NERVE ENDINGS, or receptors, are highly concentrated in the skin. When stimulated by pressure, extreme temperature, or prostaglandins (chemicals released by injured cells), they relay biochemical and electrical messages to the spinal cord and on to the brain, where they are interpreted as pain. According to the "gate control" theory, information carried on the limited number of pain nerve pathways to the brain passes through "gates." Various factors close the gates or hold them open. For example, endorphins (opiate chemicals that are the body's natural painkillers) slot into receptors located in the brain, spinal cord, and nerve endings, blocking pain impulses. How wide pain gates open and how much information reaches pain receptors partly depends on the levels of endorphins in circulation at any one time.

BIOCHEMICAL TRIGGERS
• Substances produced in tissues that are inflamed (such as arthritic joints) or congested (such as chronically tense muscles) may open pain gates

See page 108 for Biochemical Treatment Options

Realms of the Body (*see page 20*)

● **BIOCHEMICAL**
Body systems,
such as digestion

● **STRUCTURAL**
Muscles, bones,
joints, and nerves

● **PSYCHOSOCIAL**
Thoughts, feelings,
and relationships

STRUCTURAL FACTORS

ANY KIND OF STIMULATION along the path of a pain nerve will register at its tip. For example, if a finger pain nerve is pinched at the elbow, pain is felt shooting down to that finger. The pain in the finger is called "referred" pain. Continual pain can affect a pain pathway so that it becomes "facilitated," or more easily set off, long after the original problem has healed. This is thought to be caused by "pain gates" remaining open in the brain and spinal cord as a result of changes in the way the nervous system is structured. Such changes may mean that sufferers from chronic pain can sometimes become trapped in a vicious cycle. When sufferers avoid exercise, painkilling endorphins that close the pain gates are not released, and the resulting despair may keep them inactive. Inactivity weakens, shortens, and tenses muscles, creating further spasms and more pain.

STRUCTURAL TRIGGERS

• Injury or surgery • Disease, inflammation, or damage to sensory nerves (neuropathy) • Lack of movement • Postural changes • Muscle tension anticipating pain

See page 108 for Structural Treatment Options

PSYCHOSOCIAL FACTORS

TOLERANCE OF PAIN varies between individuals and also changes according to mood. Pain seems worse and is more noticeable when people are depressed than when they feel well or happy or when they are distracted by something enjoyable. Emotional states can influence the levels of painkilling endorphins in the body, which explains why soldiers have been known to carry on in the heat of battle, unaware of devastating injury. The way in which someone interprets pain, their ideas about its causes and consequences, as well as past experiences and associations with pain, will all affect the person's ability to tolerate it. Psychological states can also directly affect areas of the body that have become accustomed to sensing pain. In one experiment, just thinking about painful experiences caused the back muscles of people who complained of chronic back pain to become tense. By anticipating the worst when an attack begins, migraine sufferers were found to stiffen their muscles and restrict blood flow, thereby making the attack longer and more severe. The tendency to breathe rapidly in response to anxiety about pain can lead to hyperventilation (abnormally rapid breathing). This in turn can engender a state of panic, making muscles more prone to spasm and opening "pain gates" by altering the way nerve impulses are transmitted in the brain.

PSYCHOSOCIAL TRIGGERS

• Stress • Fear • Depression • Previous experiences of pain • Attitudes toward pain • Anticipation of pain

See page 109 for Psychosocial Treatment Options

CASE STUDY

Nancy, an aromatherapist, treated Joanna, 42, who suffered from persistent pain. Instead of gradually getting better in the normal way, a frozen shoulder became weaker, with muscle wasting and skin changes. Eventually Joanna felt pain from her head to her fingertips on one side of her body. Her doctor prescribed a tiny dose of the antidepressant amitriptyline, which dulled the pain a little, and referred her to the hospital pain clinic. Here a doctor gave her some acupuncture, which helped, and suggested she see an aromatherapist. Nancy used various essential oils according to Joanna's condition at the time of her appointment, but lavender and rosemary in particular. Joanna found that aromatherapy really made a difference and continues to have aromatherapy every three or four weeks. Nancy also gave her a relaxation tape which she found very helpful. She says can live with the pain now even though she knows she may never be entirely free of it.

PERSISTENT PAIN

BIOCHEMICAL TREATMENT OPTIONS

CONVENTIONAL MEDICINE

Painkillers

Painkillers are very helpful for acute pain but can make persistent pain worse. Five out of six people with persistent pain take painkillers, but an estimated 70 percent continue to feel severe pain. Painkillers include over-the-counter analgesics such as acetaminophen, nonsteroidal anti-inflammatory drugs (NSAIDs) such as aspirin and ibuprofen, muscle relaxants, and opioids (see Drugs Glossary, pages 177–78). The latter range from mild codeine to morphine and mimic endorphins by acting directly on the brain and spinal cord to alter perception of pain. Very severe pain arising from surgery or serious injury may be treated with injections of opioids. Morphine and diamorphine are prescribed for cancer patients. Small doses of amitriptyline, an antidepressant, seem to alter the pain experienced. The antiepileptic drug carbamazepine is useful for neuralgic pain. Research shows that cannabis may relieve muscle pain in multiple sclerosis but its prescription is a controversial issue in most countries.

COMPLEMENTARY THERAPIES

Western Herbalism ❸ (see page 127)
In clinical studies, a cream containing capsaicin has proven useful in alleviating persistent pain and is now being used in some pain clinics. Relaxant herbs valerian and scullcap are often prescribed. St. John's wort is both antidepressant and anti-inflammatory and may be useful for persistent pain.
Caution: Do not take St. John's wort with antidepressants.
Nutritional Therapies ❸ (see pages 128–29)
Practitioners find that pain tolerance is decreased if levels of magnesium are low. Supplements might be suggested.

Scullcap

SELF-HELP TECHNIQUES

• Eat a well-balanced diet rich in fruit, vegetables, and whole grains.

STRUCTURAL TREATMENT OPTIONS

CONVENTIONAL MEDICINE

In many cases, no cause for the pain can be detected by medical diagnostic tests. Sometimes persistent pain may be helped by physical therapy, massage, vibration, and the application of heat and cold. Transcutaneous electrical nerve stimulation (TENS), in which impulses are applied to nerve endings, may be given to block pain signals. Local anesthetics, or nerve blocks, can relieve pain for a time, and, in extreme cases, neurosurgery can sever nerve pathways, but it is irreversible and can mean loss of sensation and movement.
Caution: Consider structural therapies as a backup for conventional pain management, but *not* as a substitute.

COMPLEMENTARY THERAPIES

Massage ❸ (see page 116)
Therapists will aim to alleviate pain by reducing the local muscle tension that can intensify pain sensations.

Aromatherapy ❷ (see page 117)
When used with massage, essential oils aid relaxation and may even help stimulate the release of endorphins.
Osteopathy ❷ (see page 118) and **Chiropractic ❷** (see page 119)
Although manipulation alone is unlikely to cure persistent back pain, practitioners aim to relieve tension and improve posture (see also page 55).
Alexander Technique ❷ (see page 121)
Posture and chronic pain are closely linked. Improving posture may help relieve and prevent pain, especially neck and back pain.
Therapeutic Touch ❷ (see page 122)
A practitioner will pass her hands around the body to "balance energy fields." In a study,

Healing energy is directed to the patient.

therapeutic touch reduced the pain of chronic tension headaches in 90 percent of patients.
Acupuncture ❹ (see page 125)
Practitioners aim to restore the flow of qi by stimulating acupoints. Pain control is the one aspect of acupuncture that most conventional doctors accept; they believe it works by stimulating the release of endorphins and prostaglandin-suppressing corticosteroid hormones. It also appears to relieve pain from trigger points (see Glossary, pages 177–78), a common cause of persistent pain.
Hydrotherapy ❷ (see page 126)
Exercise in heated pools can ease chronic joint and muscle pain.

SELF-HELP TECHNIQUES

• Exercise to prevent muscles from stiffening.

PSYCHOSOCIAL TREATMENT OPTIONS

CONVENTIONAL MEDICINE

Pain is not measurable. Pain specialists ask about the level of pain the patient feels, what it is like, and how it restricts activities. Their aim is to improve pain tolerance. Psychologists are important members of pain management teams. It is now recognized that the experience of pain affects the entire person because of its impact on how he or she thinks, feels, and behaves.

COMPLEMENTARY THERAPIES

Psychotherapy & Counseling ❹
(*see pages 132–33*)
Our thoughts, beliefs, moods, and emotions can act as a kind of "volume control," capable of turning the pain experience up or down. Preoccupation with pain and anticipation and worry distorts thinking and raises the volume. Cognitive behavioral therapy can help replace these feelings with positive attitudes that encourage control.

Hypnotherapy ❸ (*see page 134*)
A hypnotherapist makes suggestions to help you alter pain perception and show that control of pain is possible. In studies, hypnotherapy was effective in relieving pain from fibromyalgia (muscle pain) and cancer. Self-hypnosis can be very effective for pain, although its effects tend to wear off.

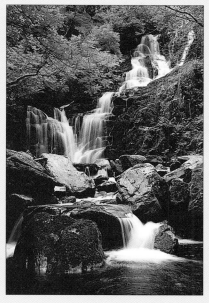
Picturing a peaceful scene can help distract the mind and reduce perception of pain.

Visualization ❸ (*see page 134*)
Guided imagery is best used alongside other techniques and helps distract from pain. You may be asked to picture yourself in peaceful, pain-free environments or to imagine your pain has a color or shape and then visualize another color or shape that will soothe or control it: a red-hot bar, for example, turning into ice cream and melting away.

Meditation ❹ (*see page 135*)
Learning to relax the body and calm and focus the mind may distract from pain.

While in a trance, the patient is told by the practitioner that he can control his pain.

After four years of mindfulness meditation, 60 percent of patients in one study said their persistent pain had decreased.

Biofeedback ❸ (*see page 136*)
Research shows that biofeedback may help 40–60 percent of people with headaches or pain in the jaw from temporomandibular joint disorder (TMJ), and can ease back pain and fibromyalgia.

Relaxation & Breathing ❸
(*see pages 170–71*)
Muscle relaxation involving diaphragmatic breathing is probably one of the most effective ways to ease and control pain. It reduces muscle spasms and helps regulate brain chemicals, blood flow, and other body processes involved in pain tolerance, and can relieve anxiety, distract from pain, and encourage sleep.

Diaphragmatic breathing reduces tension.

SELF-HELP TECHNIQUES

• To identify triggers, keep a diary to record episodes of pain and your emotional responses to them • Practice relaxation and breathing (*see pages 170–71*); imagine a warm glow entering the painful area of your body as you slowly inhale, and pain and tension carried away as you exhale • Plan any outings ahead and pace yourself to avoid fatigue • Listen to music to keep your mind occupied.

HIV & AIDS

Acquired immune-deficiency syndrome (AIDS) covers a range of diseases that usually follow infection with the human immunodeficiency virus (HIV). This destroys infection-fighting T-lymphocytes, leaving the body open to a range of potentially fatal diseases. HIV infection is symptomless at first and may take ten years or more to develop into AIDS. Although conventional treatment for HIV is effective, it is complicated and expensive, and often causes unpleasant side effects. Because complementary therapies emphasize health promotion and touch, they can integrate well into "packages" of care alongside high-tech treatments.

CASE STUDY

Stephen, a naturopath, treated Roy, 50, who was HIV-positive and had frequent infections and mouth ulcers despite conventional drug treatment. Stephen recommended a whole-foods diet high in fresh vegetables and fruit, with supplements of vitamin B-complex and the antioxidants vitamin C, zinc, and selenium. "I also suggested the amino acid lysine to balance the arginine that was provoking his mouth ulcers, plus short courses of echinacea to boost his immune system." Roy was told to take a daily long hot bath to increase his internal temperature. Stephen felt this could "burn off the viral load" and stimulate the elimination of toxins. He also suggested that Roy find an autogenics class to learn a deep-relaxation technique. After some months, Roy reported fewer infections and tests showed his disease-fighting white-cell count had improved.

BIOCHEMICAL FACTORS

HIV spreads through exchanges of body fluids and is usually transmitted sexually or by contaminated hypodermic needles and transfusion of infected blood products. The virus takes three weeks to three months from the time of infection to show in blood tests, and many people are unaware that they are HIV-positive until AIDS develops. When HIV invades the T-lymphocyte cells, it changes their genetic codes so that they make more HIV genes instead of fighting the virus. As the level of healthy T-cells falls, HIV spreads and the immune system is weakened. Infections tend to become more frequent and recovery from them harder.

BIOCHEMICAL TRIGGERS
• Recurrent infections • Poor nutrition
• Drug abuse

STRUCTURAL FACTORS

Typical early symptoms of full-blown AIDS include swollen glands, fatigue, fever, weight loss, night sweats, shortness of breath, a dry cough, and thrush. *Kaposi's sarcoma* (skin tumors that appear as purple blotches), diarrhea, and pneumonia are characteristic as the disease progresses. Finally the brain may be affected by a form of encephalitis that causes dementia.

STRUCTURAL TRIGGERS
• Unprotected sexual intercourse • Sharing contaminated needles or syringes when injecting drugs • Contaminated blood products and blood transfusion • Mother-to-child infection in the uterus or during breast-feeding

PSYCHOSOCIAL FACTORS

Some researchers believe that factors in addition to HIV may contribute to the development of AIDS. Studies show that stress, isolation, pessimism, and depression adversely affect the immune system. In HIV-positive people, this could *theoretically* promote a faster progression to AIDS. Coming to terms with being HIV-positive is unlikely to be easy, and people are led to expect a bad prognosis. The ways in which HIV is contracted, and the stigma and alienation associated with it, add an extra socially isolating dimension. As attitudes toward HIV and AIDS change with increasing survival times, the notion that being HIV-positive is a literal and social death sentence should change as well.

Realms of the Body (*see page 20*)

BIOCHEMICAL
Body systems,
such as digestion

STRUCTURAL
Muscles, bones,
joints, and nerves

PSYCHOSOCIAL
Thoughts, feelings,
and relationships

Key: Evidence of Efficacy (*see page 182*)

❶ ❷ ❸ ❹ ❺

least evidence ◄——————————► most evidence

BIOCHEMICAL TREATMENT OPTIONS

CONVENTIONAL MEDICINE

Antiviral, antibacterial, and antifungal drugs are used to prevent or combat infection. Chemotherapy involves powerful drug combinations including a protease inhibitor and AZT (*see Drugs Glossary, page 179*). These often have unpleasant side effects, but may eliminate 99 percent of detectable HIV.

COMPLEMENTARY THERAPIES

Herbalism ❸ (*see pages 125 and 127*)
Practitioners of Western and Chinese herbal medicine use a range of plant-based remedies to improve immunity

and inhibit HIV. These include artemisia, astragalus, bitter melon, echinacea, germanium-132 (a mineral found in ginseng, garlic, and watercress) and prunellin, a compound isolated from *Prunella vulgaris* (self-heal). **Caution:** Take remedies only with professional supervision.

Nutritional Therapies ❸
(*see pages 128–29*)
A diet high in immune-boosting nutrients and antioxidants will be recommended. Practitioners may suggest selenium,

zinc, bioflavonoids, and vitamins A, C, E, and B-complex to improve immunity.

SELF-HELP TECHNIQUES

• Take a high-quality antioxidant supplement • Follow a balanced (ideally, organic) diet with plenty of fruit, vegetables, and whole grains • Avoid caffeine, junk foods, alcohol, smoking, and illegal drugs.

An antioxidant diet boosts the immune system.

STRUCTURAL TREATMENT OPTIONS

CONVENTIONAL MEDICINE

A doctor will offer advice about preventing HIV transmission.

COMPLEMENTARY THERAPIES

Massage ❸ (*see page 116*)
An empathetic practitioner can provide the kind of caring touch that the stigma of AIDS denies many patients. Gentle

Regular massage can help support AIDS patients.

massage can relieve emotional distress and enhance body image and self-esteem, as well as improve circulation, lymph drainage and muscle relaxation.

Acupuncture ❷ (*see page 125*)
A practitioner will aim to alleviate symptoms and boost immune functions by reducing stress.

SELF-HELP TECHNIQUES

• Practice safer sex by using a condom • Intravenous drug users should use only new, disposable

syringes; never share a needle or syringe or use an old one • Be sure that dentists, dental hygienists, acupuncturists, tattoo artists, and body piercers have adequate sterilization procedures and use disposable needles • If you are HIV-positive and pregnant, discuss delivery and breast-feeding with your doctor or midwife
• Cover any cuts if you are HIV-positive
• In developing countries, avoid blood transfusions and carry a sterile hypodermic needle and syringe in case an injection or infusion is necessary.

PSYCHOSOCIAL TREATMENT OPTIONS

CONVENTIONAL MEDICINE

Counseling should be offered before HIV testing, and afterward to support a person whose result is positive.

COMPLEMENTARY THERAPIES

Psychotherapy & Counseling ❸
(*see pages 132–33*)
Therapists can play an important role both before and after diagnosis, not

only for basic information and advice, but also because anger, fear, denial, grief, and depression may have to be dealt with. Sharing experiences in a support group can help in a similiar way. Research has shown that appropriate support combined with a positive attitude toward the disease can raise T-cell counts, reduce symptoms, and possibly extend life span.

SELF-HELP TECHNIQUES

• Be aware of your physical, psychological, and spiritual needs
• Find a stress management technique (*see pages 168–69*) that works for you
• Supportive relationships with those who accept and understand the situation are important. Many people living with HIV say they find a new sense of meaning and purpose in life.

THE NATURAL MEDICINE CHEST

Medical emergencies require expert help and conventional treatment as soon as possible. Complementary remedies may be used to treat minor injuries. They have a role in relieving pain, calming the mind, and helping the body heal itself. Keep emergency numbers by the telephone and a first-aid kit (*see below*) in an easily accessible place, along with information on resuscitation and the recovery position, and on how to deal with choking, drowning, head and back injuries, heart attacks and stroke, bleeding, electric shock, burns, poisoning, shock, fractures, and dislocations. Organizations such as the American Red Cross provide information and first-aid courses to help you manage situations promptly and appropriately.

FIRST-AID KIT

Conventional Items
• Painkillers: acetaminophen, aspirin (also for heart attack) • Antiseptic wipes and cream • Adhesive bandages • Sterile dressings (various sizes) • Bandages: roller, triangular, tubular • Sterile eye pad
• Disposable gloves • Safety pins
• Scissors • Tweezers • Thermometer

Suggested Complementary Items
• Herbal remedies: aloe vera gel, arnica cream, echinacea tincture or capsules, pot marigold (calendula) cream, St. John's wort (hypericum) tincture or cream (with calendula), witch hazel, slippery elm powder, ginger and rosemary teas • Essential oils: camphor, lavender, tea tree, rosemary, peppermint, eucalyptus
• Homeopathic remedies (store away from essential oils): *Arnica, Aconite, Calendula, Hypericum,* and *Urtica urens*
• Bach Rescue Remedy • Nutritional: vitamin E capsules, garlic capsules

Slippery elm powder for indigestion

Vitamin E capsules to break open for burns and stings

Acetaminophen tablets ease pain.

Tea tree oil disinfects minor cuts.

Lavender oil to calm and relax

Valerian tablets for stress and insomnia

Garlic capsules help fight infection.

Witch hazel soothes stings and abrasions.

Adhesive Bandages

Roll of gauze

Thermometer

Arnica cream to relieve bruising and strains

Pot marigold cream speeds healing of minor wounds.

Urtica urens cream heals minor burns.

Bach Rescue Remedy may aid recovery from shock.

Eucalyptus oil for steam inhalation

FAINTING

First aid: If you feel faint, sit with your head between your knees or lie down. Put a person who has fainted on his side, loosen his collar, and elevate his legs to 12 in (30 cm). Be sure the airways are clear; pull the jaw forward and upward. When he recovers, give sips of water. Call an ambulance if the patient does not regain consciousness within two minutes. See a doctor if fainting is frequent or accompanied by unusual symptoms such as chest pain.
Aromatherapy (*see page 117*)
A few drops of essential oils of rosemary, camphor, or peppermint on a cloth or handkerchief held under the nose may stimulate the senses. (Do not use essential oils on pregnant women.)
Western Herbalism (*see page 127*)
After regaining consciousness, sip ginger or rosemary tea.
Bach Rescue Remedy (*see page 177*)
For emotional shock, place four drops on the tongue.

MINOR CUTS & BRUISES

First aid: Elevate the area and apply pressure for ten minutes to stop any bleeding. Clean the wound, apply antiseptic cream, and cover with a dry dressing. Ice packs or cold compresses reduce bruising. Call a doctor if bleeding cannot be controlled, if the wound is deep and may need suturing, if it becomes infected, if debris cannot be removed, or if bruising persists. Check your tetanus status: A booster injection is recommended every 5–10 years.

Aromatherapy (*see page 117*)
Tea tree essential oil is both antiseptic and antibacterial. It helps relieve pain and aid healing. Add a few drops to the water when cleaning the wound.
Western Herbalism (*see page 127*)
Pot marigold (calendula) is an antiseptic and astringent that helps

Tea tree oil will help prevent infection.

blood to clot. St. John's wort (hypericum) has astringent, sedative, anti-inflammatory, and antimicrobial properties. Add tinctures of both to warm water to wash the wound, or apply as a cream. The two are often combined in commercial preparations.
Homeopathy (*see page 130*)
Arnica (granules and cream) is recommended for bruising, *Calendula* to prevent infection and aid healing, *Hypericum* if a graze is sensitive.

BITES & STINGS

First aid: Remove an insect stinger by scraping it out with a thumbnail or blunt blade rather than tweezers. Wash with soap and water and apply an ice pack. Elevate the area to reduce swelling. Some people are allergic to insect bites so call an ambulance if the lips, tongue, or throat swell, or if breathing is difficult. Allergic reactions may lead to collapse or even to death.
Naturopathy (*see page 126*)
Apply alkaline sodium bicarbonate to neutralize acidic bee and ant stings; and acidic vinegar to neutralize alkaline wasp and hornet stings. Vitamin E oil or 3–4 tablets of vitamin C crushed with water applied to the sting may relieve pain and reduce swelling.
Western Herbalism (*see page 127*)
Onions contain enzymes said to deactivate insect poisons; place half a raw onion on the sting for ten minutes. An application of distilled witch hazel is particularly good for mosquito bites.

SHOCK

Physiological shock may follow an injury. Blood supply to the brain and gut is depleted, causing nausea, rapid pulse, clammy skin, and, in some cases, even loss of consciousness and death. Emotional shock may follow bad news.
First aid: For physiological shock, call an ambulance. Lay the patient in the recovery position (*see Fainting*). Be sure the mouth and airways are clear and turn the head to one side. Keep the patient covered and warm. Do not give food or drink.
Western Herbalism (*see page 127*)
For emotional shock only, teas and tinctures of chamomile, lemon balm, and skullcap are calming and restorative.
Homeopathy (*see page 130*)
For emotional shock, *Arnica*, *Aconite*.
Bach Rescue Remedy (*see page 177*)
Place four drops on the tongue, as required, for emotional shock.

BURNS

First-degree burns damage the skin's surface, causing redness, pain, and swelling, and second-degree burns raise blisters. Third-degree burns destroy all the layers of the skin.

First aid: Immerse first- and second-degree burns in cold water for ten minutes. Keep the area clean and cover blistered skin with a sterile, nonstick dressing. Drink plenty of fluids. Call an ambulance at once for third-degree burns. Do not put water on these or try to remove clothing sticking to the skin; instead cover the area with a

Hold the burned area under cold running water for ten minutes.

clean dry cloth. Get medical advice if a burn is larger than the patient's hand, if it is still painful after 24 hours, or if the patient is in shock or collapses.
Naturopathy (*see page 126*)
Practitioners recommend frequent applications of vitamin E oil or cream, or pure aloe vera gel, to speed healing.
Homeopathy (*see page 130*)
Urtica urens cream should be applied as necessary for first-degree burns.

chapter

3

Not all complementary therapies combine well with conventional medicine. Here we feature those that doctors who are interested in an integrative approach are likely to accept. Some, such as acupuncture, are

GLOSSARY OF THERAPIES

supported by clinically controlled trials, while others are backed by a body of anecdotal evidence. We explain each one's principles and treatments and indicate its effects on biochemical, structural, and psychosocial health. Our aim is to help you decide whether a therapy would improve your health, either on its own or as an adjunct to conventional treatment.

STRUCTURAL THERAPIES

MASSAGE

BIOCHEMICAL EFFECTS

Changes brain and tissue chemistry by encouraging the relaxation response.

STRUCTURAL EFFECTS

Pressure and stretching movements encourage muscle relaxation and improve circulation. Relieves pain by reducing the congestion of inflamed tissue.

PSYCHOSOCIAL EFFECTS

A range of feelings may be evoked, from sedation to arousal. The effect depends on the individual – one person may be reassured, another alarmed.

INTRODUCTION

Massage may be the oldest and simplest form of medical care. It has been used for thousands of years around the world to promote well-being, ease pain of all kinds, and relieve anxiety. A number of studies support its healing role in lowering blood pressure; improving circulation, muscle tone, and digestion; and promoting relaxation. Massage is an integral part of most traditional health systems around the world, and different techniques have been developed and incorporated into various complementary therapies.

HISTORY OF MASSAGE

The ancient Egyptians, Greeks, and Romans used massage for therapeutic purposes, and it has long been an important part of Traditional Chinese Medicine and Ayurveda, the traditional Indian system of medicine. For many centuries in the West, massage had a dubious connection with sin and sensuality, but at the end of the 19th century, the Swedish gymnast Per Henrik Ling made therapeutic massage respectable again. Awareness of the healing value of massage is growing rapidly. In both the US and the UK, some physical therapists and nurses are bringing

Massage can be used to promote relaxation and combat stress.

massage therapy into conventional health care. Increasingly, massage is used in intensive-care units; for children, babies in incubators, and the elderly; and for patients with cancer, AIDS, heart attacks, or stroke. It is available in some family practices, hospices, drug rehabilitation units, and pain clinics.

Babies can be soothed and calmed by gentle massage.

A head massage can relieve headaches and aid relaxation.

MAIN PRINCIPLES

Touch is our first sensual experience and, along with smell, remains the most immediate and evocative link between mind and body. The skin is the body's largest sensory organ, with millions of specialized receptors that react to heat, cold, and pressure. Massage can stimulate the release of endorphins, the natural painkillers produced by the body. It also induces a feeling of comfort and well-being that can aid relaxation and reduce levels of stress hormones, such as cortisol and norepinephrine, that may otherwise eventually weaken the immune system.

Vigorous massage can directly affect body systems that govern heart rate, blood pressure, respiration, digestion, and pain. As local circulation improves, so does the supply of oxygen and nutrients to the skin and body tissues, and excess tissue fluids are flushed away. The lymphatic system can then work more effectively to eliminate waste products

that can cause pain and stiffness in joints and muscles. Massage also relaxes tension in the muscles, improving mobility and flexibility.

Psychologically, massage can calm the mind and reduce anxiety so that people are better equipped to cope with stress. A heightened awareness of the way the mind and body affect one another may help some people take more control of their own well-being.

TREATMENT

Techniques vary according to the massage method used, but usually include stroking, where the hands glide rhythmically; kneading, in which the hands squeeze and release flesh; friction, when thumb pressure is applied to a point for deep penetration; and hacking, when the sides of the hands deliver alternate short, sharp taps to the body. Massage techniques are used in other complementary therapies, notably aromatherapy, reflexology, Rolfing, Hellerwork, and osteopathy.

MAIN USES

• Stress-related conditions, such as insomnia and headaches • Muscle and joint disorders like arthritis, sports injuries, and back pain • Pain relief • High blood pressure • Depression • Anxiety • Digestive disorders

---

PRECAUTIONS

Massage of the abdomen should be avoided in the first three months of pregnancy. Consult a doctor if you have phlebitis, thrombosis, varicose veins, acute back pain, cancer, a personality disorder, or psychotic illness. Do not massage bruises, fractures, or skin infections.
(See also page 21.)

AROMATHERAPY

BIOCHEMICAL EFFECTS

Some essential oils may have direct and specific effects on brain and tissue chemistry. The relaxation response is also encouraged.

STRUCTURAL EFFECTS

Massage with essential oils encourages muscle relaxation and improved circulation, aiding pain relief and tissue regeneration.

PSYCHOSOCIAL EFFECTS

The smells of certain oils can evoke and become strongly associated with feelings and emotions such as relaxation and well-being.

INTRODUCTION

Essential oils have been used in many cultures throughout history for healing and relaxation. Aromatherapists believe that different oils have distinct therapeutic properties. Certain oils are calming, others stimulating and uplifting. Molecules in the oils are absorbed into the bloodstream either through the skin during massage, or by inhalation of the scent through the nose and lungs. The biochemical effects on the body are not fully established, but smell is known to have psychological effects.

HISTORY OF AROMATHERAPY

Essential oils (for example, myrrh) are mentioned in the Bible, and the ancient Egyptians used them to embalm the dead. Around AD 1000, the Persian physician Ali ibn-Sina developed the method of distillation used today. Oils such as sandalwood, cedar, and rose have always been at the heart of perfumery, and highly aromatic oils like eucalyptus, mint, and camphor have long been used medicinally.

Medical interest in essential oils was rekindled in the early 20th century by French chemist Réné-Maurice Gattefossé, who applied lavender oil to a burn and was impressed by the oil's healing powers. Some French doctors now prescribe essential oils for oral use or in a vaporizer as substitutes for certain conventional medicines, for example, to control infections.

MAIN PRINCIPLES

Plant roots, flowers, leaves, and stalks (and trees, in some cases) are processed to extract the essential oils that form the basis of aromatherapy. Extraction is usually by means of distillation, in which the plant is heated by boiling or steaming until it

vaporizes. Chemicals in the scents released by the oils are thought to act on the hypothalamus, the part of the brain influencing mood and the hormonal system. Studies on hospital patients show that massage with certain oils can relieve anxiety, for example. Some oils also have obvious chemical effects when applied to the skin; tea tree, for example, is a proven antiseptic.

TREATMENT

Massage: Essential oils may be diluted in a vegetable-based carrier oil for massage. An aromatherapy massage is usually based on Swedish massage techniques that relieve tension and improve circulation.

An inhalation is an excellent way to treat respiratory problems.

Inhalation: Add 4 drops of essential oil to a bowl of steaming hot water. Cover your head with a towel, lean over the bowl with eyes closed, and inhale for 10 minutes. Alternatively, moisten a tissue with 4–5 drops of oil, hold to your nose, and inhale.
Bath: Run a warm bath and add 6 drops of essential oil. Relax in the bath for 10 minutes or more.
Vaporizers: Place 2–3 drops of essential oil in the vaporizer bowl with a small amount of water, and light a candle beneath.

Essential oils can be burned in vaporizers to fill a room with scent.

Essential oils are diluted in vegetable-based carrier oils for use in massage.

OILS AND EFFECTS

Calming: bergamot, chamomile, clary sage, geranium, jasmine, lavender
Uplifting: clary sage, grapefruit, jasmine, lavender, neroli, rose, rosemary, ylang ylang
Stimulating: black pepper, cinnamon, eucalyptus, ginger, peppermint, pine
Antiseptic, antibacterial, and antifungal: tea tree, lavender
Decongestant: eucalyptus, lavender, peppermint, pine.

MAIN USES

• Stress-related conditions, such as insomnia and headaches • Digestive disorders • Colds • During pregnancy and labor • Menstrual problems
• Relaxation and well-being

PRECAUTIONS

Take care when using inhalations if you have asthma or are prone to nosebleeds. Do not swallow oils, unless supervised by a medically qualified practitioner. Never apply undiluted essential oils to the skin (except lavender and tea tree). Keep essential oils away from open flames and out of reach of children. Consult a qualified practitioner if you are pregnant, epileptic, or have high blood pressure.(*See also page 21.*)

CHIROPRACTIC

BIOCHEMICAL EFFECTS

Improves tissue chemistry as pain and inflammatory substances and waste products disperse following local and general relaxation.

STRUCTURAL EFFECTS

Increases range of movement. Relieves muscle tension, which leads to better local circulation and reduction of swelling.

PSYCHOSOCIAL EFFECTS

By diminishing pain, increases the confidence to stretch and exercise; provides knowledge and skills to help prevent future problems.

INTRODUCTION

Chiropractors use manual techniques to diagnose and treat disorders of the spine, joints, and muscles. They treat the body as a mechanism, with the spine as its key support, linking the brain to the body. When body systems work in harmony, self-healing processes can function efficiently, and chiropractors believe that any distortion of the spine affects other parts of the body and disturbs these processes. Chiropractic is practiced in all developed countries, and a number of studies have demonstrated its effectiveness in relieving back pain.

HISTORY OF CHIROPRACTIC

Chiropractic – from the ancient Greek *cheiro*, or "hand," and *praktikos*, or "doing," – was developed in 1895 by Daniel D. Palmer, a Canadian. Palmer claimed to have restored the hearing of his office janitor, who had been deaf for 17 years following a back and neck injury. The therapy became popular throughout the West during the early part of the 20th century. Condemned as an "unscientific cult" by the American Medical Association

A practitioner examines the spine for stiffness.

(AMA) in the 1960s (the AMA lost the ensuing legal battle in 1987), chiropractic has now gained widespread recognition and is available in American and British health care systems.

Offshoots of chiropractic include Network Spinal Analysis, which concentrates on the interaction of the vertebrae and uses a sequence, or "network," of 12 adjustment techniques, and also McTimoney chiropractic, which focuses on the patient's whole body at each session and uses low-impact, relatively uncomplicated forms of adjustment.

MAIN PRINCIPLES

The spinal cord carries nerves to the whole body. Chiropractors think that any distortion of the spinal column will have an effect on other parts of the body. Accordingly, the spine should be properly aligned in order for the body systems to work in harmony and to enable the body's self-healing processes to function efficiently. Any strain, damage, or distortion of the spine is said to promote problems in the internal organs, glands, and blood vessels, and can undermine the body's self-regulating and healing processes.

TREATMENT

A chiropractor takes a detailed medical history, asks questions about lifestyle, and may perform standard diagnostic tests, including X-rays. She will maneuver you into various positions, using her hands to examine the functioning of your spinal column, joints, and muscles. Treatment of stiff or "locked" joints usually takes place on a specially adjustable chiropractic table, and consists of precise, controlled techniques known as "adjustments."

The practitioner begins by moving the joint as far as it will go (mobilization), then gives a rapid, measured thrust to move it slightly further. With any adjustment, there may be an audible but painless "click" in the joint, caused by the

Patients often lie on a special table for manipulation of the spine.

collapse of a tiny gas bubble created by the change in pressure when the joint is suddenly stretched. Initial chiropractic sessions last 30–60 minutes; subsequent ones may be brief. The total number of sessions depends on how fast the condition responds to treatment.

MAIN USES

• Spine and neck disorders • Muscle, joint, and postural problems • Sports and repetitive strain injuries • Sciatica • Headaches and migraine • Digestive disorders • Tinnitus • Vertigo • Menstrual pain • Asthma

PRECAUTIONS

If you have osteoporosis or inflammation, infections, tumors, circulatory problems, or a recent fracture, practitioners may decide not to treat you using manipulation. However, chiropractors are skilled in other pain-relief methods. Avoid vigorous manipulation if you have badly prolapsed (slipped) disks. *(See also page 21.)*

OSTEOPATHY

BIOCHEMICAL EFFECTS

Improves tissue chemistry as pain and inflammatory substances and waste products disperse following local and general relaxation.

STRUCTURAL EFFECTS

Increases range of movement. Relieves muscle tension, which leads to better local circulation and reduction of swelling.

PSYCHOSOCIAL EFFECTS

By diminishing pain, increases the confidence to stretch and exercise; provides knowledge and skills to help prevent future problems.

INTRODUCTION

The relaxed, harmonious working order of muscles, bones, and joints is held to be essential to well-being because it supports the optimum functioning of all body systems. Osteopaths use touch and manipulation to diagnose problems and to restore or improve mobility and balance. They employ a variety of therapeutic techniques, from soothing massage to high-velocity mobilization of joints. Although more clinical research needs to be done, osteopathy is well established, and its role in treating acute back pain is generally accepted by conventional medicine.

HISTORY OF OSTEOPATHY

Osteopathy, from the Greek *osteon*, meaning "bone," and *pathos*, meaning "suffering," was developed in the late 19th century by an American army doctor, Dr. Andrew Taylor Still, after his wife and three children died from meningitis. He sought ways to stimulate the body's self-healing powers and founded the American School of Osteopathy in 1892. In 1917, his pupil, Dr. John Martin Littlejohn, founded the British School of Osteopathy. Despite early opposition from conventional medicine, osteopaths were licensed in the US in 1972.

MAIN PRINCIPLES

Posture and the way we move express how we feel. Physical and emotional stress, injury, and poor posture can all adversely affect the musculoskeletal system, which supports and protects the body organs. Pain creates muscle tension, which in turn creates more pain. Osteopaths ease muscle tension and improve joint mobility in order to restore the body's ability to heal itself. While chiropractors have tended to concentrate on joint manipulation,

osteopaths traditionally focus more on "soft tissue" treatment, but today this distinction is often blurred. Practitioners are as concerned about what has triggered and is maintaining the musculoskeletal dysfunction as with the problem itself, and will look for any psychological, occupational, or lifestyle factors.

Cranial osteopathy was initially developed by American osteopath Dr. William Garner Sutherland in the 1930s and expanded by Dr. Jim Jealous of New Hampshire. It uses delicate touch around the skull and lower spine to ease the tension that is believed to disturb the flow of cerebrospinal fluid. Cranial osteopathy is claimed to be particularly successful for babies and young children and in treating problems following trauma and injury.

Practitioners believe that manipulation of cranial bones restores the flow of cerebrospinal fluid.

TREATMENT

After taking a thorough medical history, an osteopath asks about lifestyle and emotional health, performs standard medical tests, and examines posture and movements for stresses and strains.

Treatment is tailored to individual needs. It may consist simply of massage

The osteopath carefully feels each vertebra to detect problems.

and stretching techniques, or it may involve manipulation of the joints. Alternatively, the practitioner may position you in such a way that tension from areas of strain or injury is released spontaneously. Another type of treatment, known as "muscle energy techniques," involves working against resistance provided by the practitioner in order to release tension in the muscles. One visit may be enough, but three to six sessions are average, depending on your problem and state of health.

MAIN USES
- Spine and neck disorders
- Muscle, joint, and postural problems
- Sports and repetitive strain injuries
- Sciatica • Headaches and migraine
- Digestive disorders • Tinnitus
- Vertigo • Menstrual pain • Asthma

PRECAUTIONS

If you have osteoporosis or inflammation, infections, tumors, circulatory problems, or a recent fracture, practitioners may decide not to treat you using manipulation. Avoid vigorous manipulation if you have badly prolapsed (slipped) disks.
(See also page 21.)

REFLEXOLOGY

BIOCHEMICAL EFFECTS

Changes brain and tissue chemistry by encouraging the relaxation response.

STRUCTURAL EFFECTS

Encourages muscle relaxation and improves circulation; some evidence that it can relieve pain.

PSYCHOSOCIAL EFFECTS

Practitioners aim to address underlying stress-related factors that trigger or prolong health problems.

INTRODUCTION

Reflexologists believe that the feet and hands mirror the body, and stimulation of specific reflex points on them can affect associated organs and systems. The big toe, for example, reflects the head and brain. A combination of massage, pressure, and pinching over all parts of the feet (or in some cases, the hands) can bring deep relaxation. Consequently, despite a lack of evidence, reflexology is one of the most popular complementary therapies and is even offered in hospital cancer centers, pain clinics, and intensive-care baby units.

HISTORY OF REFLEXOLOGY

Foot massage dates back to ancient Egypt and China, but reflexology as practiced today was introduced in 1915 by Dr. William H. Fitzgerald, a US ear, nose, and throat specialist. Known at the time as "zone therapy," it was based on the theory that energy flows in vertical zones through the body, from the feet to the head, so that pressure

applied to a reflex point on the foot can affect all the organs, glands, bones, and muscles in that zone. In the 1930s, American physical therapist Eunice Ingham mapped the reflex points on the feet and developed techniques for stimulation. Her map is still widely used today. Ingham's student Doreen Bayley introduced reflexology to the UK in the 1960s and its popularity spread rapidly.

Practitioners stimulate reflex points on the feet.

MAIN PRINCIPLES

Zones on the left side of the body are said to correspond to reflex points on the left foot and hand, and those on the right to the right foot and hand. Practitioners believe that granular or crystalline accumulations of waste products, possibly uric acid and calcium, collect around reflex points. The more tender the points to the touch, the greater the "imbalance" in the body. The practitioner tries to break

down these deposits to free "energy flow" along the zones and stimulate circulation to clear "toxins." Mental health is also said to be reflected in the feet, so reflexology is also used to treat emotional problems.

Although similar in theory to Traditional Chinese Medicine's concept of meridians (see page 124), reflexology claims to be a separate approach. Doctors concede that pressure on the 7,200 nerve endings in each foot seems to promote feelings of deep relaxation, which may induce useful, nonspecific healing effects.

TREATMENT

Most practitioners prefer to work on the foot, so expect to take off your footwear and relax in a reclining chair with your feet raised. The practitioner stimulates the reflex points by massaging each foot with her knuckles and thumbs, observing areas of pain or tenderness. When worked on intensely, even extremely sensitive areas usually become less so. Most people find the treatment relaxing, but occasionally it is followed by a worsening of symptoms, believed to indicate that the body's natural healing processes are removing "toxins."

MAIN USES
- Stress-related conditions
- Insomnia • Back pain

PRECAUTIONS

Avoid in the first three months of pregnancy and check with your doctor before treatment if you have a long-term health problem. Tell the practitioner if you are taking medication. (See also page 21.)

REFLEX POINTS ON THE SOLES OF THE FEET

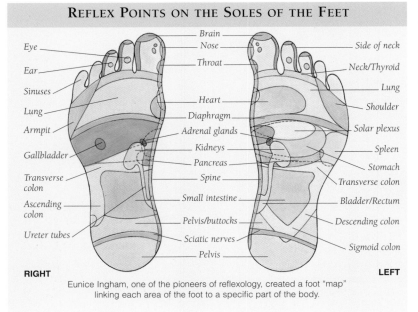

Eye, Ear, Sinuses, Lung, Armpit, Gallbladder, Transverse colon, Ascending colon, Ureter tubes

Brain, Nose, Throat, Heart, Diaphragm, Adrenal glands, Kidneys, Pancreas, Spine, Small intestine, Pelvis/buttocks, Sciatic nerves, Pelvis

Side of neck, Neck/Thyroid, Lung, Shoulder, Solar plexus, Spleen, Stomach, Transverse colon, Bladder/Rectum, Descending colon, Sigmoid colon

RIGHT

LEFT

Eunice Ingham, one of the pioneers of reflexology, created a foot "map" linking each area of the foot to a specific part of the body.

THE ALEXANDER TECHNIQUE

BIOCHEMICAL EFFECTS

Changes brain and tissue chemistry by encouraging the relaxation response.

STRUCTURAL EFFECTS

Improves posture and coordination; promotes efficient body movement; encourages the relaxation response; may improve circulation to internal organs.

PSYCHOSOCIAL EFFECTS

Promotes an attitude of active self-care; also improves self-image and esteem.

INTRODUCTION

Years of poor posture, hunching, and slumping have a detrimental effect on the working of the joints and muscles. The Alexander technique helps people stand and move more effectively, so that stresses on the body can be eased and each body system is able to function more efficiently. As the body works in a more relaxed way, the ability to cope with stress improves. Conventional medicine generally supports the use of the Alexander technique to treat persistent back pain and stress, and it has a wide international following. Many actors, dancers, opera singers, and instrumentalists say that practicing the Alexander technique improves their performance.

The practitioner corrects posture and shows how to stand in a way that exerts minimum strain on the body.

HISTORY OF THE ALEXANDER TECHNIQUE

In the late 19th century, Frederick Matthias Alexander, an Australian actor, discovered that he could prevent his voice from becoming strained by improving his posture and relaxing his muscles, especially those of the throat. He moved to London in 1904 and developed his techniques, establishing links with educators and performing artists. In 1931 he set up a training school for teachers in London. Recent studies at Columbia University in New York and at Kingston Hospital in London show that the technique can help relieve chronic back pain and improve breathing.

MAIN PRINCIPLES

Young children possess a natural grace, but years of sitting and standing in awkward positions, lifting incorrectly, and tensing the muscles at times of stress or when we are self-conscious cause us to develop poor posture, which often goes unnoticed and can be a difficult habit to break. According to Alexander, these "patterns of misuse" exert strains that inhibit optimum functioning of body and mind. By relearning basic movements, such as sitting and standing, it is possible to become aware of and to avoid postural bad habits and to align the body so that movement becomes harmonious and relaxed.

TREATMENT

The principles of the Alexander technique are best learned on a one-to-one basis from a teacher in a series of 15–30 lessons. The teacher usually begins the course by making gentle adjustments as you lie flat on a table; she will then help you to your feet. The object of this exercise is to give you personal experience of optimum "body use." Subsequent classes focus on all kinds of everyday movements – sitting, standing, walking, lifting, even ironing – while the teacher adjusts your posture and shows you how to get the fullest use from your muscles with minimum effort. She will aim to make you aware of your posture, both at rest and in activity. These so-called "thought in activity" exercises concentrate on the sensation of sitting or standing without strain, following Alexander's directions: "Free the neck; let the neck go forward and upward; let the back lengthen and widen." Postural changes can be difficult to make at first, but with practice, relaxed and effective body use can become second nature.

MAIN USES

• Back pain and other musculoskeletal problems • Stress and anxiety • Headaches • Stress-related gastrointestinal disorders • Muscle strain caused by repetitive movement • Postural pain during pregnancy

To help the cellist, the practitioner works on the head-neck-spine alignment, and the position of the wrists and elbows.

PRECAUTIONS

Always check with a doctor before consulting an Alexander teacher if you have any medical condition or symptom of illness.
(*See also page 21.*)

ENERGY HEALING

BIOCHEMICAL EFFECTS

Changes brain and tissue chemistry by encouraging the relaxation response.

STRUCTURAL EFFECTS

Can encourage muscle relaxation and improve circulation; there is some evidence that it relieves pain and helps tissue regenerate.

PSYCHOSOCIAL EFFECTS

A therapeutic relationship has potentially powerful effects and may change self-perception and improve tolerance of pain and the ability to cope.

INTRODUCTION

Energy healers claim to use an indefinable benign healing energy that can activate a patient's natural self-healing processes. They do this by laying on of hands or by offering healing at a distance through the medium of thought or prayer. Explanations for the source of healing powers vary, but most healers seem to be ordinary people who see themselves as "channels" for healing energy. While explanations elude medical science, many doctors concede that energy healing can help people, and some healers now practice in hospitals.

HISTORY OF ENERGY HEALING

Most cultures have a tradition of laying on of hands and prayers or ceremonies for recovery from illness. Usually they are linked to religious practices or to magic. Christian healing shrines such as Lourdes draw thousands of pilgrims, and some churches have revived healing services. There is active interest in energy healing in the US. Dr. Daniel Benor, an American psychiatrist and healer, published an extensive review of healing in 1993 claiming that there were enough positive results to warrant serious consideration and further research.

MAIN PRINCIPLES

The nature of the "healing energy" thought to be at work varies according to the healer's beliefs, though many believe in a divine or "higher" source. Some claim to work with the human aura, imagined as layers of color or radiance that surround each person. *Spiritualist* healers say that a spirit of the dead assists them; *spiritual* healers regard themselves as conductors of supernatural healing power.

TREATMENT

After asking questions about a client's lifestyle and complaint, typical healers will take time to "center" themselves, relaxing and focusing their minds. Most healers regard their hands as conduits of healing power and place them on or slightly above the surface of the body. By touching you lightly or making sweeping movements, healers are able to assess any "imbalances" in your "energy field." After doing this, the healer is said to be "attuned," and can then concentrate on allowing healing energy to flow into your body.

THERAPEUTIC TOUCH

Practitioners of this type of healing believe people are a unique part of a universal energy field. They use their hands in a series of sweeping movements to rebalance disruptions in the flow of "energy" with the intention of stimulating natural processes of self-healing. Therapeutic touch (TT) was developed in the 1960s by Dr. Dolores Krieger, Professor of Nursing at New York University, as a way of introducing healing techniques into the patient-nurse relationship. It is now widely practiced by nurses in American hospitals and is becoming increasingly popular in the UK and Australia. Research suggests

The practitioner passes her hands over the body without making contact.

that it can relieve anxiety, speed wound healing, decrease postoperative pain, and reduce the effects of stress on the immune system.

This reiki healer directs energy through his hands into the patient.

REIKI

Founded in the late 19th century by Dr. Mikao Usui, a Japanese theologian, and allegedly based on ancient Buddhist healing rituals, reiki is one of the fastest-growing healing therapies. The name is derived from the Japanese *rei* (universal) and *ki* (life energy). Practitioners claim to channel "reiki energy" to areas of need, both in their patients and in themselves. Reiki is said to work at an atomic level, making the body's molecules vibrate so intensely that "energy blockages" are dissolved.

MAIN USES

• As an adjunct to conventional medicine in serious, chronic, and painful conditions of all kinds • Stress-related problems • Wound healing

PRECAUTIONS

Do not consult a healer who demands your unquestioning faith in order for treatment to succeed. Healers should never offer a diagnosis or promise a cure. (*See also page 21.*)

YOGA

BIOCHEMICAL EFFECTS

Changes brain and tissue chemistry by encouraging the relaxation response.

STRUCTURAL EFFECTS

Reduces tension in involuntary muscles (such as in gut and blood vessels) and in voluntary ones (such as in back and neck); improves circulation to internal organs.

PSYCHOSOCIAL EFFECTS

Changes mood, attitude, self-image; increases the level of active self-care; improves pain tolerance and coping skills; aids mental relaxation.

INTRODUCTION

Yoga, a regime of mental and physical training, is part of Ayurveda, the traditional Indian health system, and was originally a preparation for mental and spiritual development. Various forms are now popular in developed countries, and are often initially valued for their ability to increase suppleness and relieve stress. Most doctors accept the benefits of yoga, and studies have shown it may help relieve asthma, arthritis, and heart conditions. Interest is now growing in yoga therapy, which uses specific postures to treat particular conditions.

HISTORY OF YOGA

Yoga (the word is derived from the Sanskrit for "union") was traditionally practiced by Hindu ascetics, or yogis. Originating at least 2,000 years ago, the system was introduced to the West in the 19th century and became very popular in the 1960s, along with other Eastern disciplines. It is also used as part of some US health care programs, notably Dr. Dean Ornish's regime to treat heart disease (*see page 50*).

MAIN PRINCIPLES

Yoga is a philosophy concerned with life and how it should be lived. Yogic principles can be applied to all aspects of life. At its simplest, it is a system for healthy eating habits and good personal hygiene, but it progresses through physical postures and breathing techniques to meditation, whose goal is the experience of clear consciousness. There are many types of yoga, the most popular in developed countries being hatha yoga. *Hatha* means balance of mind and body; a calm mind is achieved through regular breathing and a relaxed body. It uses *asanas*, which are postures designed to stretch and strengthen muscles and stimulate nerve centers and organs, and *pranayama*, which involves breathing techniques to influence the flow of *prana* (life energy) in the body to prepare for meditation. Popular variants of hatha yoga are Iyengar yoga, and also the flowing ashtanga developed by Patabi Jois.

TREATMENT

People of all ages can benefit from yoga, which is probably best learned in a class. Most classes last 1–1½ hours. After gentle warm-up exercises, the yoga teacher shows the correct way to perform *asanas*, which the class then practices. You should not be tempted to push yourself too far or be competitive. If you are practicing yoga for medical reasons, always consult a teacher trained in yoga therapy.

MAIN USES

• Stress, anxiety, fatigue, moderate depression • Headaches, migraine • Circulatory disorders • Asthma, bronchitis • Irritable bowel syndrome • Persistent back problems • Menstrual problems • To improve mobility • General well-being

PRECAUTIONS

Take care if you are practicing yoga during pregnancy or menstruation. The Headstand, and some other asanas, should be avoided during pregnancy; some experts also advise against this asana during your monthly period.

Consult a yoga therapist if you have neck or back problems; high blood pressure; circulatory problems; heart disease; or disorders of the brain, ears, or eyes, since some asanas are not advised. (*See also page 21.*)

PHYSICAL BENEFITS OF YOGA

Spinal muscles are toned and stretched.

HEADSTAND
This *asana* flushes blood through the internal organs, and is said to stimulate the brain.

Blood flows out from the heart via the arteries (red).

Blood flows back to the heart via the veins (blue).

The spine is gently flexed.

FORWARD BEND
Bending from the waist with the head down stretches the back, hip, and leg muscles.

SPINAL TWIST
Twisting poses increase mobility of the back muscles and help free the diaphragm.

TRADITIONAL CHINESE MEDICINE

BIOCHEMICAL EFFECTS

Plant substances, nutritional approaches, and insertion of needles into acupoints alter biochemical processes and improve organ function.

STRUCTURAL EFFECTS

Acupuncture, tuina, and exercise programs like t'ai chi and qigong can improve range of movement and lessen muscle tension.

PSYCHOSOCIAL EFFECTS

Practitioners take into account and treat stress-related factors that trigger or maintain health problems; improved well-being brings psychological benefits.

INTRODUCTION

This ancient system of healing views symptoms as signs of "disharmony" (rather than a named disease) and attributes illness to a disruption in the flow of *qi*, or "life energy." Acupressure, acupuncture, herbalism, diet, qigong, t'ai chi, tuina, and shiatsu are different aspects of Traditional Chinese Medicine (TCM), whose aim is to harmonize the flow of *qi*. Although Western doctors are skeptical about the concept of *qi*, the proven effectiveness of acupuncture in treating some conditions makes it one of the most widely accepted complementary therapies.

HISTORY OF TCM

There is evidence that acupuncture was practiced in China some 3,500 years ago. The *Nei Jing* (*The Yellow Emperor's Classic of Internal Medicine*), which dates from between 200 BC and AD 100, is one of the earliest documents to explain the principles of balance, harmony, and moderation that underlie TCM.

After its introduction to China in the 16th century, Western medicine threatened to supersede TCM. However, the establishment of the People's Republic in 1949 led to a revival of ancient medicine. In China, TCM is now taught at universities and practiced in hospitals alongside Western medicine.

New York Times journalist James Reston had an emergency appendectomy while visiting China in 1972. His account of how acupuncture relieved his postoperative pain reawakened Western medical interest. Since then, acupuncture has been widely studied, and "medical acupuncture" is now often used to help relieve pain and nausea in hospitals and pain clinics.

MAIN PRINCIPLES

TCM is about the body's processes rather than its physical anatomy. Practitioners view the body as an integrated whole, linked by energy and information transfer known as the flow of *qi*. According to TCM, *qi* moves along a network of channels, called meridians, that run through the body. Twelve meridians are named after the main internal organs through which they pass. Two further meridians, the Conception and Governing channels,

MERIDIANS AND ACUPOINTS

Bladder meridian (yang)
Triple-burner meridian (yang)
Small intestine meridian (yang)
Large intestine meridian (yang)
Pericardium meridian (yin)
Lung meridian (yin)
Heart meridian (yin)
Pericarium 6
Heart 7
Gallbladder meridian (yang)
Stomach meridian (yang)
Liver meridian (yin)
Governing vessel (yang)
Gallbladder 14
Gallbladder 20
Conception vessel (yin)
Kidney meridian (yin)
Spleen meridian (yin)

control the other 12 meridians. Disruption of *qi* on a meridian can cause a problem at any point along it; thus a disorder in the Stomach meridian, which passes through the upper gums, could cause toothache. *Qi* moves between *yin* and *yang* – opposite but complementary tendencies in the body – either to the center (*yin*) or the surface (*yang*). Factors such as diet, the strength of the organs, environment, temperament, and stress levels will determine the *yin-yang* balance. If the balance is disturbed, *yin* conditions ("hardenings," such as osteoarthritis) or *yang* conditions (inflammations) will ensue.

Yin and *yang*: opposites in harmony

Fire, earth, metal, water, and wood are the five elements (or "processes") in TCM considered to be inherent in all things in the universe, including the body's organs. Each element has a *yin* organ and a *yang* organ, as well as associated tastes and emotions. Qualities common to a given element are said to support one another. Therefore, to treat a disorder of the Spleen, which is a *yin* organ of the element earth, a Chinese doctor might prescribe sweet-tasting herbs, which are associated with earth. The 12 organs in TCM might be better translated as 12 "functions," the Chinese concept of an organ being broader and less literal than its Western equivalent. The organs are nourished by "vital substances," namely *qi*, Blood, body fluids, and *jing*, or "Kidney essence," which is a hereditary factor governing growth, sexuality, and constitutional strength.

TREATMENT

A TCM practitioner uses four methods of diagnosis to assess a patient's condition: asking, observing (this involves looking at the tongue, noting the tone of the skin and the way a patient moves), listening, smelling, and touching. The latter includes pulse-taking – checking the rhythm and strength of all 12 meridian pulses (six on each wrist). The practitioner looks for "'patterns of disharmony," for example, *yin* or *yang* excess or deficiency in particular organs, and will then suggest a program of herbal remedies, acupuncture, and other treatments.

Acupuncture
Main uses: Pain relief, anesthesia; arthritis and other musculoskeletal problems; addictions; asthma, hay

The practitioner inserts a fine needle at an acupoint on the Kidney meridian to stimulate the flow of *qi*. The procedure is usually painless.

fever; depression, anxiety; migraine; nausea and other digestive disorders; high blood pressure; women's health.
Treatment: There are about 365 acupoints along the meridians at which *qi* is concentrated and enters and leaves the body. The acupuncturist inserts fine stainless steel needles to a depth of about 4–25 mm at these sites to stimulate or suppress the flow of *qi*. Needles may be left in place for a few minutes or as long as an hour. Sometimes a practitioner will burn an herb called moxa over the acupoint to create a stimulating heat.

Acupressure and Tuina
This is acupuncture without needles. Acupressure involves the use of finger and thumb pressure to stimulate acupoints. Tuina, a vigorous form of body massage, is a popular type of massage in China. Both acupressure and tuina provide useful self-help techniques for many common ailments.

Shiatsu
Main uses: Musculoskeletal problems such as arthritis; stress, insomnia, and fatigue; headaches and migraine; asthma; digestive disorders; menstrual problems; circulatory disorders; health promotion.
Treatment: Developed early in the 20th

century from *anma*, the Japanese form of tuina, the modern therapy of shiatsu (the word means "finger pressure"), has its roots in TCM. Practitioners use fingers, thumbs, elbows, knees, and even feet in a combination of massage techniques that apply pressure to acupoints (*tsubos* in Japanese) in order to stimulate and influence the flow of *qi*.

Qigong and T'ai Chi
Main uses: Fatigue; stress-related conditions; high blood pressure, heart disease; problems of aging; musculoskeletal pain and stiffness; to promote health and well-being.
Treatment: Translating as "energy work," qigong is an ancient system of movement, breathing techniques, and meditation designed to develop and improve the circulation of *qi* around the body. T'ai chi is a dynamic form of qigong and is sometimes described as "meditation in motion" because of its sequences of slow and graceful movements.

Chinese Herbalism
Main uses: Eczema and other skin conditions; migraine; menstrual disorders; fatigue, chronic fatigue syndrome; digestive disorders including irritable bowel syndrome (IBS).
Treatment: Remedies are used to rebalance organ functions. Each herb is classified as sweet, sour, bitter, pungent, or salty, as well as "hot" or "cold." Herbs are usually prescribed in a mixture adapted to suit the

individual. They are generally taken as boiled herbal teas, but may also be prescribed as pills, powders, pastes, ointments, creams, and lotions. Western studies show that Chinese herbs can successfully treat eczema and IBS, but many doctors in the West are concerned about the possible side effects of certain remedies.

MAIN USES
• As a complete medical system, TCM claims that it can aid treatment of every type of medical problem. Chinese hospitals use it most for conditions not easily treated with Western drugs, for example, migraine and skin conditions.

Qigong exercises are designed to develop and improve the circulation of *qi*.

Bai Xian Pi
(dittany)

Huang Bai
(phellodendron)

Yin Yin Hua
(honeysuckle)

Bamboo leaf

Di Huang
(rehmannia)

Mu Dan Pi (peony)

An herbal remedy to treat eczema might include a combination of the above herbs.

PRECAUTIONS

Always consult a qualified practitioner (*see page 180*).

Make sure that your practitioner uses disposable needles. Sterilization is not foolproof, and contaminated needles can spread hepatitis and HIV.

Tell your practitioner if you are pregnant, and do not take Chinese herbs without expert advice.

TCM herbs have been known to cause liver damage. If you have had hepatitis or other liver diseases you may be at greater risk than other people.

Avoid alcohol, large meals, hot baths or showers, and strenuous exercise immediately before or after any type of TCM treatment.

Take care if you drive or do work right after acupuncture, since you may feel tired and lack concentration.

(*See also page 21*.)

NATUROPATHY

BIOCHEMICAL EFFECTS

Plant substances and nutritional therapies alter biochemical processes and improve organ function.

STRUCTURAL EFFECTS

Makes use of exercise programs, relaxation techniques, and body work therapies to improve overall movement, support, and circulatory function.

PSYCHOSOCIAL EFFECTS

Practitioners take into account and treat stress-related factors that trigger or sustain health problems.

INTRODUCTION

Naturopaths believe that the body's "vital force" strives to achieve a state of equilibrium in which all systems, especially digestion and excretion, function in harmony. An unhealthy lifestyle can disturb organ function and weaken this vital force. Practitioners use natural methods, such as whole foods, medicinal herbs, and exercise, to stimulate the body's self-healing processes. Naturopathy is practiced widely in developed countries, and many of its basic ideas have been adopted – often unknowingly – by conventional medicine.

HISTORY OF NATUROPATHY

Naturopathy grew out of the "nature cure" practiced in 19th-century Austrian and German health spas, and was introduced to the US by a German, Benedict Lust, who founded the American School of Naturopathy in 1896. John Kellogg was famous for his use of natural therapies at his Battle Creek, Michigan, sanatorium. Advances in surgery and pharmaceuticals eventually overshadowed natural methods, however, and it was not until the 1960s that interest in naturopathy revived. In some US states, naturopaths are now recognized as family practitioners and Germany has several thousand state-licensed naturopaths.

MAIN PRINCIPLES

An unhealthy lifestyle – inadequate diet; lack of sleep, exercise, or fresh air; emotional or physical stress; and environmental pollution – can allow waste products and toxins to build up in

the body and upset natural self-regulation. This overloads the immune system and weakens the organ function so that the body becomes susceptible to illness. Naturopaths believe that symptoms are signs that the body's self-healing processes are at work, and that chronic and serious diseases are the result of accumulated toxins. Rather than treating symptoms as such, they aim to build up resilience and improve elimination processes.

Herbs support the body's healing powers.

TREATMENT

At the initial visit, naturopaths build a detailed picture of the patient. As well as doing routine medical tests (such as testing blood pressure and taking blood and urine samples), they may perform less conventional tests, such as analyzing samples of blood, sweat, or hair for evidence of nutritional deficiencies. If the condition is caused by an accumulation of waste products, treatment may include fasting and other detoxifying measures. Nutritional supplements and dietary changes may be suggested if digestion is poor. Treatments vary according to the practitioner, who is often multiskilled, but generally include nutritional therapy, acupuncture, hydrotherapy, manipulation, physical therapy or massage, herbal medicine, homeopathy, reflexology, and yoga. You may need 4–30 weekly sessions, depending on the condition.

Plenty of fruit and vegetables help the body fight disease.

HYDROTHERAPY

All forms of water therapy can help cleanse, revitalize, and restore health. Hydrotherapy improves the circulation, which in turn feeds and decongests tissues, helps flush out waste products, and can even boost the immune system. Traditionally, treatment involves baths, steam rooms, and compresses, but whirlpools and water jets are now included. Cold water constricts surface blood vessels, sending blood to nourish internal organs, and relieves external inflammation. Hot water dilates surface blood vessels, reducing blood pressure and increasing blood flow to the skin.

Warm baths help relieve arthritic conditions.

MAIN USES

• Arthritis • Allergic conditions, such as asthma • Fatigue • High blood pressure, hardening of the arteries • PMS • Gastrointestinal problems • Skin conditions

PRECAUTIONS

Do not fast or follow a restricted diet without supervision of a qualified naturopath. (*See also page 21.*)

WESTERN HERBALISM

BIOCHEMICAL EFFECTS

Plant substances alter biochemical processes and improve organ function.

STRUCTURAL EFFECTS

Some herbs applied as ointments or packs have a local effect on joints and muscles.

PSYCHOSOCIAL EFFECTS

Some herbs can stimulate or calm the mind; practitioners also take into account and treat stress-related factors that trigger or sustain health problems.

INTRODUCTION

Herbal remedies have long been the most important element of folk medicine. While many conventional drugs are derived from single active chemical ingredients in plants, herbalists make use of the whole plant. They believe its components have greater therapeutic power when they work together than when used separately. Conventional medicine is showing cautious interest; evidence is mounting for some herbal treatments, but their integration with conventional drug treatments requires care.

HISTORY OF WESTERN HERBALISM

The world's ancient civilizations relied on medicinal herbs. The writings of Roman, Greek, and Arab physicians provided the basis of Western herbalism, culminating in 16th-century texts by Paracelsus, John Gerard, and Nicholas Culpeper. Herbal medicine began to decline with the growth of science in the

Berries may be dried in an oven before being used to make herbal remedies.

18th century, but the 19th century saw a revival in Europe, where it is now well established and can even be studied in university courses. In the US it is illegal to claim therapeutic uses for herbal products, so they are marketed as "food supplements." In Europe and Australia, herbal products require minimal scientific backing before medicinal claims can be made.

MAIN PRINCIPLES

Herbalism matches specific treatments to certain diseases. However, like all traditional systems, herbalism seeks to restore the body's self-healing processes, so remedies can be tailored to suit the patient's health as a whole rather than to combat individual symptoms. Practitioners look for the cause of illness, such as poor diet, an unhealthy lifestyle, or excessive stress, which may have disrupted the body's natural state of harmony, or homeostasis (*see pages 12–13*). Much of the herbalist's skill lies in knowing the action of specific plants on different body systems; for example, a plant may stimulate the circulation or or may calm the digestive system.

TREATMENT

Herbalists will take a detailed history and may give a physical examination or perform simple tests. From their conclusions they may prescribe one or more herbal remedies tailored to your individual condition; these are normally made up on the spot. Over-the-counter herbal products are useful

Aloe vera gel is scraped away from the inside of the leaf to apply to burns and chapped skin.

for common ailments. Modern production methods aim for the maintenance of consistent levels of known active constituents. Choose products from reputable suppliers and always follow the instructions on the label. Remember that herbal remedies may take longer to work than conventional medicines.

MAIN USES

- Most illnesses, including persistent conditions such as migraine and arthritis • Respiratory, digestive, and circulatory problems • Skin conditions
- Mild depression and insomnia
- Benign prostatic disease • Cystitis, PMS, and menopausal problems

An herbal gargle for laryngitis

Lady's mantle

Sage

Rosemary

PRECAUTIONS

Tell your practitioner what drugs and supplements you are taking and if you are pregnant, have heart disease, high blood pressure, or glaucoma. Remember that herbal remedies can have side effects or may interfere with some conventional drugs, so always consult a qualified herbalist.
Do not discontinue a prescribed medicine without telling your doctor.
(*See also page 21.*)

NUTRITIONAL THERAPIES

BIOCHEMICAL EFFECTS

Use nutritional approaches to alter biochemical processes and improve the function of different organs.

STRUCTURAL EFFECTS

Treat food intolerances, believed by practitioners to irritate body organs and so cause or contribute to a wide range of disease. Practitioners may suggest ways to improve fitness, strength, and flexibility.

PSYCHOSOCIAL EFFECTS

Treat physical conditions believed to affect mental states (some mental illnesses are thought to be related to allergies and intolerances). Takes into account and treats stress-related factors.

INTRODUCTION

The role of diet in causing and preventing conditions such as heart disease and cancer is well established, as is the importance of vitamins and minerals in maintaining health. Nutritionists go one step further than most conventional doctors by using diet and food supplements to *treat* as well as to prevent illness. They look for nutritional deficiencies, food allergies or intolerances, and for lifestyle and environmental factors that disturb the digestion and the full absorption of nutrients into the bloodstream.

HISTORY OF NUTRITIONAL THERAPIES

Foods such as garlic have long been valued for their therapeutic properties, but it was 19th-century naturopaths (*see page 126*) who believed in the idea of "diet as medicine." Most modern nutritionists continue in this tradition. In 1912 a Polish biochemist, Casimir Funk, coined the term "vital amines" or "vitamines" for minute substances found in food. Further discoveries in biochemistry led to a greater understanding of the need for a balanced diet and the role of different nutrients. Recognition of the importance of antioxidants (*see page 162*) in maintaining health, preventing and treating disease, and delaying aging processes is a recent development. Other landmark advances of the 1980s and 1990s have tended to support naturopathic theories about diet. They include the importance of fiber,

Vitamins are often prescribed.

Pesticides sprayed on crops can cause a buildup of toxins in the body.

the discovery of plant estrogens, and the effects of saturated fats, food additives, and pesticides on the body.

MAIN PRINCIPLES

Practitioners believe that good health is directly related to the quality of food eaten, and that an inadequate diet affects mood, fitness, and well-being and even hastens aging. These are important ideas, since crops grown in poor soil are low in essential micronutrients, and toxic chemicals in pesticides and antibiotics fed to livestock have found their way into the food chain. Highly processed "junk" foods are deficient in essential vitamins and minerals and high in refined sugar, salt, fats, and chemical additives. Many practitioners believe that even if you eat a balanced diet and have an otherwise healthy metabolism, you can be adversely affected by toxins. Industrialization and traffic pollution mean the environment contains excessive levels of heavy metals, namely lead,

The practitioner may examine the central nervous system for signs of nutritional deficiencies.

cadmium, mercury, and aluminum. Coping with these puts a strain on the body, which practitioners are convinced causes problems that range from frequent infections, vague aches and pains, and fatigue to serious conditions, including severe depression, high blood pressure, and even cancer. According to practitioners, the "toxic overload" helps upset the body's homeostatic processes (*see pages 12–13*) by overtaxing the liver and kidneys – organs responsible for detoxification and elimination – and causing problems of toxic accumulation and irritation elsewhere in the body, such as the skin and joints. A number of practitioners believe environmental factors and nutritional deficiencies are so serious that dietary adjustments alone may be insufficient. They advise high doses of vitamins and minerals, well above the accepted recommended daily levels. This practice is known as megavitamin therapy or orthomolecular therapy. Conventional doctors tend to be uneasy about the lack of research into possible side effects of such high doses.

TREATMENT

People tend to consult nutritionists when suffering from long-term health problems that have not responded to conventional treatment and for which no cause can be found, for example, fatigue, headaches, bloating, and skin or digestive problems. Practitioners take a medical history and ask detailed questions about diet and lifestyle. Some use less conventional methods of diagnosis to determine nutritional deficiencies and food sensitivities. These may include tests on samples of blood, hair, urine, or sweat, and also a procedure known as kinesiology, which tests the strength of muscles to confirm a suspected food sensitivity. Some practitioners also employ the Vega test, in which patients are connected to an electrical device designed to detect the presence of deficiencies and sensitivities.

Exclusion diets are, however, the most reliable way of detecting a food sensitivity. If the practitioner believes you have a nutritional problem, he will probably recommend and monitor one of various diets. Herbal remedies, enzymes, "live" bacteria to normalize levels of gut bacteria, and vitamin and mineral supplements may be suggested, as well as lifestyle changes or even other complementary therapies. You will probably be advised to eat high-fiber foods and organic fruit and vegetables in order to reduce your intake of toxins.

MAIN USES

- Headaches, migraine • Fatigue, CFS
- Irritable bowel syndrome, digestive disorders • Arthritis • High blood pressure • Circulatory disorders
- Menstrual problems • Asthma, eczema • Allergies and food sensitivities

PRECAUTIONS

If you are taking medication, check with your doctor before beginning a course of nutrient supplements; these may react with or counteract the effects of prescribed drugs.

Do not take high doses of vitamins or minerals without consulting a properly trained nutritionist (*see page 180*). Excessive supplementation can have adverse side effects.

Do not follow a strict diet for long periods without the supervision of a qualified nutritionist. (*See also page 21.*)

COMMON DIET THERAPIES (*see also page 165*)

Stone Age Diet
This diet is sometimes recommended for people with irritable bowel syndrome or a wheat sensitivity. The theory behind the Stone Age diet is that our digestive system has not evolved beyond the diet of Stone Age hunter-gatherers. Plain fish, lamb, vegetables, and moderate amounts of fruit are allowed, but cultivated wheat and unrefined grains, as well as dairy products, are restricted.

Raw Food Diet
This diet is based on the work of Max Bircher-Benner, a late 19th-century Swiss doctor. It includes 70 percent raw fruit and vegetables and 30 percent grains, nuts, dairy products, and meat. The "enzyme activity" of uncooked food is said to benefit the digestive system and promote well-being.

Macrobiotic Diet
Macrobiotic diets aim to balance foods according to *yin* (light) and *yang* (dense) properties (*see page 124*). The most extreme forms, intended as short-term detoxification, consist almost entirely of brown rice and vegetables, and in the long term could lead to malnutrition.

Vegan Diet
A vegan diet is entirely free of animal products – no meat, poultry, fish, eggs, milk, or honey. Adequate protein depends on a careful balance of peas, beans, nuts, grains, and seeds. Vegans need to ensure they get enough vitamin B_{12} and folate, especially during pregnancy. Nonanimal sources of calcium are available.

The Hay Diet ("Food Combining")
Dr. William Hay, an American, developed his diet in the early 1900s. He believed that protein and carbohydrates could, in the long term, cause disease if eaten together. He based this notion on the theory that proteins need an acidic environment for digestion, and carbohydrates an alkaline one. Protein and carbohydrate foods are eaten separately and "neutral" foods can be combined with either group. Although the Hay diet has no proven scientific basis – plant foods contain protein and carbohydrates and the human digestive system is

designed to cope with both – it is very popular and many followers say they feel better on it. If your resilience and energy levels are low and your digestion seems poor, the Hay diet may be worth considering.

HOMEOPATHY

BIOCHEMICAL EFFECTS

Research confirms homeopathic doses affect tissue chemistry.

STRUCTURAL EFFECTS

Practitioners may suggest ways of improving fitness, strength and flexibility.

PSYCHO-SOCIAL EFFECTS

Strong therapeutic-relationship effects. Brings about beneficial changes in mood and self-perception. Improves ability to cope with a health problem.

INTRODUCTION

Based on the theory that "like cures like", homeopathy is a system of medicine that aims to encourage the body's self-healing ability, or "vital force". This force is believed to maintain the body's health, and symptoms of illness are regarded as a sign that the body is using its self-healing powers to fight infection. Homeopathic medicines do not work in the same way as conventional drugs. Instead, they are given to boost the vital force, so that the body fights back. Remedies are repeatedly diluted to reduce side-effects but are still believed to be potent enough to trigger self-healing processes.

HISTORY OF HOMEOPATHY

Hippocrates, the "father of medicine", outlined the principle of "like curing like" in the 5th century BC. In Germany in the 1790s, Dr. Samuel Hahnemann rediscovered this principle and called it homeopathy, from the Greek *homoios* (same) and *pathos* (suffering). Using himself as a guinea pig, Hahnemann took the malaria cure quinine and developed malaria-like symptoms. He concluded that a substance that caused symptoms in a healthy person could cure the same symptoms in an ill person. He went on to test or "prove" other substances such as arsenic, and began to use them as cures. Homeopathy quickly spread across the world to Europe, Asia and the Americas, and is currently undergoing a revival in the US.

MAIN PRINCIPLES

Homeopathic remedies are derived from substances that induce symptoms similar to those of an illness. The symptoms of poisoning by deadly nightshade for

Deadly nightshade

example, resemble those of scarlet fever, so *Belladonna*, a remedy derived from deadly nightshade, was given to treat scarlet fever. Hahnemann noticed that his patients got worse before improving. To reduce the side-effects, he developed the law of "potentization", according to which doses are repeatedly diluted in the belief that the weaker the remedy, the more potent it becomes. The diluted liquid is believed to keep a "footprint-like" image of the original substance so that, even when there is no trace of the original ingredient, the liquid retains a "memory" of it. Remedies are diluted on the decimal scale (x) with a dilution factor of 1:10, or on the centesimal scale (c) with a dilution factor of 1:100.

TREATMENT

Hahnemann discovered that when he found out more about his patients, he was more likely to prescribe the correct remedy. So-called "classical" homeopaths still offer treatment based on their assessment of a patient's "constitution", taking stock of appearance, personality, likes and dislikes, among other factors.

At the initial consultation, homeopaths question their patients closely about medical health, lifestyle, moods, likes and dislikes. They then prescribe one of the 2,000 remedies available, which come in many different forms, including lactose pills, tablets and powders, as well as ointments and tinctures. Homeopaths advise taking remedies between meals so that flavours do not interfere with the remedy.

Homeopathic treatment is said to work according to the "laws of cure" – that is, symptoms getting better starting from the top of the body, improving inside before the outside and in reverse order of appearance. The longer a condition has taken to develop, the longer it takes to treat, and remedies may be changed according to how symptoms progress.

MAIN USES

• Long-term disorders, such as asthma and other allergies • Anxiety, nervous tension • Menstrual or menopausal problems • Ailments in pregnancy, including morning sickness.

PRECAUTIONS

Tell your practitioner if you are using essential oils; in certain cases they are thought to be incompatible with homeopathic remedies.

If you are allergic to milk-based products, ask for lactose-free tablets. *(See also page 21.)*

The liquid, which homeopaths call the "mother tincture", is strained into a dark glass bottle

The tincture is diluted (one drop to 99 drops of alcohol), then shaken (known as "succussion")

After repeated dilution to the required potency, a few drops are added to lactose tablets

ENVIRONMENTAL MEDICINE

BIOCHEMICAL EFFECTS

Nutritional and environmental approaches alter biochemical processes helping improve the function of different organs.

STRUCTURAL EFFECTS

Treats a wide range of diseases and food and environmental allergies and intolerances, which practitioners believe chronically irritate the organs of the body. Practitioners may suggest ways of improving fitness, strength and flexibility.

PSYCHO-SOCIAL EFFECTS

Practitioners believe that some mental illness is not "all in the mind" (e.g. that allergies and intolerances can affect how we think, feel and behave); they take into account and treat stress-related factors that trigger health problems.

INTRODUCTION

Environmental medicine, also known as clinical ecology, attributes many disorders to environmental factors. These include some types of food and the pesticides and preservatives used in food production, as well as pollen, dust and exhaust fumes. Most people are able to withstand the effects of these toxins, but in susceptible individuals they may trigger allergy-related disorders, such as eczema or hay fever, or less severe reactions, known as "intolerances" or "sensitivities". Different tests are used to identify these irritants and patients are encouraged to avoid them if possible.

HISTORY OF ENVIRONMENTAL MEDICINE

Viennese paediatrician Baron Clemens von Pirquet, working early in the 20th century, was the first person to use the word "allergy" to describe unusual responses to the environment. Allergies are now defined as immune system reactions, identified by a positive skin-prick test. More controversially, some doctors in the US went on to claim that common foods and environmental chemicals caused "delayed" or "hidden" reactions (*see pages 94–95*), ranging from headaches and fatigue to asthma and arthritis.

MAIN PRINCIPLES

Practitioners believe that we ingest a whole range of synthetic chemicals every day, in the form of unfiltered tap water and the foods that make up a typical Western diet. These chemicals are derived from pesticides, herbicides, the residues of drugs fed to the animals we eat, and also from preservatives contained in processed foods. People

who are susceptible to allergies, or who have a poor diet, may find it difficult to cope with high levels of toxins and have a tendency to develop adverse reactions.

TREATMENT

A practitioner asks questions about the patient's medical history, typical diet and lifestyle. He will then check for swollen glands and other signs of sensitivity. The patient may be given a skin-prick test, hair and blood tests to determine mineral and nutritional deficiencies. Research suggests that these methods are far from reliable for detecting food sensitivities. A radioallergosorbent blood test (RAST) reveals any immunoglobulin E, the sign of an allergic reaction. Unproven tests for sensitivities include muscle-strength testing, a Vega test (*see page 129*) and cytotoxic testing, in which a blood sample is mixed with the irritant and then checked

In an elimination diet the patient eats "neutral" foods such as cabbage, lamb, sunflower oil, pears and water

Plant pollens can trigger allergic reactions when they are inhaled

for cell damage. The practitioner may suggest an exclusion or elimination diet (*see page 129*) to identify irritant foods.

When contact is unavoidable some practitioners use desensitization treatments. These can involve placing irritants with an enzyme on the skin, or giving decreasing amounts by injection or as drops under the tongue.

MAIN USES
- Asthma, hay fever, eczema, psoriasis
- Headaches, migraines • Digestive disorders, fluid retention, weight loss
- Depression, fatigue, CFS • Arthritis.

PRECAUTIONS

Never follow an elimination diet without the supervision of a qualified practitioner. (*See also page 21.*)

In a skin-prick test, a dilution of the suspect irritant is placed on an area of scratched skin

The practitioner checks for swollen glands, which may indicate sensitivity to certain substances

PSYCHOTHERAPY & COUNSELING

BIOCHEMICAL EFFECTS

Probably helps induce helpful changes in mood-related brain chemistry.

STRUCTURAL EFFECTS

Relieves distress that can disturb body function (some therapists attribute a wide range of diseases to psychosomatic problems); some forms of psychotherapy involve body work and movement.

PSYCHOSOCIAL EFFECTS

Influences thoughts, feelings, attitudes, and behavior; allows memories to emerge and new ideas to form; changes in self-perception improve pain tolerance and ability to cope with health problems.

INTRODUCTION

In general, psychotherapy and counseling involve a "talking cure." Psychologists assess and treat problems, often working with cognitive and behavioral approaches, to change ways of thinking and behaving. Although techniques vary greatly, psychotherapy and counseling usually entail discussing with a skilled listener the thoughts, feelings, memories, and situations that contribute to a personal difficulty. Whether following loss or trauma, or triggered by unknown events, such discussions offer an opportunity for insight and resolution. Hospitals and medical practices increasingly employ psychotherapists and counselors, and your health insurance may cover some part of the treatment.

HISTORY OF PSYCHOTHERAPY & COUNSELING

Dr. Sigmund Freud developed the foundations of psychoanalysis in the 1880s. He introduced the notion of the "unconscious mind" and tried to relate disturbed thoughts, feelings, and actions to buried memories. By letting patients talk freely he hoped to help them heal lost parts of themselves.

Other therapists took up Freud's theories in various ways. Dr. Carl Jung believed in a deep human need to unify one's "essential self" and posited the existence of a "collective unconscious" shared by all human beings. In the 1920s, Wilhelm Reich explored body-centered psychotherapy, working with feelings directly through the body. Behavioral psychologists claimed that human behavior and feelings were conditioned and, once learned, could be corrected. In the 1960s, humanistic psychologists, led by Abraham Maslow, Carl Rogers, and

Psychotherapists and counselors help clients articulate their feelings.

Fritz Perls, evolved techniques to encourage personal growth. Greater understanding of how the mind uses language and relationships has led to modern short-term psychotherapy methods, which are problem-focused and solution-oriented.

PRINCIPLES & TRAINING

Analytic and psychodynamic therapies are based on the idea that thoughts and behavior are shaped by earlier experience. Traumatic memories and feelings can be repressed and return unrecognized to disturb the mind and body. Clients are encouraged to talk about their experiences and express feelings freely. *Cognitive and behavioral therapies*, on the other hand, tend not to deal with the unconscious at all, but aim to forge new ways of thinking and behaving. *Humanistic therapies* lie between these two extremes.

The distinctions between practitioners may be blurred, particularly in the case of psychotherapists and counselors, but all should have been rigorously trained and have regular professional supervision. Psychoanalysts follow the teachings of Freud, Jung, or Melanie Klein, whose theories on childhood thought processes are influential. Training lasts five to seven years, which

includes personal analysis, and some therapists may also be medically qualified. Psychologists have a science-based bachelor's degree, studying the mind and behavior. Clinical psychologists undergo further training. Psychotherapists should have trained for at least four years with a recognized institution and have experienced personal therapy. They tend to specialize in a particular technique, either psychodynamic or humanistic.

Counselors should also be highly trained. The better qualified undergo several years' training and use similar approaches to psychotherapists.

TREATMENT

It is important that you understand the therapist's approach. A session usually lasts 50–60 minutes and generally takes place once a week, but analytic sessions may be more frequent. Treatment can span a few sessions or last several years, depending on the method. Therapists encourage you to speak freely, interrupting only to help you focus on your problem; some use techniques from various approaches where appropriate. Sometimes disturbing emotions emerge, so the therapist must be trained to help you work through them.

TYPES OF THERAPY

Psychoanalysis

Treatment is usually a lengthy process, since an intense relationship with the analyst, mirroring earlier relationships in a process known as transference, must be built. Gradually the unconscious, in the form of unacknowledged and repressed ideas, feelings, thoughts, memories, and attitudes, is reowned.

Group Therapy

Clients meet in small groups (ideally the same people) over several months to share experiences and feelings with the help of a practitioner, or group facilitator. Group work can be analytical or may use a humanistic approach, such as the 12-step programs for addiction. The shared situation often intensifies the experience of the therapy.

Family Therapy

Some people become ill as a way of coping with family tensions. When a family sits down with a therapist, communication difficulties and hidden conflicts between family members can become obvious. It may be possible to resolve them and even change patterns of behavior.

Counseling

Practitioners usually focus on specific problems, such as bereavement or job loss, rather than on deep-seated personal issues. Specialized counselors deal with marital, relationship, and sexual problems, working with couples or on a one-to-one basis.

Cognitive Behavioral Therapy

This term takes in everything from basic desensitization for phobias to stress management programs and mind-body techniques like relaxation, biofeedback, visualization, and meditation. They all aim to identify and change negative thoughts, expectations, and behavior, but do not seek to understand the deeper

Group therapy enables clients to learn more about themselves by sharing feelings with others.

Neurolinguistic programming helps people connect with the world on six levels: *environment, behavior, capability, belief, identity,* and *spirituality.*

psychological origins of a problem. Such methods have proved most effective in treating stress-related conditions, phobias, obsessions, and eating disorders, and also the less severe forms of depression.

Humanistic Psychotherapy

Clients are encouraged to explore their feelings and to take responsibility for their thoughts and actions. Emphasis is on self-development and achieving one's potential. How this is defined depends on the therapist. Social or financial success, spiritual development, or emotional openness are typical goals. Techniques include experimenting with unfamiliar ways of behaving and relating to others; for instance, trying out different body language or disclosing feelings, as in Gestalt therapy (*see Glossary, pages 177–78*) and psychodrama.

Neurolinguistic Programming

This approach combines cognitive behavioral techniques and ideas from hypnotherapy. The practitioner helps you understand how you organize your thoughts, feelings, and perceptions, and assists you in reorganizing them in ways that work better.

Transactional Analysis

Not a psychoanalytic method, transactional analysis is a way of looking at the individual that encourages the recognition of potentially conflicting roles: the creative but needy child, the realistic adult, and the nurturing but judgmental parent.

Transpersonal Approaches

The therapeutic value of enhanced feelings of love, altruism, and connectedness to the universe is taken up by transpersonal approaches, such as psychosynthesis, which explore dreams, inner heroes, creativity, and aspirations.

MAIN USES

• Stress, anxiety, depression • Phobias, obsessions, compulsions • Eating disorders • Bereavement, grief • Relationship and sexual problems • Emotional instability • Psychosomatic illness • Personal development

PRECAUTIONS

Research shows people benefit most when they trust and relate to their practitioner, regardless of technique; but check his or her training and qualifications, and ask whether he or she belongs to a professional association. Shop around and remember that you are entitled to stop therapy whenever you wish.

If you have a psychotic condition, such as schizophrenia, or are manic depressive, seek psychotherapy only with the backing of your psychiatrist. (See also page 21.)

HYPNOTHERAPY

BIOCHEMICAL EFFECTS

Triggers healing processes. Causes changes in brain and tissue chemistry by inducing the relaxation response.

STRUCTURAL EFFECTS

Reduces tension of voluntary muscles, such as in back and neck, and involuntary ones, such as in gut or blood vessels.

PSYCHOSOCIAL EFFECTS

Brings about valuable changes in perceptions, attitudes, and mood, and promotes active self-care.

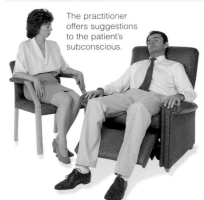

The practitioner offers suggestions to the patient's subconscious.

INTRODUCTION

When profoundly relaxed, as if in a daydream, most people become open to suggestion. Modern hypnotherapy makes use of this state of heightened susceptibility to alleviate pain, foster self-confidence, overcome phobias, or even treat conditions such as asthma.

HISTORY OF HYPNOTHERAPY

Hypnotherapy evolved from the work of the controversial 18th-century Austrian, Franz Anton Mesmer. Freud used some hypnosis in early psychoanalysis, but the modern form of hypnotherapy was developed in the 1950s and 1960s by US psychotherapist Milton H. Erickson. It is supported by clinical research and has considerable credibility – if not total acceptance – among doctors.

MAIN PRINCIPLES

After inducing a state of hypnosis in the patient, the practitioner seeks to plant positive suggestions in the subconscious mind, which is more open to influence than during normal waking life. Practitioners claim that patients are aware of their surroundings and are unlikely to do anything against their will.

TREATMENT

You will be asked about your medical history and why you are seeking help. Depending on your problem and on the practitioner's training, you may be asked to recall past experiences to help shed light on your condition, or be taken progressively deeper into a relaxed state of mind and encouraged to overcome your problem.

MAIN USES

- Pain relief • Phobias • Stress, anxiety
- Depression • Addictions • Asthma
- Skin conditions • Digestive disorders

PRECAUTIONS

Hypnotherapy may not be suitable for those with severe depression, psychosis, or epilepsy. (See also page 21.)

VISUALIZATION

BIOCHEMICAL EFFECTS

Triggers healing processes. Causes changes in brain and tissue chemistry by inducing the relaxation response.

STRUCTURAL EFFECTS

Reduces tension of voluntary muscles, such as in the back and neck, and involuntary ones, such as in the gut or blood vessels.

PSYCHOSOCIAL EFFECTS

Brings about valuable changes in perceptions, attitudes, and mood, and promotes active self-care.

HISTORY & MAIN PRINCIPLES

Also known as "guided imagery," this technique, which can be practiced either alone or with the help of a practitioner, harnesses the imagination to help people cope with stress, achieve their potential, and stimulate the body's self-healing ability. The aim is to visualize positive images and desired outcomes. Following research by US psychologist Dr. Carl Simonton in the 1960s, many cancer patients have been taught to picture the destruction of their cancer cells. Psychologists, athletes, and performers use visualization to improve motivation and change negative attitudes.

SELF-HELP

To do this exercise, you first need to learn a relaxation technique (see pages 170–71). Lie down or sit comfortably with eyes closed. Breathe slowly, relax, and mentally "let go" before focusing on your chosen image. To leave the imagery behind, simply wriggle your toes.

Fighting Illness: Create a picture of your ailment in your mind, and picture your treatment aiding your self-healing powers. Some people like to "turn down" pain on an imaginary dial.

Achieving Success: Think about your goal. Tell yourself you are in control, and picture yourself performing well.

Combating Stress: Picture yourself in a tranquil scene, making it as real as possible. Repeat phrases such as "I am relaxed and content."

MAIN USES

- Pain relief • Phobias • Stress and anxiety • Heart conditions • Cancer

Visualizing a peaceful scene aids relaxation.

MEDITATION

BIOCHEMICAL EFFECTS

Triggers healing processes. Causes changes in brain and tissue chemistry by inducing the relaxation response.

STRUCTURAL EFFECTS

Induces immediate and long-term reduction in tension of voluntary muscles, such as in the back and neck, and in involuntary ones, such as in the gut or blood vessels.

PSYCHOSOCIAL EFFECTS

Brings about valuable changes in perceptions, attitudes, and mood, and promotes active self-care. Improves tolerance of pain and ability to cope with a health problem.

INTRODUCTION

Various techniques can be used to induce "relaxed awareness," the basic meditative state of mind. All involve focusing the mind and ignoring distractions. The practice is widely recommended for stress-related conditions. People who meditate claim they have greater clarity of thought, calmness, and energy, and research suggests that it can help improve conditions including anxiety, migraine, irritable bowel syndrome, and PMS.

HISTORY OF MEDITATION

Meditation is a part of all major religions, practiced as prayer and contemplation in Christianity, Judaism, and Islam, and as a way of exploring consciousness and achieving enlightenment in Buddhism and Hinduism. The Indian yogi Maharishi Mahesh introduced transcendental meditation (TM) to the West in the 1960s, prompting scientific research in the US. From this, Dr.

Herbert Benson of Harvard University developed the idea of the "relaxation response," encouraging the practice of a nonreligious style of meditation.

MAIN PRINCIPLES

By triggering the relaxation response, meditation reverses the physiological effects of stress (*see page 84*), reducing heart rate and slowing metabolism. Brain waves change to a distinctive alpha pattern that indicates the mind and body are resting deeply, although still mentally alert. Regular meditators deal more effectively with stress and appear to maintain better health.

MEDITATION TECHNIQUES

Be prepared to try several methods until you find one that is right for you.
Mantra Meditation: A word or phrase is continually chanted or repeated in your head. The word may be an expression of your personal beliefs,

A flame may be a focus of meditation.

or simply one that holds some positive meaning for you.
Breath Awareness: You focus on your breathing and count "one," or think of a word that induces a sense of peace, each time you exhale.
Vipassana (Mindfulness): You enter a state of "diffuse openness," in which you are fully conscious of, but detached from, your immediate experience and thoughts.
Object Meditation: You focus with eyes open on an object, dwelling on its shape, weight, and texture.

A rosary can aid meditation.

MAIN USES

- Stress and anxiety • High blood pressure •Headaches • Fatigue, depression, insomnia • Pain
- Addictions • Boosting the immune system
- Personal development

MEDITATION SEQUENCE

Regular meditation relieves stress-related ailments.

IT IS POSSIBLE to learn to meditate from books, tapes, or videos, but consulting a teacher or joining a group is advisable.

1 Begin with 5–10 minutes and build up to 15–20 minutes once or preferably twice a day. To keep track of time, put a clock or timer nearby. Eventually you will not need it.

2 Sit with your back straight. You may fall asleep if slumped or lying down. A cross-legged pose can be adopted, or you could sit in an upright chair. Keep your feet firmly on the ground or on a support, and place your hands on your lap or knees. Close your eyes and relax.

3 Inhale through your nose and feel the air descending to your abdomen. Note any areas of tension in your body and, as you exhale, imagine your muscles relaxing. Notice the slow and rhythmic movement as you breathe in and out.

4 Concentrate on the focus of your meditation. This may be the rhythm of your breathing, an image,

or a word or phrase repeated silently each time you breathe out (*see above*).

5 Your attention should be relaxed but focused. If you find yourself thinking of other things, simply allow your mind to drift back to the focus of meditation.

6 Try to remain still and relaxed. You might feel restless or get the urge to move. These feelings will usually disappear.

7 When you are ready, wait for one minute before opening your eyes and for another minute before letting yourself return to full activity. Stretch and stand up slowly. If your meditation is interrupted, try to return to it later, reemerging slowly this time.

BIOFEEDBACK

BIOCHEMICAL EFFECTS

Changes brain and tissue chemistry by encouraging the relaxation response.

STRUCTURAL EFFECTS

Regulates unwanted tension in involuntary muscle (such as in the gut) or voluntary muscles (such as in the back and neck).

PSYCHOSOCIAL EFFECTS

Decreases anxiety and promotes an attitude of active self-care. Also improves ability to cope with stress.

INTRODUCTION

People can learn to control involuntary body functions such as heart rate or skin temperature using "biofeedback" machines that electronically monitor pulse rate, brain waves, skin sweat, and other physical responses. Scientific research supports biofeedback's role in teaching people to relax muscles and so relieve headaches or persistent back pain, for example, or to control pelvic floor muscles to prevent incontinence. Many doctors believe biofeedback is set to become widely available in the future.

HISTORY OF BIOFEEDBACK

In the 1960s, American scientists found that, if linked to a monitoring

device, people could learn to influence their brain waves and heart rate. Further studies showed that other biological functions could be controlled in this way. Advances in computer technology have led to increasing use of biofeedback.

TREATMENT

Different types of biofeedback devices measure changes in body functions. With the sensors in place you are taught to recognize which signals indicate relaxation or tension. Techniques such as breathing and muscle relaxation can help achieve the desired response, which might include lowered heart rate or reduced blood pressure. Mastering these takes practice, and at least six

half-hour sessions may be necessary, with further follow-up sessions at home.

MAIN USES

• Stress, tension, anxiety, insomnia
• Headaches, migraine • High blood pressure • Irritable bowel syndrome • Asthma
• Raynaud's disease
• Incontinence

Electrodes measure brain wave activity.

AUTOGENIC TRAINING

BIOCHEMICAL EFFECTS

Changes brain and tissue chemistry by encouraging the relaxation response.

STRUCTURAL EFFECTS

Regulates unwanted tension in involuntary muscle (such as in gut) or in voluntary muscles (such as in the back and neck).

PSYCHOSOCIAL EFFECTS

Decreases anxiety and promotes an attitude of active self-care. Also improves ability to cope with stress.

INTRODUCTION

A series of six mental exercises trains the mind to switch off the "fight or flight" stress response. Once learned, autogenic training (AT) offers a no-nonsense way to relax at will and stimulate the body's self-healing processes. As such, it is a useful self-help treatment for stress-related conditions. It is also claimed to have a beneficial effect on personal relationships and on performance at work, and to enhance creative skills. AT is widely available and most doctors

are comfortable with its highly structured approach to relaxation.

HISTORY OF AUTOGENIC TRAINING

In the 1920s Dr. Johannes Schultz, a German neurologist and psychiatrist, devised six silent verbal exercises to calm the mind and relax the body. Known as "autogenic" (from the Greek, "generated from within"), the exercises were further developed in Canada by Dr. Wolfgang Luthe, a colleague of Dr. Schultz.

TREATMENT

Students are carefully questioned about their medical history and psychological suitability before learning the exercises in small groups or individually over eight 90-minute weekly sessions. Each exercise aims to induce relaxation in different areas of the body: heaviness in the neck, shoulders, and limbs; warmth in the limbs; a calm heartbeat; relaxed breathing; warmth in the stomach; and coolness in the forehead. Students can enter a state similar to that of meditation.

MAIN USES

• Stress, migraine, insomnia, depression, nervous tension, ulcers • High blood pressure • Irritable bowel syndrome
• PMS • Eczema • Addictions • HIV

Autogenic training induces deep relaxation.

ART THERAPY

BIOCHEMICAL EFFECTS

Probably induces helpful changes in brain and body chemistry.

STRUCTURAL EFFECTS

Engages the body in expressing thoughts and feelings.

PSYCHOSOCIAL EFFECTS

Allows memories to emerge, ideas to form, feelings to be connected with.

INTRODUCTION

Art has the ability to promote the expression of feelings that seem too difficult or threatening to articulate verbally. Through painting, drawing, and sculpting, people may come to terms with traumatic experiences and find therapeutic relief from emotional distress. Art therapy is often available to cancer, AIDS, and Alzheimer's patients, particularly those who find it hard to talk about their concerns. The technique is also used by some psychiatrists and psychologists to treat mental and emotional disorders and addictions.

HISTORY OF ART THERAPY

Art has a long history as a vehicle of emotional expression. Sigmund Freud and Carl Jung recognized its therapeutic potential as a reflection of a patient's subconscious state. After World War II, art therapy was used in the rehabilitation of war veterans, and it is now widely practiced in the US and the UK.

TREATMENT

Sessions may be individual or in small groups, led by a therapist. Patients are encouraged to express their feelings by making images. Art therapy may help patients face issues they have repressed, since emotions can surface visually before they are verbalized. Releasing emotions through creative art is thought to be healing in itself, and the work may contain personal symbols that the patient is encouraged to interpret.

MAIN USES

• Mental and emotional problems
• Learning and communication difficulties • Eating disorders
• Stress, including stress relief in serious disease • Addictions • Bereavement
• Alzheimer's • Personal development

Images and colors often have symbolic meaning.

MUSIC THERAPY

BIOCHEMICAL EFFECTS

Probably induces helpful changes in brain and body chemistry.

STRUCTURAL EFFECTS

Engages the body in expressing thoughts and feelings.

PSYCHOSOCIAL EFFECTS

Allows feelings to be connected with; encourages communication.

INTRODUCTION

The power of music to stir and soothe the emotions and enable the expression of feelings that are too profound for words is unquestioned. Its association with healing is ancient, but music has only recently come to be employed as a therapy for those with serious disabilities, mental illness, or psychological distress. Research indicates that listening to music may stimulate neurochemicals that promote relaxation and even enhance immunity. Certainly many dentists' offices, intensive care units, and obstetric suites use music to reduce patients' anxiety.

HISTORY OF MUSIC THERAPY

Music therapy developed in the US at the end of World War II, when it was used in the psychological rehabilitation of war veterans. In the UK, the concert pianist Paul Nordoff and teacher Clive Robbins began training therapists in 1974 to work with autistic and emotionally disturbed children.

TREATMENT

Sessions are in groups or individual, and treatment varies according to the condition. Musical knowledge is unnecessary. Singing or improvising with percussion and other instruments, led by the practitioner, may help patients release tension and express emotions in a nonverbal way, enabling them to deal with problems more effectively. Listening to certain types of music can be soothing and so provide relief for those with stress-related conditions. Music can also relieve physical pain or stimulate memories, making it of particular use in work for the elderly.

MAIN USES

• Learning and communication difficulties, especially autism • Mental, emotional, and behavioral problems
• Depression • Stress, anxiety • Care for the elderly • Pain relief, especially in labor or in terminal illness

Children respond to the stimulus of music.

chapter 4

Assuming control of your health is empowering, and

active self-care is a cornerstone of integrative medicine.

The questionnaire on the following pages is

designed to help you evaluate different aspects of

YOUR HEALTH CARE PLAN

your life from diet to relationships, and to pinpoint

areas for improvement. We introduce you to a range

of health skills that improve well-being and resistance

to disease, from eating well and learning how to relax

to finding the best type of exercise for your lifestyle

and personality. Following the advice here sets you on

the road to zestful well-being and an active old age.

HOW HEALTHY ARE YOU?

Well-being depends on body and mind working in harmony, allowing you to enjoy optimum health. If you are healthy with plenty of zest for life, and if you have people to whom you can turn for support, you should find that you can meet most of life's challenges successfully.

Good health relies on biochemical, structural, and psychosocial factors. Relationships, lifestyle, environment, and the way you cope with problems can all undermine health or support it. Both psychological strain (for example, from an unhappy relationship) or a bad work environment, perhaps caused by poor air quality

or the presence of toxic chemicals, can increase susceptibility to illness, as can a diet of junk food or an aversion to exercise. If you want to strengthen your resilience, cope with disease, or just improve general well-being, then start by identifying how different factors affect you and try to change your lifestyle if necessary. Bear in mind that even if it is difficult to adjust one aspect, strengthening others can compensate. This questionnaire can help you learn about the areas of your life that influence your well-being, and identify those that may be undermining your health. The color wheel (*see page 143*) gives an at-a-glance picture of overall well-being.

BIOCHEMICAL HEALTH

A DIET LOW IN FAT and high in fruit, vegetables, and fiber can protect against disease. Many of us tend to eat too much junk and processed food, which is low in fiber and

high in fat, sugar, and chemical additives. Our genetic makeup can sometimes help us resist disease, but an unhealthy lifestyle can cancel out these inherited advantages.

GENETIC
Have you or has a close relative (parent, sibling, or child) suffered from any of the following complaints?
If you answer yes to any question, you may need to pay particular attention to your diet. In the case of questions 1–4, a doctor might recommend that you follow a low-fat diet; for questions 5 and 6, a low-sugar, high-fiber diet is likely to be advised; for questions 7 and 8, drink plenty of water.

C YES
A NO

1. High blood pressure   A   C

2. Heart attack before age 40   A   C

3. Very raised cholesterol   A   C

4. Breast cancer   A   C

5. Diabetes   A   C

6. Bowel cancer   A   C

7. Gout   A   C

8. Kidney stones   A   C

DIET/LIFESTYLE
A YES/USUALLY
B SOMETIMES
C NO/NEVER/RARELY

9. Is your diet well balanced, low in fat and high in fiber, with plenty of fresh fruit and vegetables?   A   B   C

10. Is your daily fat intake less than 30 percent of your total calorie intake?   A   B   C

11. Do you limit your salt and sugar intake?   A   B   C

12. Do you eat beans, poultry, and fish rather than red meat?   A   B   C

13. Do you drink enough water to keep your urine a pale color?   A   B   C

14. Do you avoid eating junk food and processed foods?   A   B   C

15. Do you resist the urge to eat when you're not hungry?   A   B   C

16. Do you skip meals only on rare occasions?   A   B   C

17. Do you avoid strict diets, except under medical advice?   A   B   C

18. Do you restrict your caffeine intake (coffee, tea, cola)?   A   B   C

19. Do you limit your alcohol intake (three drinks a day or less if a man, two if a woman)?   A   B   C

20. Are you a nonsmoker?   A   B   C

21. Do you avoid recreational drugs that carry a risk to health?   A   B   C

YOUR SCORE

A If you scored mostly As, your healthy diet is helping you maintain optimum well-being.

B A score of mostly Bs indicates that you should rethink your diet and pay greater attention to your general health.

C A score of mostly Cs suggests that your diet is harming your health. See your doctor for checkups and advice on diet.

STRUCTURAL HEALTH

PHYSICAL FITNESS is essential if you are to stay in good health. Regular exercise also helps prevent many serious diseases, both physical and mental. Health checkups, particularly as you get older, can identify problems before they become difficult to treat. Good living and working conditions are another important factor in maintaining well-being.

A YES/USUALLY
B SOMETIMES
C NO/NEVER/RARELY

1. Do you have plenty of energy? A B C

2. Do you get enough sleep? A B C

3. Do you get aerobic exercise for at least 20–30 minutes three times a week? A B C

4. Can you climb three flights of stairs nonstop without becoming breathless? A B C

5. Do you regularly participate in sports or exercise, either before or after work or on weekends? A B C

6. If necessary, could you run to catch a bus or train? A B C

7. Are you free of unexplained physical symptoms? A B C

8. Do you feel happy with your physical health, weight, and body shape? A B C

9. Do you use dental floss every day? A B C

10. Do you have a dental checkup at least once a year? A B C

11. Do you limit your exposure to the sun and use a sunscreen when necessary? A B C

12. Do you have a good sex life, or if celibate, are you happy to be so? A B C

13. If you use contraception and/or practice safe sex, are you happy with the form you use/practice? A B C

14. Do you work in a pollution-free environment (for example, without exposure to harmful chemicals or to excessive noise)? A B C

15. Are you able to work without physical discomfort and without placing strain on your back, joints, muscles, or eyes? A B C

16. Do you suffer from any of the following symptoms when under stress: palpitations, breathlessness, insomnia, indigestion, fatigue? A B C

WOMEN

17. Do you have a Pap test at least once every three years? A C

18. Do you regularly check (at least once a month) for lumps and other changes in your breasts? A C

MEN

19. Do you regularly check (at least once every three months) for lumps and other changes in your testicles? A C

OVER 40

20. Do you have an eye test for glaucoma at least every four years? A C

21. Do you have a checkup for abnormal blood pressure at least once a year? A C

OVER 50

22. Have you asked your doctor whether you need to be tested for bowel cancer? A C

23. Do you have a regular mammogram? A C

YOUR SCORE

A If you scored mostly As, you are maintaining a healthy lifestyle and should feel physically fit enough to lead the life you want. ☐

B A score of mostly Bs indicates that you should see a doctor for checkups and advice on starting an exercise program. Your work may be affecting your health. ☐

C A score of mostly Cs strongly suggests that you need to take better care of yourself and improve your work environment. ☐

Our genetic makeup can sometimes make us prone to disease, but a healthy lifestyle may offset these disadvantages.

PSYCHOSOCIAL HEALTH

STRESS IS A PART OF ALL OUR LIVES, but constant or excessive levels of stress undermine our physical and mental health. Remember that the degree to which pressure affects you depends on how you perceive it and how much you feel in control of it. Your reaction to stress may be influenced by your personality; those who react with aggression (called "hot" reactors) can expose themselves to heart disease, while "cold" reactors, who often suffer from low self-esteem, may deplete their immune system and so be prone to infection. People who can discuss their problems with partners or close friends are less vulnerable to stress. A life of creative and spiritual fulfillment can also help you cope with challenges.

SOURCES OF STRESS
Have you experienced any of the following life events in the past year?

C YES
A NO

1. The death of someone close to you A C

2. Major changes in close relationships (such as marriage or the birth of a baby) A C

3. A new job or home, or a change in your finances A C

4. A major illness (either your own health problem or that of a close friend or relative) A C

5. Marital or other family problems A C

6. Long-term day-to-day stress that has left you feeling exhausted: A C

ATTITUDES TOWARD STRESS

A NO/NEVER/RARELY
B SOMETIMES
C YES/USUALLY

7. Do you ever feel a compulsion to work, eat, smoke, or drink? A B C

8. Do you feel that you are no longer in control of your life? A B C

9. Do you experience any of the following problems or emotions when under stress: insomnia, fear of serious illness, lack of concentration, indecisiveness, lack of a sense of purpose, inability to enjoy life? A B C

10. Do you have problems relaxing and enjoying yourself? A B C

11. Do you find it difficult to maintain close and supportive relationships with other people, even (or especially) partners, parents, or children? A B C

"HOT" AND "COLD" REACTIONS
Questions 12 and 13 describe characteristics typical of those whose reactions when under stress are said to be "hot"; questions 14–16 describe typical "cold" reactions.

A NO/NEVER/RARELY
B SOMETIMES
C YES/USUALLY

12. When under pressure, do you become angry and blame other people? A B C

13. When under pressure, do you fume inwardly? A B C

14. When under pressure, do you deny the existence of a problem? A B C

15. Do you panic easily under pressure? A B C

16. Do you blame yourself when things go wrong? A B C

COPING SKILLS

A YES/USUALLY
B SOMETIMES
C NO/NEVER/RARELY

17. Do you laugh easily? A B C

18. Do you find it easy to express emotions? A B C

19. Do you have someone you can talk to about personal problems? A B C

20. Can you tolerate differences of opinion in your relations with others? A B C

21. Do you take time out to relax every day? A B C

22. When you're busy at work or at home, do you prioritize your tasks and plan ahead to avoid potential problems? A B C

23. Are you good at making decisions? A B C

24. Do you make your wishes and feelings known to others? A B C

25. Do you find it easy to delegate or share tasks? A B C

26. Do you feel your life has a sense of purpose? A B C

27. Is your work consistent with your values? A B C

28. Do you feel there is enough creativity and stimulation in your life? A B C

29. Does your spiritual life sustain you? A B C

YOUR SCORE

A If you scored mostly As, your self-confidence, self-esteem, commitment, sense of priorities, and assertiveness enable you to cope well with pressure. No one can afford to be complacent, however. You might wish to consider how you would react in the face of unexpected life events.

B A score of mostly Bs indicates that you can deal with some situations but not others, and would be well advised to learn strategies for coping with stress. Look at areas of conflict and self-doubt and consider making changes in your behavior and attitude.

C A score of mostly Cs strongly suggests that you could be vulnerable to illness when under stress. Are there ways you could learn to manage stress better, perhaps by avoiding over- or understimulation? What might improve your self-esteem? If you are prone to depression, consider talking with a doctor about this. Relationships and communication with others may not always be easy. Is there anything that would help to change that?

ASSESSING YOUR LEVEL OF WELL-BEING

THIS COLOR WHEEL is designed to help you identify those factors in your life that could be undermining your physical and mental well-being. The three sections of the wheel are color coded to match the three sections of the questionnaire, and the inner, middle, and outer zones of each section have been subdivided to represent your scores for A, B, and C respectively. Mark your combined score (As, Bs, and Cs) in the form of dots on the corresponding segments of the wheel.

INTERPRETING YOUR RESULTS

Together the three segments of the wheel – Biochemical, Structural, Psychosocial – make up an overall picture of your potential for well-being. By looking at the pattern of dots in each circle you can quickly assess your level of susceptibility. Is there an imbalance between the sectors? Remember that even if you can't improve in every area, steps taken in one sector probably pay dividends in the others.

INNER CIRCLE (A)

The inner circle represents the highest level of well-being that you can achieve. The higher your score here, the greater your ability to handle stressful situations and to maintain good health.

MIDDLE CIRCLE (B)

A high score in the middle circle indicates that you're doing some things right, but that there is room for improvement. Ask yourself what you can do to make your lifestyle a healthier one than at present.

OUTER CIRCLE (C)

Any dot recorded in the outer circle is a warning signal. A high score in any one section of this zone is a strong indication that you need to give particular attention to making changes in this area of your life.

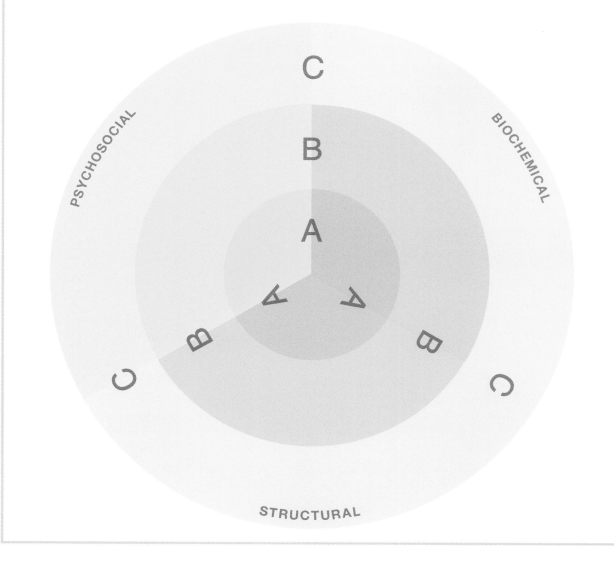

FINDING THE RIGHT THERAPY

I t is important to find a therapy with which you feel comfortable, since you are more likely to respond well to it if its approach suits your personality and views on health. Some people enjoy touch or movement therapies, for example, while others prefer those that are more mind- or emotion-oriented. Filling in the health questionnaire (*see pages 140–43*) will help you understand the factors that are influencing your health, while this questionnaire guides you toward a therapy that is most appropriate for you. There are no "right" or "wrong" answers, however, and you may prefer to use a combination of different approaches.

QUESTIONNAIRE

CIRCLE THE BOXES according to whether you agree with the statements. You should not have to spend a long time thinking about your answers. Then check whether most of your answers fall in the A, B, or C columns. Once you have read the conclusions, the flow chart opposite can help you find an appropriate therapy. For therapies, see pages 114–37.

1. Which five of the following do you think are most essential to your health?

	A	B
A diet high in fruit and vegetables	yes	no
A body structure that functions efficiently	yes	no
The ability to relax and deal with stress	no	yes
Family and friends	no	yes
Job satisfaction	no	yes
The flow of healing energy through me	no	yes
Removal of toxins and waste products	yes	no
A high standard of living	yes	no

CONCLUSION

A Mostly As: You see your health primarily in physical terms; your diet, physical condition, and environment are extremely important to you.

B Mostly Bs: You are emotionally and spiritually oriented; factors such as relationships, emotions, and spiritual harmony are central to your health and well-being.

2. How responsible do you feel about your own health?

	A	B
If I am ill, I can probably make myself well again.	yes	no
My health is largely a matter of luck; it is influenced by events and factors beyond my control.	no	yes
I am directly responsible for my own health.	yes	no
I can stay in good health only if I consult a health professional.	no	yes
My physical health depends on how well I eat, exercise, and take care of myself.	yes	no
When I am ill, I have to let nature and time heal my body.	no	yes

CONCLUSION

A Mostly As: You aim to be as healthy as possible. You take care of your health and if you are ill, you like to be actively involved in treatments.

B Mostly Bs: You see good health mostly as a matter of luck. If you are ill and need treatment, you are happy to let doctors and other health professionals take charge.

3. How do your individual preferences affect the type of therapy you choose? (For "no," circle both boxes.)

	A	B	C
I am comfortable being touched or massaged.	yes	no	no
I would like to use therapies that harness mental powers.	no	no	yes
I can swallow pills easily and can remember to take them.	no	yes	no
I am comfortable with the idea of needles stuck in me.	yes	no	no
I would change my eating habits completely if required.	no	yes	no
I am comfortable exploring my feelings with other people.	no	no	yes
I don't mind being undressed in front of a practitioner.	yes	no	no
I find it easy to picture scenes and events in my mind.	no	no	yes

CONCLUSION

A Mostly As: You are likely to be comfortable with structural therapies that involve manipulation.

B Mostly Bs: You might think about biochemical therapies, using diet, medicines, or remedies.

C Mostly Cs: You are happy exploring emotional factors, so try a psychosocial therapy.

INTERPRETING YOUR ANSWERS

USE YOUR ANSWERS to the three questions opposite to follow through the flowchart and find a therapy that may suit you. For therapies, see pages 114–37.

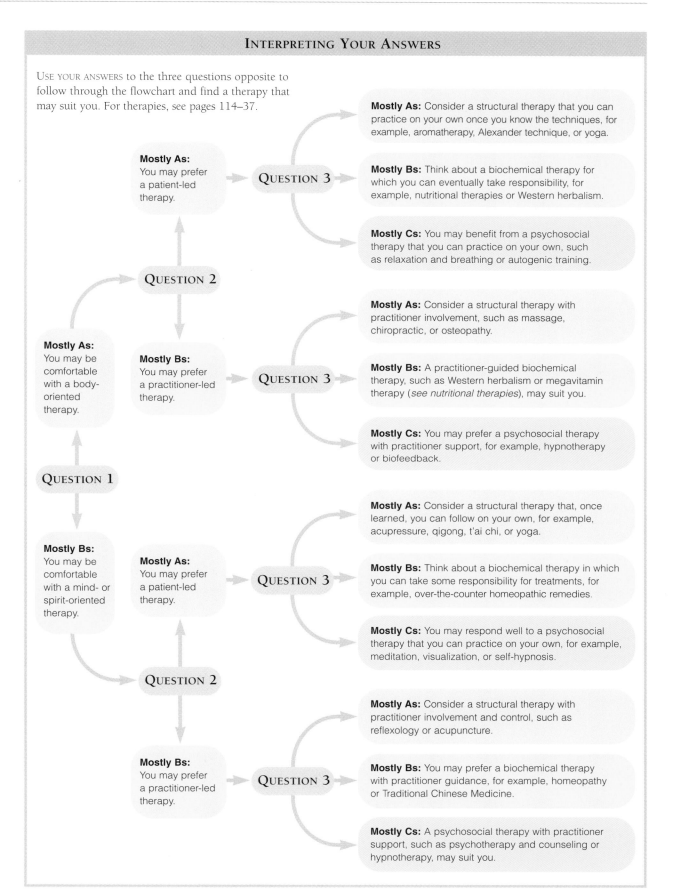

QUESTION 1

Mostly As: You may be comfortable with a body-oriented therapy.

QUESTION 2

Mostly As: You may prefer a patient-led therapy.

QUESTION 3

Mostly As: Consider a structural therapy that you can practice on your own once you know the techniques, for example, aromatherapy, Alexander technique, or yoga.

Mostly Bs: Think about a biochemical therapy for which you can eventually take responsibility, for example, nutritional therapies or Western herbalism.

Mostly Cs: You may benefit from a psychosocial therapy that you can practice on your own, such as relaxation and breathing or autogenic training.

Mostly Bs: You may prefer a practitioner-led therapy.

QUESTION 3

Mostly As: Consider a structural therapy with practitioner involvement, such as massage, chiropractic, or osteopathy.

Mostly Bs: A practitioner-guided biochemical therapy, such as Western herbalism or megavitamin therapy (*see nutritional therapies*), may suit you.

Mostly Cs: You may prefer a psychosocial therapy with practitioner support, for example, hypnotherapy or biofeedback.

Mostly Bs: You may be comfortable with a mind- or spirit-oriented therapy.

Mostly As: You may prefer a patient-led therapy.

QUESTION 3

Mostly As: Consider a structural therapy that, once learned, you can follow on your own, for example, acupressure, qigong, t'ai chi, or yoga.

Mostly Bs: Think about a biochemical therapy in which you can take some responsibility for treatments, for example, over-the-counter homeopathic remedies.

Mostly Cs: You may respond well to a psychosocial therapy that you can practice on your own, for example, meditation, visualization, or self-hypnosis.

QUESTION 2

Mostly Bs: You may prefer a practitioner-led therapy.

QUESTION 3

Mostly As: Consider a structural therapy with practitioner involvement and control, such as reflexology or acupuncture.

Mostly Bs: You may prefer a biochemical therapy with practitioner guidance, for example, homeopathy or Traditional Chinese Medicine.

Mostly Cs: A psychosocial therapy with practitioner support, such as psychotherapy and counseling or hypnotherapy, may suit you.

WORKING WITH YOUR DOCTOR

We no longer have the blind faith in the medical profession that our parents had. We expect to be involved in our own health care and are readier to provide doctors with relevant information about lifestyle, eating and drinking habits, and sexuality than generations who feared medical disapproval. We know that cures are not always possible and that a symptom could be caused by a variety of illnesses, for each of which there might be a range of treatments. Taking an active part in our own health care is an important step on the road to recovery. Studies at the Health Institute of the New England Medical Center in Boston and at Guy's Hospital in London, for example, show that if patients become involved with their care and understand what to expect, they are likely to recover faster and feel less anxious. Many people want to negotiate the kind of relationship with their doctors that will enable them to feel comfortable about asking questions and expressing worries and reservations about treatment, including discussing options connected with non-conventional therapies.

THE DOCTOR-PATIENT RELATIONSHIP

MORE AND MORE PEOPLE ARE are using non-conventional therapies – in a US study of 2,000 adults, 46 percent had visited a practitioner in 1997, up 10 percent from 1990. Yet how many tell their doctor about herbal or nutritional supplements they take or discuss their visits to a reflexologist or homeopath?

Not all doctors are happy with a "patient-centered" approach and not all are good communicators. If it is awkward to discuss conventional treatment with such practitioners, bringing up the subject of complementary therapies may be even more daunting. However, at least a third of family doctors surveyed in 15 countries have practiced therapies or referred their patients to complementary practitioners, so it is likely that if patients were more forthcoming, their doctors' reactions might surprise them, since clearly more physicians are taking an active interest in what complementary medicine has to offer.

If you enjoy a good working relationship with your doctor, the integration of conventional and non-conventional treatments could be relatively easy. But even if the physician is not enthusiastic, he or she will usually be tolerant, provided you do not abandon necessary conventional treatment. If the combination of therapies proves effective, and you find your need for drugs or other procedures diminished, then it is important to let your doctor learn from the experience.

GETTING THE BEST FROM YOUR DOCTOR
• Make a list of symptoms and questions so you will be sure to discuss them.
• If you do not understand what the doctor is saying, say so, and take notes if a consultation is likely to be complicated.
• Discuss the pros and cons of a procedure with the doctor. Ask about possible side effects and risk factors. Speak up if you are not entirely happy.
• Never use a minor complaint as an excuse to see the doctor when in reality you are worried about depression, stress, or an unexplained lump.
• Tell the doctor about any side effects of treatment before abandoning it. A switch may be possible.
• Tell the doctor about any over-the-counter medication or complementary remedies or treatments you are taking.
• Tell your doctor if a treatment worked, either conventional or non-conventional. Feedback is much appreciated.
• Make separate appointments for each family member.

• Ask for an emergency appointment only if you really cannot wait.
• When making an appointment, say if you think you will need extra time.
• Try to be punctual, but if unavoidably late call the office.
• Always keep medical appointments. Cancel them beforehand if you cannot make them.

QUESTIONS TO ASK YOUR DOCTOR
• What caused my illness?
• How is it normally treated?
• How do you intend to treat it and what are the alternatives?
• What can I do to help myself?
• Is there any danger in my trying a complementary therapy before, or as well as, the treatment you recommend?
• Are there any long-term consequences of my illness?
• Why are you sending me to that surgeon, specialized center, or hospital?
• What evidence is there that the treatment would work? What would happen if I did nothing? Are there any alternatives?

KEEPING A SYMPTOM DIARY

KEEPING A RECORD OF SYMPTOMS for any long-term health problem will enable you to track signs of improvement or decline. This will help you keep your doctor or practitioner fully informed. Note any changes in severity as well as what you ate and drank every day, and your activities and feelings. Watch out for any emerging patterns. For example, did you develop a migraine after eating cheese? Did a stressful event precede an asthma attack? Once you start a treatment, evaluate any changes in symptoms, mood, or energy levels. Progress can be slow and it may take weeks or even months before you can really be sure an improvement has taken place. In that case, use the medical outcome profile below to monitor your main problem symptoms at the end of each week.

Sample Weekly Symptom Diary

	MON	TUE	WED	THUR	FRI	SAT	SUN
Headache	3	0	4	4	0	0	0
Skin rash	2	2	2	4	1	1	1
Stressors	slept badly last night		too much cheese for supper?	ate only grapes today			

Medical Outcome Profile

1. Choose one or two problems that bother you the most. Write them on the dotted lines below. Now consider how bad each problem was over the previous week, and score it by circling the appropriate number.

2. Now choose one activity of daily living, such as walking briskly, that your problem prevents you from doing. Score how badly the problem has affected you in the last week.

PROBLEM 1

....0   1   2   3   4   5   6

PROBLEM 2

....0   1   2   3   4   5   6

ACTIVITY

....0   1   2   3   4   5   6

3. Finally, rate your general feeling of well-being during the week.

....0   1   2   3   4   5   6

Key: 0 = Not much of a problem   6 = As bad as it could be

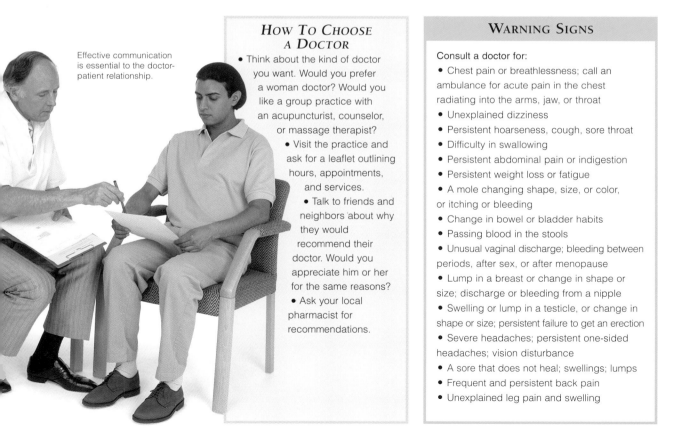

Effective communication is essential to the doctor-patient relationship.

HOW TO CHOOSE A DOCTOR

- Think about the kind of doctor you want. Would you prefer a woman doctor? Would you like a group practice with an acupuncturist, counselor, or massage therapist?
- Visit the practice and ask for a leaflet outlining hours, appointments, and services.
- Talk to friends and neighbors about why they would recommend their doctor. Would you appreciate him or her for the same reasons?
- Ask your local pharmacist for recommendations.

WARNING SIGNS

Consult a doctor for:
- Chest pain or breathlessness; call an ambulance for acute pain in the chest radiating into the arms, jaw, or throat
- Unexplained dizziness
- Persistent hoarseness, cough, sore throat
- Difficulty in swallowing
- Persistent abdominal pain or indigestion
- Persistent weight loss or fatigue
- A mole changing shape, size, or color, or itching or bleeding
- Change in bowel or bladder habits
- Passing blood in the stools
- Unusual vaginal discharge; bleeding between periods, after sex, or after menopause
- Lump in a breast or change in shape or size; discharge or bleeding from a nipple
- Swelling or lump in a testicle, or change in shape or size; persistent failure to get an erection
- Severe headaches; persistent one-sided headaches; vision disturbance
- A sore that does not heal; swellings; lumps
- Frequent and persistent back pain
- Unexplained leg pain and swelling

YOUR STRUCTURAL HEALTH

The body's flexible framework of muscles, bones, and joints protects the internal organs and allows us to move. The flow of blood, which transports nutrients, warmth, and waste products around the body, depends on the heart and its network of arteries and veins. All the body's processes are coordinated by the neuroendocrine system, which centers on the brain and spinal cord. Together, these structural systems support the health of other organs and the mind, so their optimum functioning is essential for well-being. Muscle tension, for example, can influence psychological states, and narrowed arteries can reduce the supply of blood to the tissues, adversely affecting cell biochemistry.

HEALTH OF THE MUSCULOSKELETAL SYSTEM

The spinal column consists of a stack of 33 vertebrae, which protect the spinal cord and support the entire skeleton. Many body work therapists believe that tension in the muscles attached to the spine or misalignment of the vertebrae produce pain elsewhere and can even interfere with internal organ function. The musculoskeletal system is vulnerable; accumulated postural strain, habitually tense muscles, or joints stiff from neglect can make injury and pain likely. Disorders of the musculoskeletal system are now a major cause of health problems, accounting for over a quarter of all visits to the doctor; these disorders are the most common cause of long-term disability.

MUSCLES, BONES & JOINTS

Bone is composed of a mixture of fibrous and connective tissue in which calcium is deposited. Where two bones meet is known as a joint. Some joints, such as those in the skull, are fixed, while others, such as those of the knuckles, are mobile and move within sheaths of fibrous tissue whose linings produce a lubricating fluid. Tendons attach the muscles to the skeleton, and the contraction and relaxation of the muscles enable the body to move. Voluntary muscles, such as those of the leg, are under our control, while involuntary muscles, like those of the heart or gut, are not.

An angiogram reveals the hand's structure – its bones and blood vessels.

STRUCTURAL EFFECTS OF EXERCISE

• Hand-eye coordination controls actions.

• Sweat is produced and evaporates to cool the body.

• Nervous and musculo-skeletal systems work closely to control balance and coordination.

• Blood flow to the gut decreases as more blood is directed to the muscles and lungs.

• Endorphins ("feel-good" chemicals) and epinephrine affect body systems, boosting performance.

• Blood comes to the surface of the skin to radiate away excess heat.

• Spine twists and bends and back muscles contract to increase force in hand and arm.

• Heart pumps faster, blood pressure rises, breathing rate quickens, and air flow and lung capacity increase.

• Weight-bearing joints experience high levels of "loading" and twisting.

• Metabolic rate rises, burning calories faster to provide energy.

The Heart & Circulation

In an 80-year life span, the heart beats more than three billion times. It pumps blood around the body through a network of arteries and veins, which are linked by tiny capillaries with walls thin enough to allow oxygen and nutrients to pass from the blood to the cells, and waste products to pass back into the blood. Deoxygenated blood flows to the heart from which it is pumped through the pulmonary artery to the lungs. Here, carbon dioxide diffuses into the alveoli – tiny sacs linked to the smallest air tubes (bronchioles) – and is exhaled. At the same time, oxygen passes into the capillaries, oxygenating the blood. The blood then returns to the left side of the heart to be pumped out around the body via the aorta, the body's largest artery.

The circulatory and respiratory systems face a number of hazards. In urban areas, the air may be so laden with industrial chemicals and traffic fumes that the respiratory system's mucous membrane defenses are overwhelmed and environmental toxins can enter the bloodstream. In addition, damage to the artery walls – made worse by poor diet, chemicals, smoking, stress, and high blood pressure – can lead to atherosclerosis (*see pages 48–51*). In this, toxins and calcium are deposited on the damaged lining of blood vessels, narrowing them, which is especially dangerous in the arteries supplying the heart muscle (coronary arteries) and in the brain because elasticity is reduced and vital circulation is impaired. These fragile, narrowed arteries can also be blocked by a blood clot, or can leak. The result may be a heart attack, or a stroke, which can lead to brain damage.

The Brain & Nervous System

The human brain has been called the most complex object in the known universe. Together with the spinal cord, it comprises the central nervous system, which is composed of billions of interconnecting nerve cells, or neurons, that process information from sense organs and receptors throughout the body. Nerve fibers fan out from the central nervous system, networking to the muscles, internal organs, and glands. The somatic nervous system controls muscles involved in voluntary movement, and the autonomic nervous system controls unconscious functions, such as the contraction of the gut. The autonomic system has two functions. Its sympathetic nerves stimulate glands and involuntary muscles, while its parasympathetic nerves reduce activity in the same tissues. The regulation of blood pressure, heart and breathing rates, muscle tension, and the secretion of intestinal juices and enzymes depends largely on the balance between the two.

Strain & Pain

When a muscle is strained or otherwise irritated, pain nerves fire off messages to the spinal cord, which sends back "reflex nerve impulses" that make the muscle tense up further (*see below*). At the same time, chemicals released by the inflammatory process and other waste products build up in the tense muscle, producing more pain. Just how susceptible a muscle is to such strain and how long it needs to recover depend on a number of factors, but especially on preexisting bone and joint problems, postural and occupational "loading," and the general degree of psychological tension and stress.

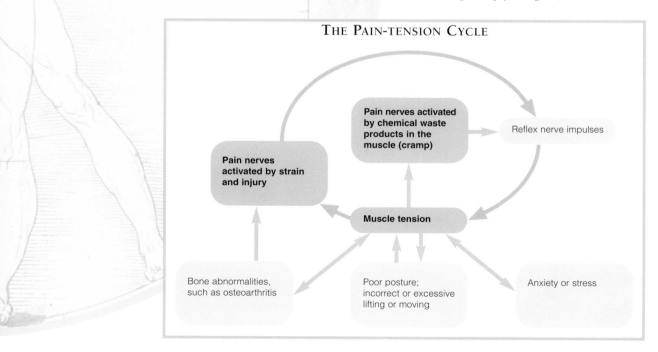

THE PAIN-TENSION CYCLE

Pain nerves activated by chemical waste products in the muscle (cramp)

Reflex nerve impulses

Pain nerves activated by strain and injury

Muscle tension

Bone abnormalities, such as osteoarthritis

Poor posture; incorrect or excessive lifting or moving

Anxiety or stress

BODY WORK

Daily activities like sitting and bending expose joints and muscles to all sorts of mechanical strain. This may be harmful if movements are sudden, awkward, repetitive, or unaccustomed, or if muscle weakness and tension have made the body susceptible to damage. Chronic back pain (*see page 52*) and repetitive strain injury (RSI) are just two of the conditions that can result from poor posture and inappropriate body use. Sitting exerts even more pressure on the back than standing; as the upper body shifts forward, the back muscles strain to keep the body upright. Fortunately, good posture, back fitness, and well-designed furniture can distribute pressure so that strain is taken off the back.

In evolutionary terms, standing upright is very recent. To avoid problems, the vulnerable back needs all the care it can get.

EVERYDAY GOOD POSTURE

THE BACK IS HELD TOGETHER by hundreds of muscles that not only move it but keep it from overstretching by protectively tensing. Twisting, swiveling, and bending put the back muscles and joints under strain, especially if these are already sensitized by slouching. Learning how to stand, bend, lift, and carry objects correctly will prevent future problems.

Neck is relaxed; shoulders are dropped

Lower back is slightly curved

Weight is evenly distributed

Good Posture

STANDING

Good posture distributes pressure so that the back does not take all the strain. Try standing against a wall so that your head, upper back, and buttocks are touching it. Your hand should be able to slide easily into the space between your lower back and the wall, yet should almost be touching both surfaces.

CARRYING

Distribute full shopping bags and other heavy loads evenly between both hands. To carry only one item, do not arch your back or twist your body. The bend-and-twist combination is the worst possible position for the lower back. Try to take the weight in your arms and abdominal muscles and alternate the load from one side to the other. Better still, carry the object in a backpack, where the weight is more evenly placed, or pull it behind you on wheels.

BENDING AND LIFTING

When you lift a heavy object, do not bend at the waist. Bend at the knees and let the leg muscles do the work. If the object is heavy, squat with a straight back and your legs apart; tighten your stomach muscles and hold the object close to your body.

Box is carried close to the body

Spine stays in a straight line

1 Place your feet apart. Crouch down, bending the hips and knees, but avoid bending the back.

2 Stand up, taking the strain in the legs. Carry the load close to your body without twisting the back.

DESK SENSE

IF YOU WORK AT A DESK or a computer terminal, you may find yourself perched on the edge of your seat leaning forward to read, with your neck bent and shoulders hunched. To maintain this position for the 35–45 hours a week expected of the average office worker requires a lot of what is known as "static" effort. Muscles in the back, arms, head, and shoulders are forced to contract for long periods, causing tension and pain. Blood flow may be congested so muscles are fatigued, and breathing can be restricted because the stomach is compressed (*see Relaxation & Breathing, pages 170–71*). Adjustable chairs and desks should prevent much of this discomfort.

THE PERFECT CHAIR

If possible, try out a new chair for a day before buying. Choose one with a five-legged base and an adjustable back and seat, and make sure that all knobs and levers are easily reachable when you sit down. The chair should support the small of your back and you should be able to place both feet flat on the floor (if not, use a foot rest). The keyboard should be at, or just below, elbow height. A seat that tilts forward is more comfortable for working at a computer or a desk. The seat of the chair should have a curved "waterfall" edge, be wide enough so that you can change position comfortably, and be deep enough to support the full length of the thighs, but not so deep that there is pressure behind the knees when you lean back.

THE IDEAL WORK STATION

Many office workers complain of fatigue, but a well-designed chair and the positioning of your keyboard and screen can prevent most of these problems. Arrange your work station to conform to your body by adjusting the chair, screen, keyboard, and phone, and place documents so that the most important task is directly in front of you. Try not to hunch over books; instead, prop them up on an adjustable desk stand. (A work table that slopes upward is best.)

SCREEN TIPS

• The top of the screen should be at or just below eye level.
• Keep the screen at a comfortable distance.
• Adjust contrast and brightness to avoid eye fatigue.
• To reduce reflection, tilt the monitor and use an antiglare screen.
• Avoid having an unshielded window either in front of or behind you.
• Make sure that overhead lighting does not reflect on the screen.
• Keep the screen clean.
• Have your eyes tested if you suffer from fatigue, headaches, and eyestrain.
• Take regular breaks. Get up and walk around every hour or so, and stand up and stretch every 20 minutes.

KEYBOARD TIPS

• Hold your wrists straight, with elbows at approximately 90 degrees.
• Adjust seat and keyboard positions to be comfortable.
• Do not hammer the keyboard.
• Do not overstretch your fingers.
• Do not rest your wrists on the keyboard or desk while typing. (Use a special wrist rest if necessary.)
• Limit repetitive mouse movements by learning shortcut keystrokes.

DESK EXERCISES

• Alternately stretch out your fingers and clench your fists to combat stiffness and improve circulation in your hands.
• Relax your neck by rolling your head across your shoulders from side to side.
• Keeping your arms by your sides, roll your shoulders forward and backward to loosen a stiff neck and shoulders.
• Relieve aching eyes by looking away from the screen and focusing on more distant objects. For relief from screen glare occasionally cover your eyes.

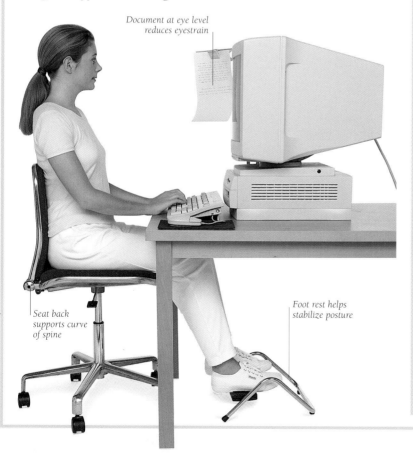

Document at eye level reduces eyestrain

Seat back supports curve of spine

Foot rest helps stabilize posture

BENEFITS OF EXERCISE

Regular exercise does more than keep you fit. It makes the heart and lungs work better, tones muscles, and strengthens bones and joints. It stimulates the circulation to the brain and internal organs, boosts the immune system, and helps protect against insomnia, depression, heart disease, high blood pressure, cancer, and osteoporosis (brittle bone disease). Exercise also triggers the release of endorphins, brain chemicals that lift mood and generate a sense of glowing well-being. What's more, it is not necessary to spend hours pounding machines in the gym to benefit from exercise. As little as 15 minutes of moderate physical activity twice a day, five days a week, can make a big difference to your health and will make you look better too, with glowing skin and a leaner body.

"My quality of life has been so much better since I started skating. I feel healthier, more energetic, and no longer get tension headaches."

WHAT CAN EXERCISE DO FOR YOU?

THE SEDENTARY LIFE OF MOST PEOPLE in developed countries is bad for health. For example, exercising less than 30 minutes a week doubles the risk of dying from coronary heart disease. Activity is powered by energy from food and the oxygen we breathe. Overweight, sedentary people often lack energy because of sluggish circulation and an oxygen deficit in their muscles. Exercise raises the heart rate so blood circulates more efficiently around the body, increasing the number of capillaries (tiny blood vessels) that feed the muscles. Muscle fibers, including those of the heart, flex and become stronger. The metabolic rate increases and bone density improves. Exercise can also:

LOWER THE RISK OF CANCER
According to a study at the University of California, women under 40 who exercise for at least four hours a week are half as likely to develop breast cancer as those who do not. Exercise also seems to help protect against colon cancer, probably by stimulating the immune system and speeding up digestion.

WARD OFF HEART DISEASE & STROKE
Brisk walking for three hours a week can lower cholesterol and reduce the risk of stroke. Recent research suggests that strength training can lower blood-fat levels.

SHORTEN COLDS
Exercise tones up all body systems, including those that fight infection. In one study, walking briskly for 45 minutes five days a week halved the duration of colds.

EASE BACK PAIN
Weak back muscles are vulnerable to strain. Exercise, particularly swimming, yoga, and Pilates, can treat and prevent backache by helping the muscles supporting the spine become stronger. Improving physical fitness is the single most helpful approach for chronic back pain.

BUILD BONE
Weight lifting, as well as weight-bearing exercise such as walking and jogging, increase bone density among people of all ages.

BOOST BRAIN POWER
Improved circulation carries oxygen and glucose to the brain cells more efficiently. Exercise that requires coordination and mental agility – for example, tennis – may generate nerve cell connections in the brain.

IMPROVE SLEEP
Walking or low-impact aerobics for 40 minutes four times a week may help you fall asleep faster and for longer, according to studies.

LIFT PMS AND MENSTRUAL PAIN
Moderate to vigorous exercise produces sweat, which offsets water retention, a symptom of PMS. It also promotes blood circulation and increases the production of mood-enhancing endorphins.

ENHANCE MOOD
Exercise releases endorphins, the body's natural opiates, and mood-enhancing neurotransmitters such as serotonin. As body temperature rises, stress chemicals are burned off, making you feel relaxed.

HELP YOUR SEX LIFE
Exercise encourages the endocrine glands to produce more testosterone, the sex hormone in both men and women. In studies, people who exercise three times a week reported greater arousal, more frequent sex, and more satisfaction.

EXTEND LONGEVITY
A Finnish study found six 30-minute brisk walks a month cut the risk of premature death by 44 percent. Inactivity is even more life-threatening than smoking, according to the Cooper Institute for Aerobics Research in the US.

TYPES OF EXERCISE

THERE ARE THREE TYPES OF EXERCISE: aerobic, anaerobic, and stretching. You should aim to include all three in a fitness program, but it is important that you choose an appropriate activity, according to your age and ability, and build up levels of intensity gradually.

AEROBIC EXERCISE is any vigorous activity sustained for at least 12 minutes without a break. It should make you puff, but not so hard that you cannot carry on a conversation. During aerobic exercise, the heart pumps faster, forcing the lungs to work harder to bring in more oxygen. Blood is pumped faster around the body to nourish the cells, burn fat, and carry away waste products. As muscles are developed, both stamina and energy are increased so you can go longer without becoming exhausted. **Examples:** aerobics classes such as step; brisk walking, jogging, swimming, inline skating, dance, cycling, rowing.

Rowing is an excellent form of aerobic exercise.

ANAEROBIC EXERCISE, or strength training, develops muscular strength and "resistance," which is the ability to carry, lift, push, or pull a heavy load, or give extra power to a tennis serve or football kick. These are brief, intense bursts of action in which there is no time for the muscles to draw on oxygenated blood for energy. They rely instead on other chemical processes that produce lactic acid, a waste product, which can cause muscle fatigue and cramps unless muscles are strong and toned. **Examples:** weight lifting, push-ups, resistance bands, abdominal crunches, leg raises.

Push-ups develop arm, stomach, and shoulder muscles

STRETCHING improves the ability of the joints to move through their full range of motion. If muscle fibers are too tight, the ability to stretch, twist, and turn with ease is hindered. Stretching exercises can prevent muscle tissue from shortening and stiffening; avert pulled or torn muscles; relieve pain; improve muscle strength, length, and tone; and enhance body awareness and appearance. Suppleness can reduce stiffness after exercise, improve your posture, keep you active as you age, and even prevent falls. **Examples:** yoga, Pilates, t'ai chi.

Yoga is an effective way for people of all ages to improve their flexibility.

Use two fingers to locate the pulse on the side of your neck.

YOUR PULSE RATE

The number of times your heart beats per minute can be measured by taking your pulse. During aerobic exercise your heart rate should be 60–90 percent of its maximum; to establish the maximum, subtract your age from 220.

To take your pulse, place two fingers on the pulse at the side of your neck or on your wrist. Count the beats that occur within 15 seconds, then multiply the number by four to arrive at the number of beats per minute. Avoid obsessively taking your pulse unless you have high blood pressure or heart disease or you are a competitive athlete. As you become fitter, you will need to step up the intensity of exercise to maintain your optimum heart rate.

YOUR EXERCISE PROGRAM

Beginning an exercise program is the best lifestyle change you can make for your health. However, embarking on an exercise program will also be a challenge. It is easier to sustain enthusiasm if you choose an activity that you enjoy and which suits your personality, age, and way of life. Set yourself realistic goals and begin gradually. There are many ways to incorporate exercise into your life: using the stairs rather than the elevator; walking to the store instead of driving; joining in a vigorous game with the children, or doing housework energetically. Remember anything that makes you feel out of breath counts as exercise.

"Now that I go to salsa classes, exercise is no longer a chore. I love dance and it's a great way to meet new people."

BECOMING MOTIVATED

It is never too late to start exercising. Even in your 70s, regular, moderate exercise can add a year to your life. However, the less active you have been, the less energy you are likely to have, so starting an exercise program can initially seem difficult. Remember you are bound to feel some muscle soreness and fatigue at first and it may take up to six weeks to stop feeling lethargic. But once you are fit enough to enjoy exercise, you will begin to experience the feelings of well-being, calm, and relaxation that follow a session. The key is to find an activity that you enjoy, which gives you an immediate payback in terms of having fun or learning new skills. Studies show that if you can keep exercising regularly for six months, you are likely to start thinking of yourself as an active person and continue.

EXERCISE GUIDELINES

• Make exercise part of your routine so that you spend less time thinking about it.

• Write upcoming fitness sessions in your diary as if they were business meetings.

• Choose a form of exercise that is convenient for your lifestyle and budget. Traveling an hour each way to a swimming pool four times a week will soon become difficult and tedious.

• Set sensible goals, especially if you have not exercised for a while. Attempting to do an hour of aerobics every day could leave you feeling tired and dispirited. Aim instead simply to complete a certain number of sessions a month.

• As you get fitter, notice how your heart and breathing rates take less time to settle down after exercise. After two months of exercising three times a week, you will feel noticeably fitter.

• Plan fitness sessions with a friend, so that exercise becomes more of an enjoyable social occasion and is harder to cancel.

• Try different forms of exercise to prevent boredom. Change your schedule each week or try something innovative like inline skating, Pilates exercises, or salsa dancing.

Exercising at home to music is a good way to start a program.

AEROBIC EXERCISE TIPS

• Begin by aiming to do 15–30 minutes of moderate exercise every other day.

• Warm up for 5–10 minutes before exercise with gentle stretches and walking in place to stimulate heart rate and blood flow, and stretch muscles to reduce the risk of injury.

• Stop exercising if you feel any pain.

• Slow down if your muscles are sore after exercise.

• Wear appropriate clothing and footwear. The wrong kind of shoe can put strain on the knees, feet, ankles, hips, and back. If you exercise outdoors, dress in light layers to remove as you warm up.

• Drink plenty of fluids before, during, and after exercise to prevent you from becoming dehydrated.

• At the end of the workout, slow down gradually to let your heart rate return to normal.

• Stretch muscles after exercise to prevent cramps and stiffness. Hold each stretch for at least six seconds.

• Give your body a rest at least one day a week, since excessive exercising can depress the immune system.

PRECAUTIONS

Consult a doctor before starting an exercise program if you are over 45, obese, or have a history of heart disease, high blood pressure, back pain, or dizziness.

WHICH EXERCISE SUITS YOU BEST?

1. During exercise, do you like to:
- A *Push yourself to your limits?*
- B *Keep pace with a companion?*
- C *Work at your own pace?*

2. Do you see exercise as an opportunity to:
- A *Let off steam?*
- B *Socialize?*
- C *Be reflective?*

3. When exercising, is the presence of other people:
- A *An inducement to perform as well as you can?*
- B *Enjoyable, challenging, or exhilarating?*
- C *Daunting, disconcerting, or distracting?*

4. Does most of the fun of exercising come from:
- A *Competing against others?*
- B *Improving on your last performance?*
- C *The delight of physical activity?*

5. Is your main reason to exercise to:
- A *Improve your overall physical zest?*
- B *Look and feel good?*
- C *Enhance your sense of control?*

YOUR SCORE

MOSTLY As:
You like to test yourself and thrive on competition. Consider squash, tennis, marathon-running, and triathlons.

MOSTLY Bs:
You are most likely to enjoy exercise that has a sociable element. Think about joining a gym, health club, or a walking or cycling group, and playing regular tennis or badminton for a taste of competition.

MOSTLY Cs:
For you, exercise is a chance to escape, to meditate, and enjoy a peaceful period of physical activity. Consider a regular program of repetitive exercise that you can practice alone, such as walking, running, or swimming.

Tennis is a good form of competitive exercise.

WHICH ACTIVITY?

AEROBICS includes step, jazz, kick-boxing, or even dynamic yoga. Take care if you are out of condition. Low-impact aerobics, where one foot stays on the floor, is easier on joints.

AQUAROBICS, or workouts in water, is one of the safest forms of aerobic exercise. It works the heart, lungs, and muscles without straining the joints.

CROSS-TRAINING, including biathlons and triathlons, combines two or three sports to overcome boredom and exercise more muscle groups.

CYCLING is excellent aerobic exercise and puts little stress on the joints.

DANCING – whether tango, salsa, jazz, Middle Eastern, or whatever – is excellent aerobic exercise, with socializing an added bonus.

PILATES, which is fast becoming popular, claims to rebalance the body and develop strength, muscle tone, flexibility, and mental concentration.

RACKET SPORTS, including tennis, squash, and badminton are good for improving agility and coordination. Playing singles is more aerobic than playing doubles.

ROWING can improve overall strength and endurance and gives the aerobic benefits of running. It puts little strain on the back, joints, and muscles.

RUNNING AND JOGGING are excellent forms of aerobic exercise, but don't attempt either until you can walk two miles briskly without difficulty.

SKIING can be expensive but develops balance, agility, and coordination. Cross-country skiing offers a more complete aerobic and muscle workout than almost any other sport.

SWIMMING works two-thirds of the body's muscles as well as the heart and lungs, and improves muscle strength, endurance, posture, and flexibility. The water takes 90 percent of your weight so it is good for people with arthritis and asthma. If you do the breaststroke, try to immerse your head to avoid neck and back damage.

WALKING is safe, simple, and cheap and can be incorporated into any routine. It is both aerobic (provided your pace is at least four miles an hour) and weight-bearing (so it is good for increasing bone density).

WEIGHT- AND STRENGTH-TRAINING are usually done with machines. They strengthen all major muscle groups and can increase bone density. The metabolic rate also increases, so more calories are burned.

YOGA is excellent for flexibility, breathing, muscle coordination, circulation, and relaxation.

Weight-training strengthens muscle groups.

EXERCISES

Key

A ACUTE
For acute pain and stiffness

R RECOVERY
For when acute pain has worn off

P PREVENTIVE
For long-term prevention

Many muscle and joint problems can be prevented by developing strength and flexibility. Everyday activities such as housework and gardening, as well as sports, can cause stresses and strains, but the more supple you are the more protected you will be from injury. Exercise routines can target specific muscle groups to sculpt your shape and improve posture. The back has to support the entire weight at all sorts of angles and cope with different loads, so strong, supple abdominal and lower back muscles are vital. Avoid exercises that might strain the spine, such as straight-leg toe touches or backward bends, and always stop and rest if you feel any pain when exercising – pushing through the pain only risks injury.

Strong and supple abdominal and lower back muscles will help prevent joint problems and back pain.

BASIC EXERCISES

THESE EXERCISES are useful for strengthening and stretching the muscles that support and align the spine. Make them part of your regular routine if you are prone to back pain. If you do them each day they will strengthen the abdominals and keep the back and leg muscles from becoming tight and sore.

R **P** SIDE STRETCH

1 With your feet at shoulder-width apart, stretch your right arm straight upward with your left arm relaxed by your side.

2 Slide your left arm down your leg as far as you can and hold the position for 7 seconds.

3 Slowly return to the upright position. Repeat 3 times on each side.

P HAMSTRING STRETCH

1 Lie on your back with a leg raised and the knee bent at right angles.

2 Slowly straighten your leg as much as you can, keeping the thigh vertical. Hold for 10 seconds. Repeat 3 times with each leg.

Keep this leg flat on the floor.

P CALF STRETCH

1 Stand facing a wall at an arm's length away with your right foot in front of the left. Place your hands on the wall at shoulder height.

2 Bend your elbows and lean toward the wall, keeping your back straight and your left heel on the ground. You should feel a stretch in your left calf.

3 Hold this position for 15 seconds. Repeat 3 times on each leg.

P ABDOMINAL STRENGTHENING

1 Lie on your back with your legs bent and your hands by your side.

Reach forward with your arms.

2 Raise your head and shoulders off the ground. Hold for 7 seconds, then release carefully. Repeat up to 10 times.

BACK & NECK EXERCISES

THE FOLLOWING EXERCISES ease stiff joints slowly and gently. If you have acute back pain, use them as a first-aid measure; rest in bed only if it is impossible to move, and then for no more than two days. Consult a doctor and start to mobilize the back and joints as soon as you can, because prolonged inactivity results in stiffness, loss of strength, and more pain.

A PELVIC TILT

1 Lie on your back with knees bent and feet flat on the floor.

2 Press the back of your waist against the floor, tighten your abdominal and buttock muscles, and tilt your pelvis up and forward. Hold for at least 6 seconds, relax slowly, and repeat up to 10 times.

A R P GENTLE TWISTING

1 Lie on your back with knees bent and feet flat on the floor.

2 Keeping your knees together and your shoulders flat on the floor, let your legs fall gently over to one side as far as they will go. Hold this position for one minute. Repeat the exercise, twisting to each side, up to 5 times.

A R P CAT STRETCH

If it is painful, raise the back a little.

1 Position yourself on all fours. Look straight ahead, and arch your back downward. Hold for 5 seconds.

Keep hands and knees at shoulders' width apart.

2 Curve your spine upward until it forms an arc. Hold for 5 seconds. Repeat the whole exercise 10 times.

Slowly drop your head.

A LOWER BACK STRETCH

1 Lie on your back with knees bent and feet flat on the floor. Grasp your knees with both hands, and draw them up toward your chest.

2 When you feel a slight stretch in your lower back, inhale deeply and hold this position for 10 seconds. Slowly lower your legs, being sure that your back stays pressed against the floor. Repeat 3 times.

A PASSIVE EXTENSION

1 Lie on your belly, looking straight ahead, with your hands flat on the floor on either side of your head.

2 Slowly straighten your arms, lifting your shoulders and chest off the ground. Repeat 5 times, allowing your spine to arch more each time.

A NECK RETRACTION

1 Sitting upright, look straight ahead; pull your chin back to straighten your neck and elongate your spine.

2 Pull your chin back and raise your shoulders until they feel relaxed. Keep your neck straight. Repeat 3 times.

YOUR BIOCHEMICAL HEALTH

The nutrients we absorb are crucial to biochemical health, and scientists are discovering that the foods we eat and how we prepare them can either help prevent disease or directly contribute to poor health. The average Western diet is unhealthily high in refined and preserved foods. In developed countries, soaring rates of heart disease, gastrointestinal disorders, and certain cancers result from our appetite for foods high in fat and sugar. We should know better; one of the great nutritional discoveries of the last 15 years has been the role of antioxidants. These nutrients in fruit and vegetables actually seem to protect against disease and premature aging. And continuing research reveals the unexpected importance of substances in such ordinary foods as broccoli and garlic. The adage "you are what you eat" is proving more true and more complex than anyone ever suspected.

DIGESTION & STRESS

Many practitioners pay close attention to diet and digestion. Clearing the gut of toxins and unfriendly bacteria so it can eliminate waste products, and a well-functioning liver, are considered vital for good health. The inability to cope with stress can have an adverse effect on these processes. Digestion begins when the anticipation and smell of food trigger the secretion of saliva, which moistens food so that it is easier to chew. However, the "fight-or-flight" response to stress dries the mouth and reduces the production of digestive enzymes and juices that break down food. Stress also slows down digestion so that energy can be diverted to the muscles for action. Less blood circulates to the stomach and to the intestines, and the rhythmic contractions of the gut become slower, faster, or irregular (*see below*). Constant stress sustains these reactions, so that food remains inadequately digested and absorbed, with damaging effects on health.

WHAT IS A BALANCED DIET?

Carbohydrates
50%

Fats
30%

Proteins
15%

In broad terms, a balanced diet consists of 50 percent carbohydrates, 15 percent protein, and no more than 30 percent fats, with plenty of fiber, vitamins, minerals, and water (*see pages 160–61*). Many people are hazy about nutrients such as different types of carbohydrates or essential fatty acids, let alone newly relevant nutrients such as lycopene (found in red vegetables and thought to prevent prostate cancer). Fortunately, most dieticians agree on easy-to-follow guidelines (*see right*), which concur with the so-called Mediterranean diet. (People in Greece and Italy have low rates of chronic diseases, which is thought to be linked to their diet rich in fruit and vegetables, olive oil, and red wine.)

STRESS & DIGESTION

STRESS

Toxin-induced ailments lead to more stress and undermine the body's ability to cope.

Toxins cause problems in other parts of the body (for example, in joints and skin).

• Fewer digestive enzymes
• Poor circulation to the gut
• Irregular peristalsis (contractions of the gut that push food through it)

Toxins overload the liver and kidneys.

Food is not properly broken down or absorbed, and the gut lining may become too absorbent.

Leaky gut: Toxins from poorly digested food "leak" from the gut into the bloodstream.
Dysbiosis: Poorly digested food in the gut encourages overgrowth of "unfriendly" bacteria (candidiasis).

A shared meal offers a chance to relax and communicate.

HEALTHY EATING HABITS

Many of us in developed countries have fallen into bad habits, grabbing meals on the run and wolfing junk food that lacks essential nutrients and is full of preservatives. With more people going out to work, there is an understandable trend toward relying on convenience foods. This is not intrinsically wrong, but it does mean that we must become aware of what we are eating and compensate for any dietary inadequacies.

Eating "little and often" is a worthwhile axiom. Although short periods of fasting seem to sharpen mental alertness, persistent low blood sugar causes irritability, depression, and mood swings. Several light meals a day with fruit and nut snacks maintain stable blood-sugar levels, and are easier to digest and less likely to make you sleepy than a hefty lunch and dinner laden with sugar and saturated fat. To avoid an energy slump after lunch, eat a midday meal of protein and complex carbohydrates, such as lean chicken or fish with pasta or whole-grain bread.

Breakfast is worth making time for, no matter how busy your schedule, since it is necessary to stir the metabolism and restore energy after the overnight fast. Studies show that children who eat breakfast are mentally more alert later in the morning than those who do not. But choose foods that are high in complex carbohydrates, like toast, cereals, and fruit, rather than high-protein and fatty foods such as fried eggs and bacon or cheese and ham. It is important to remember that eating should be enjoyable. The whole process of preparing and consuming a meal ideally should be be a social event, shared with family and friends. Perhaps if we sat down to enjoy at least one meal together every day, without watching television at the same time or rushing off afterward, not only would our digestive systems be under less strain, but we might also communicate better and feel less stressed.

MOOD FOODS

Certain foods are known to affect mood. Bananas and some high-protein foods, including meat, milk, and eggs, contain the amino acid tryptophan, for example, which is metabolized to serotonin, a brain chemical that induces calm and sleep. Lowered levels of serotonin are linked to depression and hostility. A mid-morning cup of coffee whets concentration thanks to its caffeine, a stimulant also found in tea, chocolate, and cola. However, six or more cups a day raises blood pressure and stress-hormone levels and can cause tremors, palpitations, insomnia, and accelerated bone calcium loss. More positively, cocoa and chocolate contain phenylethylamine, a chemical associated with mood enhancement.

12 WAYS TO IMPROVE YOUR DIET

- Be sure half your daily calorie intake comes from starchy foods like bread, pasta, rice, and potatoes.
- Eat at least five portions of fruit and vegetables every day.
- Limit your intake of saturated fat (found in meat and dairy products).
- Steam or stir-fry vegetables rather than frying or boiling them.
- Cook with pure, unrefined vegetable oils such as olive oil rather than with animal fats.
- Use skim milk and low-fat dairy products instead of full-fat versions.
- Get more of your protein from poultry, fish, beans, cereals, and low-fat dairy products, rather than from red meat.
- Eat oily fish, such as salmon, twice a week for their essential fatty acids.
- Reduce your intake of coffee, tea, and cola drinks. Drink herbal teas, fruit juices, and water instead.
- Replace butter with a low-fat spread, high in polyunsaturated fats and low in trans-fats (look for "nonhydrogenated fat" on the label) and spread thinly.
- Avoid "junk" and processed foods loaded with preservatives, colorings, and flavorings.
- Limit alcohol intake to no more than 14 units a week for women and 21 for men (a unit = 1 glass of wine, ½ pint of beer, or 1 jigger of hard liquor). A daily glass of red wine may lower the risk of heart disease.

Probably the best single way to improve your diet is to increase your intake of fruit and vegetables.

NECESSARY NUTRIENTS

All foods contain proteins, carbohydrates, and fats in varying combinations. These molecular compounds are essential for good health, providing energy and playing a vital role in the growth and maintenance of body cells. Food is also a source of vitamins and minerals, each necessary only in tiny amounts, but with a specific part to play in the body's metabolism. Fiber, from plants, is another essential nutrient, helping the digestive system function efficiently. Our most precious nutrient, however, is water – nearly two-thirds of the human body is made up of it. Without water, our body systems would stop working and we would die within days.

Most people in the Western world get more protein than they need. The excess is used for energy or converted into fat.

PROTEIN

THE PROTEIN WE EAT is broken down into its component amino acids, used by cells as building blocks for growth, maintenance, and repair. The body can make some amino acids itself, but there are nine (the so-called essential amino acids) that can be obtained only from food. In addition, amino acids are used to produce enzymes, catalysts that allow complex chemical processes to take place, and also DNA, which carries the genetic information controlling all metabolic activity. Ideally, around 10–15 percent of our diet should be in the form of protein. If we don't get enough protein, the body will break down cells in order to provide it. In fact, most people in the Western world get more protein than they need. The excess is used for energy or converted into fat and stored.

Sources Meat, fish, poultry, eggs, dairy foods, and soybeans are sources of the range of amino acids, and one helping a day is sufficient. Low-quality sources, such as peas, beans, bread, rice, pasta, potatoes, and nuts, must be combined in meals to provide the whole range. Rice and lentils, baked beans on toast, and cereals with milk are all examples of protein-rich combinations.

CARBOHYDRATES

CARBOHYDRATES are our most readily available source of food energy and should account for 50 percent of our diet. The body transforms them into glucose (the body's basic fuel) and glycogen, which is stored in the liver and muscles for conversion to glucose. Carbohydrates fall into two categories: *complex,* which are broken down slowly to provide energy over a long period (these should form two-thirds of carbohydrate intake), and *simple* (sugars), which provide instant energy. Some types, such as cane sugar, are known as "empty" calories since they lack extra nutritional value.

Sources *Complex:* starchy foods – bread, pasta, rice, potatoes, peas, beans, whole grains, and cereals. *Simple:* fruit, vegetables, and honey (glucose and fructose), milk (lactose), sprouting grains (maltose), and cane or beet sugar (sucrose).

WATER

ALL THE BODY PROCESSES, including digestion and elimination, need water – ideally, three to four quarts a day. The best way to get enough water is to drink about two quarts every day, or enough to keep your urine pale yellow. In hot weather, if exercising, or during a fever, you may need more water, since your body loses fluid by sweating. Tap water may be preferable to some bottled waters, which can contain bacteria, nitrates, and chemicals. When buying bottled water, read the label carefully.

Sources Fruit, vegetables, dairy products, bread, cereals, and meats provide one-third of daily intake. The rest can be made up with plain water, juice, milk, and other drinks.

Caution Alcohol, tea, coffee, and colas are diuretics and actually expel more water from the system than they contain.

FAT

FATS, OR LIPIDS, ARE THE MOST CONCENTRATED source of food energy. High-fat foods are therefore high-calorie foods. A certain amount of fat is necessary for the body to function healthily, but too much can lead to health problems. In the US, the recommended maximum level is 30 percent of total calorie intake, although experts suggest this should be as low as 10 percent for those who have a problem metabolizing fats. Fats are also important for storing energy, for transporting fat-soluble vitamins (A, D, E, and K) and for producing hormones. They also provide essential fatty acids (EFAs) that the body cannot produce by itself.

Fats make food palatable and delay its exit from the stomach. A balance of EFAs and the prostaglandins they produce (see Glossary, page 178) is vital for good health. EFA deficiencies have been linked to arthritis, allergies, and atherosclerosis, or narrowing of the arteries.

According to their chemical composition, fats are classed as saturated or unsaturated (see below). Unsaturated vegetable oils are converted to saturated fats (such as margarine) by a process known as hydrogenation. This creates trans-fatty acids, linked to heart disease. Vegetable oils are thus considered a healthy alternative to margarine.

SATURATED FATS

Mainly associated with meat and dairy produce, saturated fats are not an essential part of a healthy diet. High intakes raise blood cholesterol levels, and increase the risk of obesity, heart disease, atherosclerosis, and cancer of the bowel, breast, and pancreas.
Sources Butter, dairy products, coconut and palm oil, fatty meats, hard margarine, solid cooking fats, cakes, and cookies

UNSATURATED FATS

Monounsaturated fatty acids can replace saturated fats in the diet.
Sources Peanut oil, canola oil, avocados, nuts, seeds, and – especially – olive oil. The latter also contains polyunsaturated fatty acids (see right); it is a strong feature of the diet in Mediterranean countries that have low rates of heart disease. Where possible, use cold-pressed, unrefined olive oil from a single source.

Polyunsaturated fatty acids, or PUFAS, contain essential fatty acids, which the body cannot produce and so must be obtained from the diet. They are important in maintaining cell membranes, transporting fats around the body, and forming prostaglandins. These chemicals are produced as and when required for numerous body functions, including circulation, water balance, and maintaining the immune system. Essential fatty acids are grouped into two families (see below).

Omega–6 polyunsaturated fatty acids are derived from linoleic acid.
Sources Seed oils such as sunflower oil, corn oil, peanut oil, olive oil, and evening primrose oil

Omega–3 polyunsaturated fatty acids are derived from alpha-linolenic acid. They are important in early brain development and protect against heart disease and cancer of the breast, bowel, colon, and pancreas. They may also be used to treat arthritis and psoriasis.
Sources Leafy vegetables, oily fish, fish oils, and shellfish

FIBER

DIETARY FIBER IS THE TERM used to describe a complex group of substances found in the cell walls of plants. Fiber is resistant to digestive enzymes, and so passes through the gut without being absorbed. This softens and increases the bulk of feces, preventing constipation and allowing the digestive enzymes time to work. Fiber also absorbs the toxic by-products of digestion. Low-fiber diets are linked to bowel and gallbladder

cancer and other intestinal diseases. The normal daily fiber intake of most adult Americans is around 11 grams. However, many experts recommend up to 35 grams. The two main groups of fiber are soluble and insoluble. Insoluble fiber speeds the passage of food through the intestines and reduces the buildup of carcinogens that can cause colon cancer. Soluble fiber lowers blood cholesterol levels and

inhibits the absorption of glucose.
Sources
Insoluble fiber: rice, bran, nuts, wheat bran, whole grains, dried fruit
Soluble fiber: oat bran, peas, beans, fruit, vegetables

VITAMINS & MINERALS

Vitamins and minerals are essential to our diet, since the body is unable to manufacture them for itself. Each vitamin has specific functions in the body, while at least 16 minerals are vital for life, growth, or reproduction. Ideally, we should obtain all the vitamins and minerals we need from our food, especially if we eat a well-balanced diet.

However, scientific evidence increasingly suggests that the mass production of food may deplete some of these nutrients and that supplements may therefore be beneficial. Supplements should be taken with care, however, since research also suggests that the key to optimum nutrition lies in the way food components work together, rather than in isolated vitamins or minerals.

SUPPLEMENTS

THE WORLD HEALTH ORGANIZATION and other agencies have established guidelines for daily levels of nutrients, known as RDAs (recommended daily allowances) or RNIs (reference nutrient intakes), but many nutritionists claim these are only minimum levels to prevent disease and not enough for optimum health. In any case, individual needs vary according to age, gender, and state of health. Nutritional supplements can certainly be of benefit in some situations.

Some people need extra vitamins and minerals.

For example, the occurrence of spina bifida and other birth defects is dramatically reduced when pregnant women take additional folic acid. In all adults, folic acid seems to protect against heart disease. Vitamin E supplements may reduce the risk of heart attack by up to 75 percent. Vegans, those on a diet, and heavy smokers may all be advised to take B complex vitamins. On the other hand, iron can cause health problems if taken in excess, as can vitamins A and D.

If you have cut corners nutritionally, a good antioxidant-rich multivitamin and mineral supplement may be useful until you improve your diet. Always consult your doctor before taking supplements if you are pregnant or on medication.

ANTIOXIDANTS

OVER 100 ANTIOXIDANTS have been discovered (see below). These nutrients are able to "scavenge" (seek out and destroy) potentially harmful molecules known as free radicals. The body produces free radicals as part of its normal metabolism and as a defense against infection but, in the few seconds they exist, they can damage DNA and cell membranes and affect cholesterol so that it "furs up" arteries. If unchecked, these reactions contribute to heart disease, cancer, premature aging, and other health problems. Eating an unhealthy diet (especially fried or burned food), exercising excessively, and being exposed to environmental chemicals, cigarette smoke, sunlight, and radiation can all raise levels of free radicals.

VITAMINS	Vitamins A (beta carotene, *see below*), C, and E
MINERALS	Selenium, zinc, manganese, and copper
BIOFLAVONOIDS	These are plant chemicals that boost vitamin C activity and appear to have anti-infective and anticarcinogenic properties. They are found in prunes, citrus fruit, cherries, berries, plums, rosehips, grapes, papaya, melon, broccoli, tomatoes, tea, and red wine.
CAROTENOIDS	These yellow and red pigments are present in many plants. The best known is beta carotene, which the body converts to vitamin A. Others include lycopene (found in tomatoes) and lutein and zeaxanthin (found in spinach, kale, broccoli, turnip and mustard greens), which also prevent age-related macular degeneration.
GLUTATHIONE	This enzyme is produced by the body from foods rich in amino acids L-cysteine and L-methionine (red peppers, garlic, onions, broccoli, sprouts, yogurt, egg yolks, wheat germ, and poultry).

Good sources of antioxidants include citrus fruit, tomatoes, and spinach.

VITAMINS

VITAMIN D, PRODUCED NATURALLY when the skin is exposed to sunlight, is the only vitamin the body can make efficiently on its own. All the others must be obtained from the food we eat. The fat-soluble vitamins A, D, E, and K can all be stored in the body, unlike the B complex vitamins (with the exception of B_{12}) and vitamin C, which are water soluble (dissolvable in water). Stress, antibiotics, and alcohol can all affect the body's absorption of water-soluble vitamins.

VITAMIN	MAIN USES	GOOD SOURCES	RDA
VITAMIN A	Antioxidant (*see left*); necessary for good vision; maintains skin and mucous membranes. In excess, can cause birth defects, blurred vision, and headaches.	Present as retinol in animal foods (liver, butter, cheese, eggs, oily fish) and as beta carotene in plant foods (carrots, tomatoes, spinach, broccoli)	Women, 600 mcg; breast-feeding women, 950 mcg; men, 700 mcg
VITAMIN B_1	Helps convert food into energy; prevents the buildup of toxic substances.	Whole grains, brown rice, nuts, whole-wheat pasta and bread, fortified white bread and breakfast cereals, dried beans, lean meats, fish	Women, 0.8 mg; men, 1 mg
VITAMIN B_2 (RIBOFLAVIN)	Helps convert food into energy.	Nuts, dairy products, liver, yeast extract, eggs, lean meat, leafy vegetables, lentils, breakfast cereals	Women, 1.1 mg; men, 1.3 mg
NIACIN	Involved in the synthesis of DNA; helps convert food into energy; supports the nervous and digestive systems.	Dairy products, liver, oily fish, chicken, turkey, whole-wheat bread, brown rice, yeast extracts, nuts	Women, 13 mg; men, 17 mg
VITAMIN B_6 (PYRIDOXINE)	Promotes brain activity; stimulates production of antibodies and formation of red blood cells; helps release energy from protein.	Whole grains, dried beans, eggs, nuts, oats, fish, liver, brown rice, bananas, green leafy vegetables, yeast extracts, whole-wheat bread, soybeans	Women, 1.2 mg; men, 1.4 mg
VITAMIN B_{12}	Protects the nerves; important for cell division, formation of red blood cells, and enzyme function; involved in production of DNA and RNA.	Foods of animal origin, such as meat, poultry, fish, eggs, dairy products; some fortified breakfast cereals	Men and women, 1.5 mcg
BIOTIN	Stimulates body to produce energy; maintains enzyme function, healthy skin, hair, and bone marrow; supports glands producing sex hormones.	Almost all foods, especially liver, peanut butter, egg yolk, yeast extracts	Men and women, 150 mcg
FOLIC ACID (FOLATE)	Works with B_{12} to form new cells, especially blood cells; important in making DNA and RNA; helps prevent birth defects such as spina bifida, and is therefore essential for pregnant women.	Wheat germ, liver, broccoli, green cabbage, peas, beans, nuts, yeast extract, and fortified bread and breakfast cereals	Men and women, 200 mcg; pregnant women, 300 mcg (400 mcg in first 12 weeks)
PANTOTHENIC ACID	Converts food into energy; promotes synthesis of cholesterol, fat, and red blood cells, as well as antibody formation; supports nervous system and skin.	All meat and vegetable foods, especially liver, yeast extracts, kidney, nuts, wheat germ, soy flour	Men and women, 3–7 mg
VITAMIN C	Antioxidant; makes collagen (important for healthy gums, teeth, bones, and skin) and neurotransmitters (serotonin, norepinephrine, *see Glossary, pages 177–78*); aids absorption of iron and helps skin heal; protects against infection.	Oranges and other citrus fruit, blueberries, strawberries, kiwi fruit, tomatoes, spinach and other dark green vegetables, potatoes, mango, papaya	Men and women, 40–60 mg; smokers, at least 80 mg
VITAMIN D	Important for absorption of calcium and phosphorus essential for healthy bones and teeth.	Made by the skin in response to sunlight; also found in milk, oily fish, brown rice, eggs, butter, margarine	Produced by the body when skin is exposed to sun
VITAMIN E	Antioxidant; prevents formation of free radicals following ingestion of polyunsaturates; proven ability to protect against heart disease.	Nuts, vegetable oils, whole grains, olives, asparagus, spinach, tuna, eggs, avocado, blackberries, whole-wheat bread, brown rice, salmon	Women, at least 3 mg; men, at least 4 mg
VITAMIN K	Helps body digest certain proteins and prevents blood clots from forming.	Green leafy vegetables (green cabbage, broccoli, brussels sprouts)	Women, 65 mcg; men, 70 mcg

MINERALS

ALTHOUGH MINERALS ACCOUNT for only 3–4 percent of body weight, some, such as calcium and iron, which are necessary for healthy bones and red blood cells respectively, are required in fairly large quantities. Others, such as iodine, zinc, molybdenum, and chromium, are needed in such tiny amounts they are known as trace elements, but are, nevertheless, essential constituents of particular enzymes or hormones. If you take supplements, consult a nutritionist or doctor, since there is a delicate balance between different minerals and an excess of one can affect the efficacy of others. An excess of iron in the diet, for instance, inhibits the absorption of zinc.

MINERAL	MAIN USES	GOOD SOURCES	RDA
CALCIUM	Growth and maintenance of bones and teeth; blood clotting, muscle function, and heartbeat regulation; especially important in women to prevent osteoporosis after menopause.	Milk and dairy products (including low-fat items), canned sardines, eggs, spinach and other green leafy vegetables	Ages 11–18, 800–1000 mg; over 18, 800 mg
CHROMIUM	Regulation of blood sugar and cholesterol.	Red meat, liver, egg yolks, seafood, whole-grain cereals, cheese	Men and women, 25 mcg
COPPER	Building bones and connective tissue; aids absorption of iron.	Organ meats, shellfish, nuts and seeds, mushrooms	Men and women, 1.2 mg
FLUORIDE	Protection against tooth decay.	Tap water, toothpaste, tea	no RDA
IODINE	Hormone production by thyroid gland.	Iodized table salt, seafood, seaweed	Men and women, 150 mcg
IRON	Carrying oxygen to body cells.	Liver, shellfish, dried fruit, dark green leafy vegetables, whole-wheat bread, peas, beans, red meat, fortified cereals	Women, 14.8 mg; men, 8.7 mg
MAGNESIUM	Bone growth and nerve and muscle function.	Wheat bran, whole grains, raw leafy vegetables, almonds, cashews, soybeans, bananas, apricots	Men and women, 300 mg
MANGANESE	Bone growth and cell function.	Nuts, whole grains, vegetables, fruit, tea, egg yolks, peas, beans	Men and women, 1.4 mg
MOLYBDENUM	DNA production.	Organ meats, yeast, peas, beans, whole grains, leafy vegetables	Men and women, 50–400 mcg
PHOSPHORUS	Release of energy from food; nutrient absorption; maintenance of healthy bones and teeth.	All protein foods – meat, poultry, fish, seafood, egg yolks, milk, dried peas, beans, nuts	Men and women, 550 mg
POTASSIUM	Regulation of heartbeat; muscle contraction; transference of nutrients to cells; regulation of fluids and electrolyte balance (see Glossary, pages 177–78); nerve function.	Citrus fruit, bananas, dried fruit, avocados, peanut butter, dried peas and beans, potatoes	Men and women, 3500 mg
SELENIUM	Works with vitamin E as an antioxidant (see Glossary, pages 177–78); involved in sexual development and may help prevent cancer.	Organ meats, white fish, tuna, shellfish, red meat, egg yolks, poultry, garlic, tomatoes, muesli, whole-grain cereals, whole-wheat bread, dairy foods, lentils, avocados, Brazil nuts	Women, 60 mcg; men, 75 mcg
SODIUM	Regulation (with potassium) of fluid balance; nerve and muscle function.	Table salt, anchovies, yeast extracts, processed meats	Men and women, 1600 mg
SULFUR	Protein production.	All protein foods – meat, poultry, fish, seafood, egg yolks, milk, dried peas, beans, nuts	no RDA
ZINC	Antioxidant; growth and sexual development; immune function; enzyme action.	Liver, red meat, oysters, peanuts, sunflower seeds, cheese, eggs	Women, 7 mg; men, 9.5 mg

SPECIAL DIETS

For various health or ethical reasons, some people need to modify their diet. Increasing numbers, for example, are giving up meat for health reasons or a concern about the treatment of animals reared for consumption and about the levels of antibiotics, hormones, and other drugs given them. Other people need to adapt their diet to lose weight, or to take a food intolerance (*see pages 92–95*) into account. Followers of rigorous regimes such as the "Stone Age" diet (*see page 129*) claim special benefits, and certain regimes such as the Pritikin diet or Gerson therapy aim to prevent or cure particular diseases, notably heart disease and cancer. Always consult a doctor before following a strict diet, since restricted diets risk malnourishment in the long run. This is especially important for children.

Studies quite clearly show that people who eat a vegetarian diet run less risk of heart disease and colon cancer.

VEGETARIANISM

Studies show that vegetarians run less risk of contracting heart disease, gallbladder problems, diabetes, high blood pressure, osteoporosis, diverticular disease, and colon cancer; vegan diets have been prescribed for high blood pressure, arthritis, angina, and asthma with some success. If you are vegetarian, it is essential to eat alternative sources of protein and, if vegan, of vitamin B_{12} (*see page 129*).

WEIGHT LOSS

Obesity is common in industrialized countries and is clearly linked to diabetes, high blood pressure, heart disease, joint problems, and, indirectly, to some forms of cancer; an obsession with weight can lead to anorexia, bulimia, and fad diets that risk malnourishment. To find out if your weight is healthy, assess your body mass index (*see below*). If under- or overweight, keep a food diary for a week. On average you should eat 1,800–2,200, calories a day depending on gender, age, and activity levels. The secret to increasing your weight healthily is to eat more complex carbohydrates (*see page 160*). To lose weight, reduce fat consumption (*see right*) to no more than 30 percent of total calorie intake. In addition, get aerobic exercise for 30 minutes and anaerobic exercise for ten minutes three times a week (*see pages 152–53*). There is no evidence that "wonder" pills cure obesity, although there are prescription drugs that inhibit nutrient absorption, reduce appetite, and increase metabolic rate.

Regular exercise helps control weight.

TIPS TO HELP REDUCE FAT INTAKE

- Remove fat from meat and skin from poultry before eating, or better still, avoid red meat.
- Grill or roast meat on a rack.
- Avoid frying but if you do, drain food on paper towels before eating.
- Skim fat from casseroles while cooking and when cool.
- Remember that even low-fat margarine contains unhealthy fats; spread thinly.
- Switch to low-fat milk, cheese, and yogurt.
- Use herbs and spices to add flavor to food.
- Avoid cake, cookies, pastry, candy, and desserts made with fat or shortening.

BODY MASS INDEX

THE EASIEST WAY TO ESTIMATE if you are the correct weight for your height is to work out your body mass index.

Note: If you exercise frequently, the calculation may be distorted by your increased muscle mass.

Divide your weight in kilograms by your height in meters squared (round up to the nearest decimal point).
For example, you are 5 ft 4 in tall and weigh 130 lb:

1.6 x 1.6 = 2.6   58.5 ÷ 2.6 = 22.2

To convert pounds to kilos, multiply pounds by 0.45 (130 lb x 0.45 = 58.5); to convert feet to meters multiply feet by 0.3 (5.3 ft x 0.3 = 1.6)

SCORE	
Under 20	underweight
20–25	healthy weight
25–30	overweight
Over 30	obese

Spicy stir-fried dishes are excellent for those who wish to lose weight.

HEALTH & THE ENVIRONMENT

The quality of food is a growing concern in industrialized countries and is one aspect of the fear that the natural world is under threat from pollution. Many people worry, for instance, about genetically modified crops and the effects of additives, pesticides, and other environmental toxins on the body. The scare in the UK over beef infected with BSE (bovine spongiform encephalopathy) is just one example of incidents that leave consumers skeptical about official reassurances and anxious to find food that is as unprocessed and pure as possible. Environmental factors are thought to have wide-ranging effects. In some individuals they may be a factor in food sensitivity (*see pages 94–95*), and they can interfere with the way the hormones work or affect how well the immune system responds to infection.

CHEMICALS IN FOOD

BOTH NATURAL and chemical substances are widely used in agriculture and food processing. While some are harmless, others can affect health.

ADDITIVES
Substances are added to food to preserve it and provide flavor and color. In the US, the actual name of all additives, except for flavorings, must be included in the list of ingredients. Not all of these additives are necessarily bad, and some are necessary to prevent food from spoiling. Ascorbic acid (vitamin C) for example, is used to prevent fruit juices from turning brown and fatty foods from going rancid. The following, however, can cause problems:
Monosodium glutamate (MSG) can make some people ill or trigger food intolerance symptoms.
Nitrites and nitrates, used to preserve processed meats and fish, may convert to potentially carcinogenic nitrosamines in the body.
Benzoic acid, added to soft drinks and beer, can cause adverse reactions.
Sulfur compounds in dried fruit and relishes may trigger asthma and other allergic reactions.
Colorings such as Yellow Dye No. 5, found in soft drinks and sweets, are said to contribute to allergic and behavioral problems in some children.

Crops are sprayed with a variety of insecticides.

Guar gum and gum arabic, used to improve texture and smoothness, may cause gas in some people.

CHEMICALS IN FARMING
Pesticides are used in agriculture to kill insects, weeds, and fungi, while antibiotics are routinely added to feed to prevent the infections prevalent when livestock are raised intensively.
Pesticides such as organophosphates and dioxin may affect the body,

especially the central nervous system, in various ways.
Antibiotics and antifungals are linked with antibiotic-resistant bacteria.
Growth hormones may affect the body in ways we do not yet understand.
Heavy metals, such as cadmium, mercury, and lead are found in fish and shellfish from rivers and coastal waters polluted by industrial waste. These metals interfere with immune responses and affect the central nervous system.

ORGANIC PRODUCE
Where possible, it is wise to reduce the danger from chemicals by choosing organically produced foods. Although such foods are more expensive, demand for them now outstrips supply, and intensive farming methods for the time being may still be the only way to feed the world's population.

"Those suspicious of of genetically modified food and the consequences of consuming crops laden with pesticides insist that long-term scientific testing is necessary."

Organic vegetables are better for health.

THE IMMUNE SYSTEM

THE BODY'S DEFENSES PROTECT it from invading foreign substances – viruses, bacteria, pollen, dust, and toxic chemicals – which could inflict damage, ranging from an infected cut to cancer. The frontline defenses are the skin, mucous membranes (of the respiratory system, gut, and genitals), small hairs in the nose and ears, and acid juices in the stomach.

If invaders breach these barriers and enter the bloodstream, they are met by defensive white blood cells called lymphocytes. These are formed in the bone marrow and circulate around the body in the lymphatic system, which is a network of vessels that filters debris and toxins out of body tissues. Lymphocytes engulf the invading microbes.

Antibodies are produced by a special kind of lymphocyte in response to a specific invader. A flu antibody, for example, is produced to attack a flu virus. Once programmed, the lymphocyte recognizes the invader if it appears again and rapidly produces more targeted antibodies. This is the principle behind immunization. Although some immunity is passed on from mother to child in the womb and in breast milk, we acquire most of it by dealing with invading microbes as we grow up. It is widely accepted that exposure to infection develops a competent immune system.

IMMUNE DISORDERS

Special "suppressor" T-cells switch off antibodies when there are enough to fight invaders. Too many can block antibody production so the system is "immunodeficient." This may happen naturally, as in HIV (human immuno-deficiency virus) or with the use of drugs, after an organ transplant.

"Helper" T-cells prompt production of antibodies. If they dominate, the body no longer recognizes the difference between invading substances and itself. It starts to attack its own cells in what are called autoimmune diseases, which include multiple sclerosis and rheumatoid arthritis.

Finally, the immune system can become hypersensitive and react against normally harmless substances, such as grass, dust, pollen, and certain foods (see pages 92–99).

DAMAGE TO THE IMMUNE SYSTEM

Malnutrition and vitamin deficiency are linked to poor immune function. Environmental chemicals and toxic heavy metals such as cadmium, lead, and mercury damage the immune system (see left) as do tobacco smoke and certain drugs. Stress (see pages 84–85), excessive exercise, aging, and certain infections (most notably HIV) reduce immune competence.

A lymphocyte engulfs an invading flu virus.

HOW TO PROTECT THE IMMUNE SYSTEM

• Eat a balanced diet with plenty of fruit and vegetables, nuts, seeds, and whole grains, and cut down on saturated fats, sugars, processed products, and chemical additives.
• Limit caffeine and drink alcohol in moderation. (One or two drinks a day are not harmful).
• Stop smoking, since it increases susceptibility to infection.
• Improve your diet with a good-quality antioxidant supplement on a "bad nutrition day."
• If you are elderly, pregnant, or suspect your immune system is struggling because of an infection, environmental pollution, or stress, consider taking a multivitamin and mineral supplement.
• Include in your diet herbs that stimulate the immune system: garlic, ginger, thyme, sage, and rosemary.
• Participate in aerobic exercise for 30 minutes three times a week.
• Practice stress-reducing techniques such as meditation (see page 135).
• Avoid environmental chemicals, such as gasoline exhaust fumes, wherever possible.
• Enjoy social interaction with friends and family.
• Be sure you get enough rest and sleep to repair your body.
• Develop positive beliefs and attitudes toward life and other people. Research shows that optimism and altruism actually promote health.
• If you get an infection, fight it with over-the-counter herbs such as echinacea, garlic, or astragalus.

HORMONES

HOW WELL THE BODY can cope with stress, environmental change, and fluctuating amounts of sleep and food depends on the interweaving processes in the brain, nervous system, and endocrine (hormone) glands.

The endocrine system and the brain secrete chemicals, known as hormones, that influence mood and vitality and regulate all body functions from digestion to the menstrual cycle, blood

circulation, and the "fight or flight" response (see page 84).

The pituitary gland orchestrates all hormonal activity. It produces growth hormones as well as substances that control the output of other hormonal glands. These include the thyroid gland in the neck, which regulates metabolism; the adrenal glands above the kidneys, which coordinate the body's chemical balance and response to stress, physical

injury, and infection; and the pancreas, which secretes insulin to regulate blood-sugar levels. The pituitary gland also regulates the ovaries' production of estrogen and progesterone and the testes' output of testosterone.

Endocrine disorders usually require conventional treatment. But if hormone levels are only mildly disturbed, complementary approaches might, with your doctor's support, be worth trying.

YOUR PSYCHOSOCIAL HEALTH

Dealing with crises, life events, and conflict is part of the constant adaptation to change that is essential to well-being. We tend to think about managing stress in purely psychological terms, but the process also requires energy, so it puts a strain on the body. How well we cope will depend on how much energy, support, and information are available. Certain challenges are inescapable, but difficulties arise when challenges are severe and sudden, such as injury or shock, or persistent and drawn out – the effects of poor nutrition, perhaps, or of an impossible job or relationship. Stress management techniques can help us adapt to and control stress.

WHAT IS STRESS?

We feel stressed in situations that tax our ability to cope and/or endanger well-being. These prompt the instinctive stress, or "fight or flight," response, which was originally intended to be an immediate and short-term reaction to an external danger, such as a predatory wild animal. The physical act of running away or fighting would naturally absorb the stress hormones, expend the energy generated, and resolve the feelings of anger or fear aroused. After the crisis, a set of calming-down reactions, known as the "relaxation response," would reverse the arousal, preventing it from becoming harmful.

In the modern world, however, our challenges tend to be more mental and emotional, often involving successive episodes of psychological tension (for example, a delayed train, being late for

RECOGNIZING THE SYMPTOMS OF STRESS

Often people who suffer from stress are unaware of just how stressed they are, and even rely on a constant epinephrine surge to keep going. They have forgotten what it feels like to be relaxed and ignore the signs that their coping mechanisms are beginning to burn out. Key signs of too much stress include:
- Irritability
- Sleeping badly
- Constant tiredness
- Inability to wind down even on weekends or during a vacation
- Finding it difficult to concentrate or to make decisions
- Tense muscles
- Skin irritations
- General aches and pains
- Frequent infections

If you suspect you are suffering from stress, see pages 84–85.

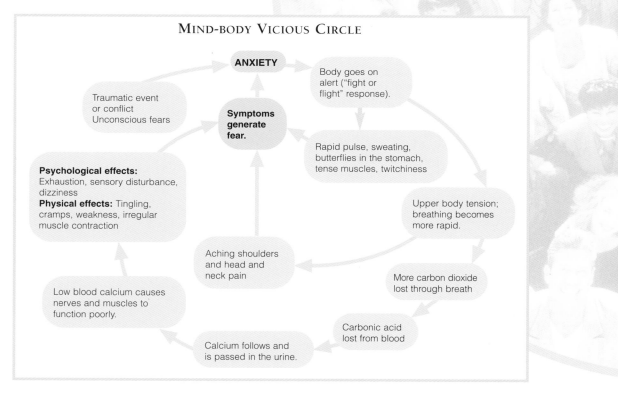

MIND-BODY VICIOUS CIRCLE

ANXIETY

Body goes on alert ("fight or flight" response).

Traumatic event or conflict Unconscious fears

Symptoms generate fear.

Rapid pulse, sweating, butterflies in the stomach, tense muscles, twitchiness

Psychological effects: Exhaustion, sensory disturbance, dizziness
Physical effects: Tingling, cramps, weakness, irregular muscle contraction

Upper body tension; breathing becomes more rapid.

Aching shoulders and head and neck pain

Low blood calcium causes nerves and muscles to function poorly.

More carbon dioxide lost through breath

Carbonic acid lost from blood

Calcium follows and is passed in the urine.

a meeting, arguing with a partner). Stress chemicals have no chance to dissipate, and the body and mind may begin to act and feel as if in continual physical danger. Exhaustion and jitters from tense muscles, overactive circulation and senses, and, finally, damage to the immune system, are all likely outcomes.

Causes of stress, known as stressors, range from the life-threatening (mugging) to the trivial (a ringing phone). Between the two extremes is a spectrum of potential stressors, both external (life events like bereavement, or an environmental stimulant such as noise) and internal (memories, expectations, and feelings such as shame and rage). As stressors multiply in number and grow in magnitude, the ability to cope diminishes. Sometimes we are able to handle major issues but fall apart over interminable daily hassles, which are now understood to be as likely as major life dramas to provoke unhealthy coping strategies, such as turning to alcohol and "comfort" foods.

WHY LEARN TO RELAX?

The stress response should naturally be followed by the relaxation response, in which heart and breathing rates are lowered and stress hormone levels are reduced. However, if you are constantly in a state of arousal, you can forget what deep relaxation and calm awareness feel like. Learning to switch on the relaxation response at will is an essential part of managing stress and it enables the vicious cycle of stress responses (*see left*) to be broken. See over for instructions on deep breathing and muscle

relaxation. It may also help to buy a relaxation tape that will talk you through the steps.

Breathing calmly and relaxing the mind and body are integral elements in many stress management techniques, such as t'ai chi, yoga, meditation, autogenic training, visualization, and self-hypnosis (*see Glossary of Therapies, pages 114–37*). Which one you follow is very much an individual choice and you may have to sample several. Some people also find that they relax deeply only after aerobic exercise so take time to discover the strategy that works for you.

AN ANTISTRESS PACKAGE

Relaxation techniques are not the whole answer. If your mind is buzzing with worries, conflicts, negative attitudes, and prejudices, you may need to consider counseling or psychotherapy. Cognitive behavioral therapy (*see pages 174–75*) is a potent tool for changing the way you think and feel about stressors. Time management techniques can clear the internal (and external) clutter and enable you to prioritize tasks, while assertiveness training and learning social skills may help you deal with people and gain control over situations in which you felt vulnerable. Self-confidence and self-esteem are important, but if a problem seems bigger than you are, it could be because it is. Seek help. Major crises always require support, help, and energy to move forward. If you feel exhausted, it is important to get some rest. You need respite and recuperation before you can begin to make sense of your situation.

Meditation is one of many techniques that induce the relaxation response.

12 WAYS TO CONTROL STRESS LEVELS

- Allow at least 20 minutes a day for the relaxation technique of your choice, even if you have to mark it in your diary.
- Eat a healthy balanced diet (*see pages 158–61*).
- Exercise for at least 20 minutes four times a week.
- Be assertive. Decide what it is you want or feel and say so specifically; say no to unnecessary requests.
- Delegate. Hand over jobs that other people can do, so that you are not overcommitted.
- Organize your day and prioritize tasks to make the most efficient use of your time.
- Make your workplace as comfortable as possible (*see page 151*).
- Try to avoid working late. Long working hours have been linked to mental and physical health problems.
- In the hour before bedtime detach yourself from the day's events with music, a book, or some visualization. Aim for 6–8 hours sleep every night.
- Find time in the week for pleasure and creativity. Go to the theater, the movies, or an art gallery; have dinner with friends; paint, sing, or garden.
- When you go away on vacation, leave work behind. Several short breaks can be more restful than one long vacation that includes stressful traveling.
- Seek help when you need it. Open up to friends, family, and professionals who act as listeners. Being able to make use of social support in times of stress is good for mental and physical well-being.

Getting adequate sleep is a powerful way to cope with stress.

RELAXATION & BREATHING

Simple breathing exercises and muscle-relaxing techniques can alleviate the physical and mental effects of stress by lowering heart rate, reducing blood pressure, and lowering levels of stress hormones. Such techniques have been used for thousands of years in Eastern health systems and form part of many complementary therapies. Western medicine is finding relaxation techniques increasingly valuable and they are now often taught in health centers and hospitals.

THE MIND-BODY CONNECTION

Breathing is involuntary, but when consciously controlled, it forms a link between the mind and body. Yoga postures (*asanas*) and breathing techniques (*pranayama*) are used to calm body and mind (*see page 123*). Traditional Chinese Medicine uses breathing and movement exercises in T'ai chi and Qigong to control the flow of *qi*, or "life energy," through the body (*see pages 124–25*).

PROGRESSIVE MUSCLE RELAXATION

In the 1930s, American physiologist Dr. Edmund Jacobson developed one of the earliest relaxation techniques practiced in the West. He called his systematic approach to relaxing "progressive muscle relaxation" (*see opposite*). In the 1960s, Dr. Herbert Benson of Harvard Medical School found that simply sitting in a quiet environment, breathing calmly, and focusing the mind could reverse the physiological effects of stress. He called this state of relaxed awareness the "relaxation response" (*see right*).

FIGHT OR FLIGHT

When stress triggers the "fight or flight" response (*see pages 84–85*), breathing becomes quick and shallow, reinforcing the messages of alarm being sent to the brain. If this type of breathing continues, too much carbon dioxide is removed from the blood, which then loses its proper acidity. This directly affects the body's nerves and muscles, prompting symptoms such as faintness, palpitations, and panic attacks. Calm abdominal breathing, particularly when practiced with muscle relaxation and visualization (*see page 134*), may alleviate this condition by "turning off" the "fight or flight" response.

HOW TO CONTROL YOUR BREATHING

ABDOMINAL, OR DIAPHRAGMATIC, breathing is a gentle, relaxing technique that allows the lungs to fill and empty with minimal effort. The diaphragm is the sheet of muscle between the chest cavity and the abdomen. When you breathe in, the diaphragm contracts and moves down, the abdomen rises, and the chest expands slightly. When you breathe out, the diaphragm relaxes and rises, making the chest cavity smaller and expelling air from the lungs.

1 Remove your shoes and loosen any tight clothing. Sit in a comfortable position with your back supported, either cross-legged or on a chair. Alternatively, you can lie on a mat or firm bed with a small pillow supporting your head.

2 Place one hand on your upper chest and the other on your abdomen, below your breastbone. Note which hand moves when you breathe. If the hand on your chest moves more than the one on your abdomen, you breathe mainly in the upper chest. Try to breathe so only your lower hand moves.

3 Place both hands on your abdomen below the ribs. Breathe in slowly through your nose, allowing your abdomen to rise as your diaphragm moves downward.

4 Pause for a few seconds between breaths, then breathe out slowly through the nose, feeling your abdomen fall as your diaphragm relaxes. Let as much air out of your lungs as possible.

5 Repeat three or four times. Try to relax your muscles and concentrate on your breathing, not on any thoughts that come to you.

Aim to keep this hand motionless.

TRY TO PRACTICE FOR
10–15 MINUTES A DAY.

HOW TO RELAX YOUR MUSCLES

DURING STRESSFUL PERIODS, we tend to tense our muscles, resulting in aches, pains, and fatigue. A practitioner trained in massage therapy (see page 116) or an osteopath (see page 119) can help you become aware of tension patterns in your body. Relaxation classes usually include the following progressive muscle relaxation exercise. It involves tensing and relaxing all the major muscle groups. As you release each muscle, repeat to yourself, "relax and let go." Each time you tense and relax a muscle group, take time to feel the difference. If thoughts or worries drift into your mind, return to focusing on your breathing and how your body feels. Avoid holding your breath.

Making time to relax each day reverses the effects of stress, calms the mind, and encourages peaceful sleep.

1 Remove your shoes and loosen any tight clothing. Lie on a mat placed on the floor, or on a firm bed with your head supported by a small pillow. Your head, torso, and legs should be in a straight line, with your feet apart and your hands by your sides.

2 Close your eyes and become aware of the weight of your body. Focus on the rhythm of your breathing and the rise and fall of your abdomen. Try to breathe more slowly than usual, emphasizing the "out" breath and pausing before you breathe in again.

3 Tense the muscles in your right foot, hold for a few seconds, then release. Tense and release the calf, followed by the thigh muscles. Repeat the process with the left foot and leg.

4 Tense and relax each buttock in turn, then your stomach muscles. Clench and release your right fist, then all the muscles in your right arm. Repeat with the left arm.

5 Lift your shoulders up to your ears, hold for a few seconds, then lower them again. Repeat two or three times. To free the neck, rock your head gently from side to side.

6 Yawn and then relax your face. Twist your mouth into a pout, and release. Frown, then scrunch up your nose and let go. Raise your eyebrows, then release and relax all the muscles in your face.

7 Focus on your breathing again, and tell yourself you feel peaceful and warm. When ready, wriggle your toes and fingers and ease your back muscles. Bend the knees, roll onto one side for a while, then slowly get up.

> **TRY TO PRACTICE FOR 10–15 MINUTES A DAY.**

YOUR EMOTIONS

Tears at losing a loved one, joy at a reunion, anger when hurt or frustrated – these powerful emotions are all a normal part of life. They also show how intimately the mind and body are interconnected. Pleasure triggers waves of endorphins that influence all the body's systems; fear releases stress chemicals that speed up heart rate and cause the muscles of the gut to contract. The ability to deal with feelings is essential to the management of challenging situations such as having a baby or losing a parent or a job. How individuals respond to life's demands depends partly on their genetics, physical makeup, and brain chemistry, but also on their personality and culture. Whereas some people might view crying as a sign of weakness, people from another culture may be more likely to regard the same display of emotion as entirely normal. Childhood experiences are also a factor; children who are bullied, for example, often grow up to bully in turn.

Feelings of mistrust and aggression have been compared to a slow drip of poison.

COPING WITH DIFFICULT EMOTIONS

IT IS ENTIRELY NATURAL to be anxious or apprehensive, or to feel angry and guilty at times. Denying negative feelings can lead to problems, and one reaction may predominate, distorting your way of coping with stress and emotions. For example, you may adopt a self-blaming style whenever life becomes difficult, or you may always blame others.

Anger is potentially one of the most difficult emotions to handle, and those who are dominated by it tend to overreact to any form of stress. While the occasional explosion of righteous anger may be cathartic, violent outbursts of temper over everyday annoyances simply reinforce inappropriate behavior and usually provoke unconstructive responses from other people.

Talking about disagreements can help dissipate anger.

Your way of coping with your emotions affects your health. For example, pessimists are more likely to suffer from poor health; optimists, who interpret events in the best light, enjoy greater well-being.

A personality profile known as "type A" – driven, tense, competitive, angry, and aggressive – has been directly linked to heart disease (*see page 49*). The American research scientist Dr. Redford Williams has defined the relevant trait as "hostility," a combination of cynical mistrust, anger, and aggression. He compares it to a slow drip of poison, especially when partnered with other negative emotions such as jealousy and resentment. In hostile people, angry reactions provoke strong physiological responses – extra stress hormones flood the system and blood pressure soars, straining the body and endangering long-term health.

If you think you are prone to anger, ask yourself the questions in "Are You Hostile?" (*page 49*) and follow the advice in "Tips to control anger" (*right*) and in "Steps to a trusting heart" (*page 51*). It is also important to learn stress management techniques (*see pages 170–71*).

TIPS TO CONTROL ANGER

- Breathe slowly for several minutes to calm down (*see pages 170–71*).
- Walk away from a situation or mentally distance yourself. The old adage "count to ten" still holds true.
- Reframe the trigger event. For example, if annoyed by a rude sales-person, tell yourself, "She must be under terrible pressure," and remind yourself, "I am not the target."
- Listen to the other person, who may need to vent feelings. Hold your tongue if necessary. Express your views calmly.
- Don't demonize your attacker. Remember that most arguments are about values, and the issues involved may not be black and white.
- Don't blame others for your anger. Apologize or compromise if appropriate.
- Don't endlessly replay events that have provoked you to anger.

There are various long-term measures you can take to help control anger:
- Practice stress management techniques to reduce tension and promote well-being (*see pages 170–71*).
- Practice a relaxation technique to help calm yourself at will.
- Exercise regularly (*see pages 152–53*) to relieve stress and alleviate feelings of frustration.

SELF-ASSERTIVENESS

LEARNING SKILLS that enable you to be more assertive is an effective way to overcome feelings of self-blame and depression. This type of psychological training will make you aware of your real needs and ways to express them, and will encourage you to expect these needs to be met.

Long-term poor health can sometimes be traced to humiliating experiences never brought into the open but continually replayed at an unconscious level; they may be a source of distressing negative self-talk. According to one study, finding a way to recount the shaming event can have real health benefits. Counseling might be a solution, but even writing about the event can improve well-being. American students who practiced creative writing were found to enjoy significantly better health than those who did not. Ideally, you should set down not only what happened but also how it made you feel, what you wish you had said or done, how you would have liked it to turn out, and how you feel it has affected you.

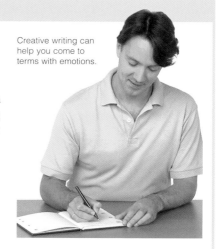
Creative writing can help you come to terms with emotions.

POSITIVE EMOTIONS

HAPPINESS HELPS THE HEALING process along. Laughter and optimism, for example, have been linked to rises in antibody levels in the saliva and in hormones that boost the immune

Laughter has positive physical effects.

system, increasing the activity of natural killer cells, which fight infection. Laughing, like exercise, also eases muscle tension, encourages diaphragmatic breathing (*see pages 170–71*), improves circulation, and releases endorphins, the body's natural pain-relieving opiates. People with a good sense of humor tend to experience less fatigue, anxiety, anger, and depression when under pressure.

Humor implies an exchange of feeling with others. It is no surprise that "connectedness" – a network of friends and family, a readiness to find emotional support, and to give and receive love – seems to encourage

good health. Lonely, isolated people are vulnerable to illness; people who maintain caring relationships throughout their lives are likely to live longer than those who do not. Perhaps that is why some studies have found that those who go to church appear healthier than those with no religious belief. Other studies, however, suggest that health benefits derive from spiritual awareness and from active involvement in the community, rather than from organized religion. In a recent study, women with breast cancer who joined support groups were found to live twice as long after diagnosis as those who did not. This result can be attributed to the expression and sharing of emotions, encouraging feelings of optimism and a sense of control over the illness.

Sometimes it is difficult to express feelings in words. Music, art, and dance can help us touch our emotions directly and intuitively without having to pin them down verbally.

Sharing your emotions can help promote a positive outlook.

WAYS TO ENCOURAGE POSITIVE EMOTIONS

- Visualize yourself at a time when you were happy, relaxed, and full of energy – try to recall your emotions and reexperience how you felt.
- Develop your sense of humor.
- Practice looking on the bright side.
- Work on closeness. If you are glad to see someone, or grateful for an act of kindness, say so enthusiastically.
- Let those who are dear to you know how much you love them.
- Learn yoga, qigong, or meditation (*see pages 123, 125, and 135*) to help still the mind and focus thoughts.
- Altruism is healthy. Do something to help other people, whether voluntary work or visiting a sick neighbor.
- Link up your thoughts with feelings. Try writing an account of unpleasant or traumatic events, describing your emotions.

IMPROVING WAYS OF THINKING

Some people, by virtue of their psychological and physical makeup, seem to handle stress more effectively than others. In a study of American executives involved in a company reorganization, some succumbed to stress-related diseases, while others seemed to thrive. Researchers attributed the difference to characteristics that together constitute "hardiness": a sense of commitment to themselves, families, and jobs; a feeling of being in control of their lives; and a belief that change is a challenge and an inevitable part of life.

The "hardy" executives had a flexibility and readiness to adapt, which seemed to give them better physical and mental health than that of the rigid, black-and-white thinkers, and they were also able to communicate more effectively. Fortunately, it is possible to change attitudes, beliefs, and behavior and to improve communication and reactions to events so that stress becomes easier to deal with.

Adapting to life's events and accepting change are key to stress-free living.

STRESS MANAGEMENT

MONITORING EVENTS IN A STRESS DIARY (*see opposite*) can help define the kind of pressures that are stressful for you, and filling in the questionnaire (*see page 142*) identifies how you react to stress. Particularly if you are a silent, obsessive worrier or a hot-tempered blusterer, it is important to learn how to adapt your response to stress. Researchers at the Mind/Body Medical Institute of Harvard Medical School have devised the following approach to managing stress.

1 STOP!
When confronted by a stressful situation, think "STOP!" before your imagination runs amok in expectation of the worst possible scenario. Picture a big red STOP! sign, if you like. "Thought-stopping" helps to break the panic cycle.

2 BREATHE
Breathing diaphragmatically (*see page 170*) helps diffuse tension immediately.

3 REFLECT
When panicking, people stop thinking logically. Ask yourself why you are so distressed. Is it really a crisis? What is the worst thing that can happen? Will worrying help? Reflecting calmly will help to identify irrational thinking and eliminate knee-jerk responses.

4 CHOOSE
Deciding what to do involves choosing an appropriate response.

5 TAKE ACTION
Depending on the situation, you could:
- Tackle the problem at once.
- Put it on hold until you are able to deal with it effectively.
- Make a full list of possible solutions to discover options and compromises.
- Relax and do something enjoyable to put yourself in a better, calmer mood.
- Look at the problem from a different perspective (sitting in a traffic jam, for example, might give you the opportunity to do some forward planning or breathing exercises).
  - While you are considering what to do, repeat words or phrases with a particular positive meaning, for example "I am peaceful" or "I can organize my life."
  - Talk to yourself constructively. For example, rather than worryng about a speech ("I hate talking in public," "I'll fluff my words and look silly"), try saying to yourself, "I'll take a deep breath and relax" and "They'll enjoy what I have to say."
  - Talk about the problem. An amazing amount of stress can be eliminated simply with better communication.

COMMUNICATING WELL

VERBAL COMMUNICATION includes what you say, how you say it, and how you listen and understand. Nonverbal communication encompasses your body language, eye contact, and actions. If you communicate well, others will respond better to you, which in turn raises your self-esteem, improves your relationships, and can actually prevent stressful situations. Here are some simple rules to sum up the essence of good communication.

• Maintain eye contact during a conversation (but avoid staring).

• State your message clearly and specifically. "I'm unhappy because the arrangements haven't allowed enough time for traveling" is more accurate than "I'm not happy about this."

• Support your words with appropriate nonverbal behavior. Do not say, "It's OK, no problem" when you're frowning, biting your lips, and drumming your fingers.

• Listen to what the other person actually says. Give him or her your full attention, don't interrupt, don't jump to conclusions or put your own interpretation on their words.

• Clarify any areas of doubt by reiterating what you think they said. "You want me to double-check these figures with the marketing department."

• Accept other people's opinions and feelings as genuine, even when they are different from your own.

Plenty of eye contact aids communication.

ACHIEVING HIGH SELF-ESTEEM

OVERCOMING POOR SELF-ESTEEM gives you the emotional "hardiness" to deal with stressful events. Even quite tiny shifts in how you perceive yourself can bring about profound changes. The Mind/Body Institute at Harvard University suggests you try to become aware of the origins of low self-esteem. Think of your life as a bus with every significant person from your past on board. When they make criticisms such as "Why are you so clumsy?" ask yourself: "Who is driving this bus? Who is in control?" Taking over the driver's seat yourself might entail putting some of the passengers off the bus – and out of your mind – permanently.

BUILDING CONFIDENCE

CONFIDENT, OPTIMISTIC PEOPLE take a positive approach to life and do not interpret events negatively. If an acquaintance suddenly crosses the road as they approach, for example, they attribute it to being unseen rather than deliberate avoidance. Sometimes behaving in a confident manner generates real confidence. If you hide your anxieties and act with self-assurance, people often respond by listening and assuming you know what you are talking about, which in turn reinforces your confident behavior.

Behaving confidently builds self-esteem.

KEEPING A STRESS DIARY

Every week (or every day) describe in a diary a situation that caused you to feel stressed:

• How did you feel physically?
• What were your first thoughts?
• What emotions did you feel?
• What distorted beliefs may have been behind your thoughts (for example, "Nobody loves me," "I'm always the one who gets dumped on," "I'm trapped in a situation that won't ever get better")?
• How did you behave during or immediately after the situation?
• What could you think or do differently to cope better next time?
• How might this make you feel and behave?

TIPS FOR CONFIDENT BEHAVIOR

• Visualize yourself behaving in a confident manner (see page 134) and practice deep breathing when you feel stressed (see pages 170–71).
• When you meet someone, look at the person long enough to acknowledge him or her and then look away again.
• Watch your body language. Confident people take up space and look relaxed. They don't twitch or fiddle, hunch their shoulders, or cross their arms and legs defensively.
• When you speak, take time to pause and breathe evenly throughout.
• Lower your voice if you hear it rising.
• Be prepared. Make notes and know your facts before going into a meeting or a difficult interview, for example.
• If you make a mistake, ask yourself "Will this matter in ten years' time?" Most things won't.
• Remind yourself that the other people have better things to do than analyze your shortcomings.

RESEARCH INTO THERAPIES

DESPITE THEIR POPULARITY, more research into complementary therapies is needed. Most conventional practitioners, quite rightly, want evidence that a complementary approach is safe and effective before using it or recommending it to their patients, and trials are under way in a number of areas.

Even in conventional medicine, "evidence-based" treatments are an increasingly important goal. With so many demands on funds, doctors and health care providers are reluctant to support treatments that are not proven to be effective. Since the development of new high-tech drugs and procedures is extremely expensive, their cost effectiveness and patient acceptability have become big issues.

Complementary therapies will always be the alternative of choice for some people but, if they are to become truly integrated with conventional medicine, they will have to prove their worth. This may not be easy. Some practitioners argue that it is impossible to measure something as subtle as qi, "life energy," or "the healing process." In addition, how do you devise a trial to take into account the treatment that has been tailored to a specific individual? And how do you judge the result of a treatment that might not cure someone, but makes them *feel* better? Although many complementary practitioners maintain simply that there are enough reports from patients to support their claims, contemporary medical research in complementary medicine uses the tool of outcomes research, which evaluates patient outcomes of actual medical treatments.

Most research into complementary medicine has been done by doctors with an interest in the field, but few have the expertise to conduct a scientifically acceptable study. Colleges that train practitioners of complementary medicine have only just begun to include research as part of the curriculum, and few have linked up with university- or hospital-based researchers.

Part of the problem is funding. Research organizations are often unwilling to make grants in unusual or controversial areas, and drug companies are unlikely to invest in research due to few financial incentives. A second difficulty is a lack of subjects. A trial with 30 people, no matter how promising the results, is not as impressive as one of 300 or 3,000. Large numbers of patients are usually available only through big organizations like the US National Institutes of Health or a group of university hospitals, but ailments typically treated by complementary therapists are seldom seen in hospitals.

Much of the necessary research into complementary medicine will therefore be done in collaboration with family doctors and with the participation of patients. Mobilizing the person's own efforts to become well is one of the most important aspects of integrative health care, so ways must be found of doing research *with* people, rather than *on* them.

Fortunately the situation is changing. US Food and Drug Administration and European Community regulations now demand that products making medicinal claims must provide proof, and growing consumer awareness is encouraging investment in research. More complementary practitioners and their professional organizations are realizing the importance of submitting their therapies to scientific evaluation and exploring ways of doing so.

In the US, the National Center for Complementary and Alternative Medicine (NCCAM), funded by the National Institutes of Health, currently supports 12 centers conducting complementary and alternative medicine research with an annual budget of more than $50 million. In 1998, the November issue of the *Journal of the American Medical Association* was devoted to complementary and alternative research studies and found, just as in the case of conventional medicine, that some treatments worked and some did not.

Other organizations, such as the UK's Research Council for Complementary Medicine and the Cochrane Collaboration are establishing a database of randomized controlled trials involving complementary treatments. Peer-reviewed journals, such as the American *Alternative Therapies in Health and Medicine,* publish research studies. Pages 182–85 list some of the better studies that support complementary therapies.

TYPES OF STUDIES

The most rigorous engine for scientific proof is the clinical trial, which was originally devised to test pharmaceutical drugs. To be reliable it should contain all the following elements:

Controlled trial At least two groups are compared. The experimental group receives the treatment; the other group (the control) receives none.

Randomized trial Large numbers are used in the trial to cancel out individual differences. Bias is also overcome by assigning patients at random into experimental and control groups.

Randomized double-blind study If practitioners and researchers know which is the active treatment and which the placebo, their behavior can be affected so that the patient may guess which is which. In this ultimate test, neither the patients nor the practitioners know who is receiving which treatment.

Placebo-controlled trial Any treatment, even a sugar pill, tends to make about a third of people feel better. This is known as the placebo effect and indicates the psychological power of belief over physical function. In fact, skeptics attribute much of the success of complementary therapies to this effect. In a clinical trial, the placebo is a treatment that appears indistinguishable from the experimental one but is inactive. The experimental treatment must perform significantly better than the placebo to be considered valid. Finding a placebo can be a challenge, especially with a therapy like acupuncture. Researchers either have to insert needles into sham, or non-acupuncture, points or use a plastic tube that feels like a needle insertion.

Meta-analysis, or systematic review These methods collect and analyze the results of a number of studies. Each study is assigned points according to its scientific reliability. The mathematical analysis of a whole group of trials gives a more accurate picture of the total evidence available.

GLOSSARY OF TERMS

Words in CAPITAL LETTERS are defined elsewhere in the glossary.

ACUPOINT Term used in Traditional Chinese Medicine for a point along a MERIDIAN at which the flow of QI is accessible. Acupoints are stimulated by acupressure or by acupuncture needles.

ACUTE Describes a disorder or symptom that comes on suddenly. See also CHRONIC.

AEROBIC Designed to increase oxygen uptake (when used in the context of vigorous exercise).

ALLERGEN An environmental or dietary irritant that triggers an allergic reaction in sensitive people.

ANAEROBIC Not designed to increase oxygen uptake (when used in the context of exercise such as lifting weights and performing stretches).

ANTIBODY Protein in the blood responsible for destroying invading substances that the body considers harmful.

ANTIFUNGAL Substances that destroy or inhibit fungal infections.

ANTIOXIDANTS Substances capable of neutralizing FREE RADICALS.

APPLIED KINESIOLOGY Detection of body system imbalances and food and environmental sensitivities by muscle-resistance testing.

ARACHIDONIC ACID Derivative of an essential fatty acid that produces substances causing inflammation.

ARGININE Amino acid essential for sperm formation. It appears to encourage the growth of the *herpes simplex* virus.

ASANA Physical posture adopted in yoga.

AUTOIMMUNE DISEASE Disorder in which the immune system fails to distinguish between substances that are "self" and those that are "non-self," and produces ANTIBODIES to attack the body's own tissues.

AUTONOMIC NERVOUS SYSTEM Part of the nervous system that controls body functions such as breathing and heart rate that are not under conscious control.

BACH FLOWER REMEDIES Infusions of plant materials in spring water, often taken to ease emotional problems.

BARIUM X-RAY Procedure to detect and monitor diseases of the gastrointestinal tract in which the element barium, opaque to X-rays, is either swallowed (barium meal)

or introduced into the lower intestine through the rectum (barium enema).

BIOPSY Removal of a small piece of living tissue for examination in a laboratory.

BODY CLOCK The system that regulates eating, sleeping, metabolism, and attention span. It is also known as the circadian rhythm because it is primarily set by sunlight and darkness.

BODY WORK Term used to describe manipulative therapies or techniques, such as massage.

CANDIDA Common but incorrect term for candidiasis, an overgrowth of *Candida albicans*, a yeastlike microorganism that occurs naturally in the mouth, gut, and vagina and on the skin, and which is normally controlled by "friendly" bacteria.

CENTRAL NERVOUS SYSTEM Brain and spinal cord; receives and analyzes information and initiates a response.

CHOLESTEROL Fatlike substance in the blood and most tissues. High levels in the blood can damage artery walls.

CHRONIC Term used for conditions of long duration and slow changes. It is the opposite of ACUTE.

COENZYME Q10 Made by the body, this ANTIOXIDANT nutrient (also known as ubiquinone) helps release energy from food. It is also available as a supplement.

COGNITIVE BEHAVIORAL THERAPY Form of psychotherapy pioneered in the 1960s and based on a belief in the ability of the mind to change negative patterns of thinking and behavior.

COLONOSCOPY Examination of the inside of the colon, the major part of the large intestine, by means of a flexible fiber-optic instrument called a colonoscope.

CT (COMPUTED TOMOGRAPHY) SCAN Diagnostic technique that uses X-rays and computers to produce a cross-section view of the tissue being examined.

CYTOTOXIC TEST Diagnostic technique in which damage to white blood cells when mixed with extracts of a possible ALLERGEN is said to suggest sensitivity.

DIURETIC Stimulates urine production.

DNA (DEOXYRIBONUCLEIC ACID) Principal molecule found in the cells of living organisms; carries the genetic information that controls all metabolic functions.

DYSBIOSIS Condition in which poorly

digested food in the gut encourages overgrowth of unfriendly gut bacteria.

ELECTROLYTE BALANCE Electrolytes, or body salts, are minerals present in body fluids and within cells that regulate water balance, blood acidity, nerve impulses, and muscle contraction. Diarrhea, vomiting, and certain drugs can upset the balance between various salts and cause problems.

ENDOCRINE SYSTEM Collection of hormone-producing glands in the body.

ENDORPHINS Morphinelike substances produced naturally by the body to relieve pain; known as the body's natural opiates.

ENDOSCOPY Examination of a body cavity by means of an endoscope, a tubelike viewing instrument used for diagnosis and treatment.

EPISIOTOMY Surgical procedure in which an incision is made in the perineum (tissue between the vagina and anus) to facilitate delivery of a baby.

FIGHT OR FLIGHT RESPONSE Physiological response to what the body sees as a threat. Chemicals are produced to make the body more efficient in either fighting or fleeing from the apparent danger.

FLAVONOIDS Chemicals with strong ANTIOXIDANT properties thought to help prevent certain forms of cancer. (Bio)flavonoids are found in fruits such as lemons, plums, and blueberries.

FREE RADICALS Potentially harmful molecules, produced naturally in the body, which can damage DNA and cause a range of physiological problems. They are linked to various health problems, including cancer and heart disease.

GESTALT THERAPY Method of psycho-therapy that helps clients gain self-awareness by analyzing their thoughts, feelings, and behavior in a variety of scenarios and situations.

HAIR ANALYSIS Diagnostic technique used by nutritional therapists and environmental medicine practitioners in which strands of hair are analyzed in a laboratory to assess deficiencies or excesses of minerals in the body that might contribute to illness.

HOLISTIC Term used to describe an approach to treatment in which the "whole" person is taken into account rather than just his or her symptoms.

177

HOMEOSTASIS Processes by which the body maintains a constant internal environment (*see pages 12–13*).

HRT (HORMONE REPLACEMENT THERAPY) Treatment of menopausal symptoms using hormones, often administered in the form of skin patches and/or pills, to counteract falling levels of estrogen.

HYPERVENTILATION Very deep or rapid breathing, usually caused by anxiety. It can lead to abnormal loss of carbon dioxide from the blood, the symptoms of which include numbness of hands and feet, faintness, muscle spasms and twitches, and feeling unable to breathe properly.

ILEOSTOMY Operation in which the lower part of the small intestine (ileum) is severed and the end brought through the abdominal wall to allow the discharge of feces into a bag attached to the skin.

IMMUNE SYSTEM Body organs responsible for resisting infection.

LYMPH Body fluid that contains lymphocytes (a type of white blood cell); has an important role in the IMMUNE SYSTEM, bathes all body tissues, and is circulated into the bloodstream.

LYSINE One of the eight essential amino acids, obtainable only from food. It is seen as instrumental in preventing and treating cold sores and herpes infections.

MERIDIANS Energy channels that are considered in Traditional Chinese Medicine to run up and down the body transporting *QI* (vital energy). Each meridian is related to a *YIN* or *YANG* organ.

METABOLISM General term for the chemical processes that take place in the body, governing all body functions.

MIND-BODY TECHNIQUES Approaches that harness thoughts, feelings, imagination, and actions in order to influence biochemical and structural processes.

MOXIBUSTION An acupuncture procedure in which the herb moxa (mugwort) is burned over acupoints to create heat.

MRI (MAGNETIC RESONANCE IMAGING) Diagnostic technique exposing body tissue to high-frequency radio waves; it is used particularly for examining the central nervous system.

NEBULIZER Device used to administer a drug in aerosol form through a mouthpiece or face mask.

NEEDLING Insertion and tweaking of acupuncture needles to stimulate ACUPOINTS.

NEUROTRANSMITTER Chemical released from nerve endings that transmits impulses to another nerve cell or to a muscle cell.

NITROSAMINES Substances formed when nitrites (chemicals used as meat preservatives) react with amines (nitrogen compounds in food); they have been shown to cause cancer in laboratory animals.

NOSODE Homeopathic remedy originally made from bodily secretions and now made from many body tissues.

PELVIC FLOOR EXERCISES Precise exercises that strengthen the muscles surrounding part of the vagina, rectum, and urethra.

PERISTALSIS Involuntary wavelike action of muscles in certain tubular structures of the body (for example, in the intestines) that causes the contents to move forward.

PHYTOESTROGENS Chemicals of plant origin that have an action similar to that of the female hormone estrogen; they are found in soybeans and other legumes.

PILATES A body-conditioning technique that increases flexibility and strength.

PLACEBO Chemically inert substance given in place of a drug; often used in scientific studies as a control.

PRANAYAMA Breathing techniques in yoga that aim to regulate *prana* ("vital life energy" in Ayurvedic medicine, akin to *QI*).

PREECLAMPSIA Serious condition in which high blood pressure, an accumulation of fluid in the tissues (edema), and protein in the urine develops in the second half of pregnancy.

PROBIOTICS "Friendly," disease-destroying bacteria in the digestive tract that aid the manufacture of vitamins and enzymes, improving digestion.

PROSTAGLANDIN Drug or naturally occurring substance within the body that has several actions, including causing muscle contractions and producing mucus in the stomach lining.

PULSE-TESTING Diagnostic technique that uses the pulse in the radial artery of the wrist. Western practitioners feel one pulse point to check the rate blood pumps from the heart. Traditional Chinese and Ayurvedic practitioners monitor nine pulse points, the strength of which are said to reflect the flow of "life energy."

QI "Life energy" force of Traditional Chinese Medicine that enters and can be accessed at ACUPOINTS on the body. It is said to be inherited at conception and is also derived from food and air.

RADIATION THERAPY The use of X-rays or other sources of radioactivity to treat cancer and occasionally other diseases.

REFERRED PAIN Sensation experienced as a result of spinal problems that can affect nerves and muscles linked to other parts of the body, causing pain in those areas.

SEROTONIN Substance found particularly in the blood, intestinal wall, and central nervous system that acts as a NEUROTRANSMITTER, relaying information across nerve endings.

SICK-BUILDING SYNDROME Condition in which symptoms such as fatigue, lack of concentration, and recurrent infections are attributed to poor ventilation and chemical fumes from furnishings and office machines.

SIGMOIDOSCOPY Examination of the rectum and lower parts of the large intestine (sigmoid colon) with a viewing instrument called a sigmoidoscope.

TENS (TRANSCUTANEOUS ELECTRICAL NERVE STIMULATION) Stimulation of body tissue with pulses of low-voltage electricity; used for pain relief.

TRANS-FATTY ACIDS Fats occurring naturally in meat and dairy products and artificially in foods such as margarine, where edible oils are treated to become solid (hydrogenation). Research links artificial trans-fatty acids to heart disease.

TRIGGER POINTS Areas of muscle tension caused by pain from the spine and connected tissue; they feel like hard nodules when pressed.

ULTRASOUND Sound with a frequency higher than the range of the human ear, used to scan internal organs and the fetus in the womb, and to treat soft-tissue injuries.

UVA LIGHT Natural or artificial light containing ultraviolet wavelengths; its antiviral, antifungal, and antibacterial properties make it effective in the treatment of psoriasis and other skin problems.

VEGAN Person who eats only foods of plant origin.

VEGA-TESTING Diagnostic technique in which a machine measures electrical resistance at various points on the body to homeopathic dilutions of suspect substances.

YIN and **YANG** Opposing but complementary energies in Traditional Chinese Medicine; all things are said to be a manifestation of *yin* or of *yang*.

DRUGS GLOSSARY

ACE INHBITORS Powerful VASODILATORS that block an enzyme involved in blood vessel constriction; often prescribed for angina and high blood pressure.

ACETAMINOPHEN A nonopioid analgesic that does not cause stomach upset or bleeding, but can damage the liver and kidneys if taken in overdose.

ACYCLOVIR Antiviral for herpes infections.

ALBUTEROL A bronchodilator used to treat asthma, bronchitis, and emphysema.

ALPHA BLOCKERS Relieve urinary retention by relaxing the muscle of the sphincter.

ALPROSTADIL A PROSTAGLANDIN used to treat male impotence.

AMITRIPTYLINE A tricyclic ANTIDEPRESSANT used to improve mood, activity levels, and encourage sleep in long-term depression.

ANALGESICS Drugs that relieve pain.

ANTACIDS Mildly alkaline compounds that neutralize excess stomach acid.

ANTIBIOTICS Bacteria-destroying drugs used to treat bacterial infections. Broad-spectrum antibiotics such as penicillins and tetracyclines can treat many common infections but increasing bacterial resistance is limiting their use.

ANTICONVULSANTS Inhibit excessive electrical activity in the brain. They are used to prevent and stop epileptic fits.

ANTIDEPRESSANTS Drugs used to treat moderate to severe depression.

ANTIFUNGALS Drugs used to treat fungal infections, particularly of the skin, mouth, throat, and vagina.

ANTIHISTAMINES Drugs that counter the effects of histamine, a chemical released in the body during an allergic reaction.

ANTIHYPERTENSIVES Drugs used to reduce high blood pressure.

ANTI-INFLAMMATORIES Drugs to relieve inflammation; the two major groups are NONSTEROIDAL ANTI-INFLAMMATORY DRUGS (NSAIDS) and CORTICOSTEROIDS.

ANTIRHEUMATICS Drugs used to treat various rheumatic disorders, most commonly rheumatoid arthritis.

ASPIRIN An ANALGESIC and NSAID, used to relieve pain, reduce fever, and alleviate arthritis symptoms. In low doses, it helps prevent blood clots in people with coronary artery disease and reduces the chance of heart attacks and strokes.

AZT Also known as Zidovudine, an antiviral drug used to treat AIDS.

BARBITURATES Sleep-inducing drugs. Rarely used because of risk of dependence and overdose.

BENZODIAZEPINES Antianxiety drugs that reduce excessive activity in the part of the brain that controls emotion.

BENZOYL PEROXIDE A topical preparation that treats acne and fungal skin infections by removing the top layer of skin and unblocking sebaceous glands.

BETA BLOCKERS Blocks norepinephrine, the main "fight or flight" hormone, reducing heart rate and preventing dilation of blood vessels. Used mainly for heart disorders, but also for migraine, anxiety, overactive thyroid, and glaucoma.

BIPHOSPHONATES A group of drugs (such as Etidronate) that treats bone disorders such as osteoporosis.

BROMOCRIPTINE Inhibits excessive secretion of the hormone prolactin. It can be used to treat female infertility and to relieve symptoms of Parkinson's disease.

CALCIUM CHANNEL BLOCKERS Help blood vessels dilate by preventing the movement of calcium in muscles that make the vessels contract. Treats angina, abnormal heart rhythm, and high blood pressure.

CHLOROQUINE Antimalarial and antirheumatic drug.

CLOMIPHENE Drug used to treat infertility by increasing the output of pituitary gland hormones that stimulate ovulation.

CLOTRIMAZOLE An ANTIFUNGAL drug.

CORTICOSTEROIDS Often referred to as steroids, these are used to control inflammation (for example, in eczema, inflammatory bowel disease, rheumatoid arthritis), and for conditions caused by deficiency of adrenal gland hormones.

CYCLOSPORIN Immunosuppressant drug used to treat severe cases of psoriasis.

DIFLORASONE Treats psoriasis by reducing inflammation.

DOMPERIDONE An antiemetic used for treating nausea caused by gastrointestinal disorders such as gastroenteritis.

ERGOTAMINE A vasoconstrictor used to treat headaches and migraine.

ERYTHROMYCIN Broad-spectrum ANTIBIOTIC.

FINASTERIDE An enzyme inhibitor used to treat benign prostatic enlargement.

FLUCONAZOLE An ANTIFUNGAL drug.

GONADOTROPIN Human chorionic gonadotropin (HCG), a hormone produced by the placenta and extracted from the urine of pregnant women; used to treat infertility by stimulating the ovaries to produce estrogen and progesterone.

H2 BLOCKERS Antiulcer drugs (such as Cimetidine, Ranitidine) that help healing by preventing the release of histamine in the stomach, so reducing acid production.

HYDROCORTISONE A CORTICOSTEROID identical to the hormone cortisol produced by the adrenal glands.

IBUPROFEN An ANALGESIC and NSAID similar to ASPIRIN but less likely to cause bleeding in the stomach.

IDOXURIDINE Antiviral drug commonly used to treat herpes infections.

INDOMETHACIN An NSAID used to treat arthritic conditions, including gout.

LITHIUM A metallic element used to treat manic and severe depression.

MEFENAMIC ACID A NONSTEROIDAL ANTI-INFLAMMATORY DRUG.

MESALAZINE Drug used to treat ulcerative colitis and sometimes Crohn's disease by relieving inflammation in the large intestine.

METHOTREXATE Cancer-therapy drug that inhibits the metabolic functioning of cells. It is also used to treat psoriasis.

MONOAMINE OXIDASE INHIBITORS (MAOIS) Antidepressant drugs that increase levels of serotonin and other mood-enhancing brain chemicals; they are quite effective for people with anxiety and phobias.

MONTELUKAST Prevents and treats asthma by preventing contraction of the airways. Brand name: Singulair.

NONSTEROIDAL ANTI-INFLAMMATORY DRUGS (NSAIDS) A group of drugs used to relieve pain, stiffness, and painful inflammation affecting the muscles, bones, and joints.

NOREPINEPHRINE REUPTAKE INHIBITORS Antidepressants that increase levels of norepinephrine, a chemical affecting mood.

NORATRIPTAN A serotonin-inhibiting drug used to treat headaches and migraine.

NYSTATIN An ANTIFUNGAL drug.

OPIOIDS A group of drugs (also known as narcotics) that relieve pain, treat diarrhea, and suppress coughs. Codeine (in over-the-counter preparations) is a mild opioid.

PROGESTOGEN Synthetic form of the female sex hormone, progesterone.

PROTEASE INHIBITORS Drugs that treat HIV by preventing formation of HIV proteins.

PROZAC Brand name for fluoxetine, one of the SSRIs (selective serotonin reuptake inhibitors), a group of antidepressants that boost levels of serotonin, the mood-enhancing brain chemical.

RANITIDINE An antiulcer drug. Brand name: Zantac.

RETINOIC ACID A form of vitamin A.

SALMETEROL One of a group of broncho-dilator drugs used to treat asthma and bronchitis by relaxing the muscles around the bronchioles (narrow lung airways).

SERMS (Selective Estrogen Receptor Modulators) A form of HRT that mimics estrogen's effects in some parts of the body but blocks it in others.

SILDENAFIL A drug to treat erectile dysfunction (impotence) by increasing blood flow to the penis to establish and maintain erection. Brand name: Viagra.

SODIUM CROMOGLYCATE An antiallergy drug that prevents the release of histamine; inhaled to prevent asthma attacks.

STATINS Drugs that lower blood cholesterol, used to prevent stroke and heart atttack.

SUMATRIPTAN A serotonin-inhibiting drug used to treat headaches and migraine.

SULFASALAZINE Treats symptoms of ulcerative colitis, Crohn's disease, and rheumatoid arthritis.

TETRACYCLINE Broad-spectrum ANTIBIOTIC used to treat chlamydia and nonspecific urethritis.

TRANQUILIZERS Sedative drugs. Minor tranquilizers, such as benzodiazepines, are given in short courses to treat anxiety without risking dependence. Major tranquilizers control psychotic symptoms.

TRICYCLICS A group of antidepressant drugs (such as Amitriptyline) that raise levels of serotonin and norepinephrine, brain chemicals involved in mood.

VASODILATORS Widen blood vessels; used to treat angina and high blood pressure.

ZOLMITRIPTAN A serotonin-inhibiting drug used to treat headaches and migraines.

FINDING A PRACTITIONER

BEING ABLE TO TRUST YOUR PRACTITIONER and feeling a sense of rapport with him or her are vital factors in the healing process and should be considered when looking for a complementary practitioner. Competence is another key factor. Since finding a good practitioner can be a matter of trial and error, many people prefer word-of-mouth recommendations.

Establishing adequate standards of training, ethical practice, and disciplinary procedures for complementary therapies has always been a problem. While some practitioners complete 3–4 years of full- or part-time degree studies, others operate on the basis of a weekend correspondence course.

This lack of regulation means you have little means of redress if anything goes wrong or you are dissatisfied. At the very least, you need to feel confident that your practitioner would be able to recognize any undiagnosed serious condition and would advise you to seek medical help if the problem appeared to lie beyond his or her expertise.

If you are considering chiropractic, osteopathy, acupuncture, psychotherapy, counseling, or hypnotherapy, it is worth asking your doctor if he or she can recommend a practitioner, since these therapies are becoming more accepted in mainstream medicine. Some conventional health professionals may also be qualified practitioners of acupuncture or homeopathy.

If you are choosing a complementary practitioner for yourself, you should consider the following issues:

TRAINING AND CREDENTIALS
Always be sure that the practitioner is adequately trained and reputable, especially if the therapy involves the use of either physical manipulation or invasive techniques (for example, if you swallow medication or have needles inserted into you); these procedures can be harmful. Ask the following questions:
• What are the practitioner's qualifications?
• What sort of training was undertaken, and for how long?
• Is the practitioner licensed in your state (if appropriate)?

• For how many years has the practitioner been in practice?
• Does the practitioner advise your doctor of any treatment?

PROFESSIONAL ORGANIZATIONS
Some disciplines have professional associations to regulate training, provide a code of conduct, and maintain a register of members. For others, particularly noninvasive therapies, standards vary greatly and there may be more than one representative body. You should ask the following questions:
• Is the practitioner registered with a recognized organization, and does this organization have a public register of practitioners?
• Does the organization have a code of practice specifying the professional conduct required?
• Does the organization have a grievance system, and an effective disciplinary procedure and sanctions?
• Can the practitioner give you the address and telephone number of the organization?

FINANCIAL CONSIDERATIONS
• Is treatment available at little or no personal cost on referral by your doctor? Some therapies, such as chiropractic, osteopathy, homeopathy, acupuncture, and psychotherapy, may be available through a limited number of mainstream health practices.
• Can you claim for the treatment through your health insurance plan, if you have one?
• What is the cost (both short- and long-term) of treatment?
• How many treatments might you require?
• Does the practitioner have malpractice insurance so that you receive compensation if he or she is negligent?

PRECAUTIONS
Avoid any practitioner you feel uncomfortable with. Trust and empathy are important, and treatment is unlikely to succeed without them. Treatment is often conducted on a one-to-one

basis, and may involve removing clothes and being touched. Also avoid any practitioner who seems to be making excessive claims about the treatment or who guarantees a cure. No form of treatment – either conventional or complementary – is perfect, and miracles should be neither expected nor promised. After your initial consultation, ask yourself the following questions:
• Was the practitioner's conduct entirely professional?
• Did the practitioner answer any questions clearly and thoroughly?
• Were you given information to read on your own time?
• What was the practitioner's attitude toward any conventional medicine you may be receiving? Avoid any practitioner who suggests changing your conventional medicine without first consulting your doctor.

FINDING OUT MORE

KNOWING WHERE TO GO FOR INFORMATION and help enables you to become more actively involved in your own health care. When you understand the causes of illness, the meaning of symptoms, and what treatment options are available, you may feel more in control of your well-being; this is therapeutic in itself.

Good information is not always easy to find, but the following sources are good starting points:

ONLINE SITES

Although the Web is brimming with advice on health matters, much of it can be ill-informed, biased, or downright wrong. This is especially true of interactive sites. If you ask an "expert" a health question, make sure you check the expert's credentials or know how much privacy you can expect. Be suspicious of "miracle cures" and note any sponsorship or advertising deals that could indicate a conflict of interest.

The following are reputable medical sites that provide reliable information and links to related sites, including complementary medicine.

www.healthfinder.gov/
Developed by the US Department of Health and Human Services, it directs visitors to selected online publications, databases, websites, and support and self-help groups.
www.omni.ac.uk
Organizing Medical Networked Information, from Nottingham University, is the nearest UK equivalent to healthfinder, though mostly aimed at medical professionals.
www.intelihealth.com
Includes advice on self-care and diagnoses, as well as drug and research databases.
www.nlm.nih.gov
Basic information and up-to-date research from the US National Library of Medicine.
www.ncbi.nlm.nih.gov/pubmed
Medline is the world's largest database of medical papers at the US National Library of Medicine.
www.ama-assn.org
The American Medical Association site includes a consumer-health area.
www.oncolink.upenn.edu
The University of Pennsylvania's online site provides information on all types of cancer.
cancernet.nci.nih.gov
Current information on cancer, sponsored by the US National Cancer Institute.
www.patient.co.uk
UK patient information and links to relevant organizations and support groups.
www.altmedicine.com
Alternative Health News Online covers major topics and offers links to other sources of information.
www.hon.ch
Internationally selected guidelines for responsible medical and health information on the Internet.
www.nhsdirect.nhs.uk
Health information and advice from the UK National Health Service.

BOOKS

The following books provide basic information to enable an understanding of the structural, biochemical, and psychosocial approach to integrative health care:
Benson, H. & Stuart, E. *The Wellness Book* (Fireside, Simon & Schuster, 1992)
Benson, H. *Timeless Healing: the Power and Biology of Belief* (Scribner, 1996)
Chevallier, A. *Encyclopedia of Medicinal Plants* (Dorling Kindersley, 1996)
Daniel, R. *Healing Foods: How to Nurture Yourself and Fight Illness* (Thorsons, 1996)
Gawain, S. *Creative Visualization* (Bantam, 1982)
Goleman, D. *Emotional Intelligence* (Bantam, 1995)
Goleman, D. & Gurin, J. *Mind/Body Medicine* (Consumer Reports Books, 1993)
Kabat-Zinn, J. *Full Catastrophe Living* (Piatkus, 1996)
LeShan, L. *How to Meditate* (Thorsons, 1995)
Lockie, A. & Geddes, N. *Complete Guide to Homeopathy* (Dorling Kindersley, 1995)
Maxwell-Hudson, C. *The Complete Book of Massage* (Dorling Kindersley, 1988)
Moyers, B. *Healing and the Mind* (Doubleday, 1993)
Nagarathna, R., Nagendra, H.R., & Monro, R. *Yoga for Common Ailments* (Gaia, 1990)
Ornish, D. *Dr Dean Ornish's Program for Reversing Heart Disease* (Ballantine Books, 1990)
Reader's Digest *Foods that Harm, Foods that Heal* (Reader's Digest Association, 1996)
Smith, T. (ed.), *The British Medical Association Complete Family Health Encyclopedia* (Dorling Kindersley, 1995)
Tanner, J. *Beating Back Pain* (Dorling Kindersley, 1987)
Williams, R. & Williams, V. *Anger Kills* (Times Books, 1993)
Woodham, A. & Peters, D. *Encyclopedia of Healing Therapies* (Dorling Kindersley, 1997).

BIBLIOGRAPHY

Therapies: Evidence of Efficacy
In *Treating Ailments (see pages 24–111)*, the efficacy of each therapy for a particular ailment is rated 1–5 based on the available research.
Key to Ratings:
1 *Rumored to be effective* (traditionally used but efficacy doubted; no research)
2 *Effective in practitioners' opinion* (practitioners are convinced, but no reliable research studies)
3 *Possibly effective* (some research, but results are inconclusive or conflict)
4 *Probably effective* (positive evidence from randomized and/or controlled trials)
5 *Definitely effective* (good evidence available from several sound randomized controlled trials or a meta-analysis – *see page 176*)

HEADACHES
Chiropractic Boline P.D. *et al.* "Spinal manipulation vs. amitriptyline for the treatment of chronic tension-type headaches: a randomized clinical trial" *J. of Manipulative Physical Therapy* 1995, 18(3):148–54
Osteopathy Schoensee S.K. *et al.* "The effect of mobilization on cervical headaches" *J. of Orthopaedic & Sports Physical Therapy* 1995, 21(4):184–96
Visualization Blanchard E.B. *et al.* "The role of regular home practice in the relaxation treatment of tension headache" *J. of Consulting & Clinical Psychology* 1991, 59(3):467–70
Biofeedback Zitman F.G. "Hypnosis and autogenic training in the treatment of tension headaches: a two-phase constructive design study with follow-up" *J. of Psychosomatic Research* 1992, 36(3):219–28
Kuile M.M. *et al.* "Autogenic training and cognitive self-hypnosis for the treatment of recurrent headaches in three different subject groups" *Pain* 1994, 58(3):331–40
Therapeutic Touch Keller E., Bzdek V.M. "Effects of therapeutic touch on tension headache pain" *Nursing Research* 1986, 35(2):101–105
Hypnotherapy Melis P.M. *et al.* "Treatment of chronic tension-type headache with hypnotherapy: a single-blind time-controlled study" *Headache* 1991, (10):686–89

MIGRAINE
Nutritional Therapies Mansfield L.E. *et al.* "Food allergy and adult migraine: double-blind and mediator confirmation of an allergic etiology" *Annals of Allergy* 1985, 55:126–29
Western Herbalism Murphy J.J. "Randomised double-blind placebo-controlled trial of feverfew in migraine prevention" *Lancet* 1988, 2(8604):189–92
Chiropractic Parker G.B. *et al.* "A controlled trial of cervical manipulation for migraine" *Australian and New Zealand J. of Medicine* 1978, 8(6): 589–93
Acupuncture Tavola T. *et al.* "Traditional Chinese acupuncture in tension-type headache: a controlled study" *Pain* 1992, 48(3): 325–29
Vincent C.A. "A controlled trial of the treatment of migraine by acupuncture" *Clinical*

J. of Pain 1989, 5(4): 305–12
Hypnotherapy Olness K. "Comparison of self-hypnosis and propranolol in the treatment of juvenile classic migraine" *Pediatrics* 1987, 79(4): 593–97
Biofeedback Blanchard E.B., Andrasik F. "Biofeedback treatment of vascular headache" in *Biofeedback: Studies in Clinical Efficacy* ed. Hatch, J.P. *et al.*(1987, Plenum, New York) 1–79
Relaxation & Breathing Sorbi M. *et al.* "Long-term effects of training in relaxation and stress-coping in patients with migraine: a 3-year follow-up" *Headache* 1989, 29(2): 111–21

ACNE
Aromatherapy Bassett I.B. *et al.* "A comparative study of tea-tree oil versus benzoyl peroxide in the treatment of acne" *Medical J. of Australia* 1990, 153: 455–58

PSORIASIS
Western Herbalism Gieler U. *et al.* *J. of Dermatological Treatment* 1995, 6: 31–34
Wiesenauer M., *et al.* *Phytomedicine* 1996, (3) 231–35
Galle K. *et al.* *Phytomedicine* 1994 (1) 59–62
Syed T.A. *et al.* "Management of psoriasis with aloe vera extract in a hydrophilic cream: a placebo-controlled, double-blind study" *Tropical Medicine and International Health* 1996, 1:505–509
Biofeedback Winchell S.A. *et al.* "Relaxation therapies in the treatment of psoriasis and possible pathophysiologic mechanisms" *American J.of Academic Dermatology* 1988, 18:101–104

ECZEMA
Traditional Chinese Medicine Atherton D.J. *et al.* "Treatment of atopic eczema with traditional Chinese medicinal plants" *Pediatric Dermatology* 1992, 9:373–75
Sheehan M.P. *et al.* "Efficacy of traditional Chinese herbal therapy in adult atopic dermatitis" *Lancet* 1992, 340:13–17
Nutritional Therapies Soyland E. *et al.* "Dietary supplements with very long-chain-3 fatty acids in patients with atopic dermatitis: a double-blind, multicentre study" *British J. of Dermatology* 1994, 130:757–64
Sampson H.A. "Role of immediate food hypersensitivity in the pathogeneses of atopic dermatitis" *J. of Allergy & Clinical Immunology* 1983, 71:473–80
Hypnotherapy Ehlers A. *et al.* "Treatment of atopic dermatitis: comparison of psychological and dermatological approaches to relapse prevention" *J. of Consulting & Clinical Psychology* 1995, 63(4):624–35

HERPES
Western Herbalism Wolbling R.H., Leonhardt K. "Local therapy of herpes simplex with dried extract from *Melissa officinalis*" *Phytomed* 1994, 1:25–31
Visualization Kiecolt-Glaser J.K. *et al.* "Psychosocial enhancement of immunocompetence in a geriatric population"

Health Psychology 1985, 4(1):25–41
COLDS & FLU
Traditional Chinese Medicine Kong X.T. *et al.* "Treatment of acute bronchiolitis with Chinese herbs" *Archives of Disease in Childhood* 1993, 68:468–71
Naturopathy Mossad S.B. *et al.* "Zinc gluconate lozenges for treating the common cold. A randomized double-blind placebo-controlled study" *Annals of Internal Medicine* 1996, 125:81–88
Ernst E. *et al.* "Regular sauna bathing and the incidence of common colds" *Annals of Medicine* 1990, 22:225–27
Western Herbalism Melchart D. *et al.* "Echinacea root extracts for the prevention of upper respiratory tract infections" *Archives of Family Medicine* 1998, 7:541–45
Zakay Rones Z. *et al.* "Inhibition of several strains of influenza virus *in vitro* and reduction of symptoms by an elderberry extract (*Sambucus nigra L.*) during an outbreak of influenza B in Panama" *J. of Alternative & Complementary Medicine* 1995, 1:361–69
Homeopathy Ferley J.P. *et al.* "A controlled evaluation of a homoeopathic preparation in the treatment of influenza-like syndromes" *British J. of Clinical Pharmacology* 1989, 27(3):329–35
Papp R. *et al.* "Oscillococcinum in patients with influenza-like syndromes: a placebo-controlled double-blind evaluation" *British Homeopathic J.* 1998, 87:69–76
Aromatherapy Saller R. *et al.* "Dose dependency of symptomatic relief of complaints by chamomile steam inhalation in patients with common cold" *European J. of Pharmacology* 1990, 183:728–29

IRRITABLE BOWEL SYNDROME
Naturopathy Nanda R. *et al.* "Food intolerance and the irritable bowel syndrome" *Gut* 1989, 30(8):1099–104
Western Herbalism Lech Y. *et al.* "Treatment of irritable bowel syndrome with peppermint oil: a double-blind study with a placebo" *Ugeskrift For Laeger* 1988, 150(40):2388–89
Psychotherapy & Counseling Read N. "The role of psychological and biological factors in postinfective gut dysfunction" *Gut* 1999, 44:400–406
Hypnotherapy Whorwell P.J. *et al.* "Hypnotherapy in severe irritable bowel syndrome: a further experience" *Gut* 1987, 28(4):423–25

INFLAMMATORY BOWEL DISEASE
Nutritional Therapies Riordan A.M. *et al.* "Treatment of active Crohn's disease by exclusion diet: East Anglian multicentre controlled trial" *Lancet* 1993, 342:1131–34
Beluzzi A. *et al.* "Effect of an enteric-coated fish-oil preparation on relapses in Crohn's disease" *New England J. of Medicine* 1996, 334:1557–60
Loescheke K. *et al.* "n-3 fatty acids only delay early relapse of ulcerative colitis in remission" *Digestive Diseases & Sciences* 1996, 41:2087–94

Massage Joachim G. "The effects of two forms of stress-management techniques on feelings of well-being in patients with inflammatory bowel disease" *Nursing Papers* 1983, 15:(5)18
Biofeedback Marzyk P.M. "Biofeedback for gastrointestinal disorders: a review of the literature" *Annals of Internal Medicine* 1985, 103:240–44
Milne B. *et al.* "A stress-management programme for inflammatory bowel disease patients" *J. of Advanced Nursing* 1986, 11(5):561–67

HIGH BLOOD PRESSURE
Nutritional Therapies Witteman J.C.M. *et al.* "Reduction of blood pressure with oral magnesium supplementation in women with mild to moderate hypertension" *American J. of Clinical Nutrition* 1994, 60:129–35
Margetts B.M. *et al.* "A randomized control trial of a vegetarian diet in the treatment of mild hypertension" *Clinical and Experimental Pharmacology and Physiology* 1985, 12(3):263–66
Auer W. *et al.* "Hypertension and hyperlipidaemia: garlic helps in mild cases" *British J. of Clinical Practice* 1990; (supplement 69):3–6
T'ai Chi Jin P. "Efficacy of T'ai Chi, brisk walking, meditation and reading in reducing mental and emotional stress" *J. of Psychosomatic Research* 1992, 36(4):361–70
Meditation Patel C. *et al.* "Controlled trial of biofeedback-aided behavioural methods in reducing mild hypertension" *British Medical J.* 1981, 282:2005–08; 2081–122
Biofeedback Glasgow M.S., Engel B.T. "Biofeedback and relaxation therapy" in *Biofeedback: Studies in Clinical Efficacy*, ed. JP Hatch, *et al.* (Plenum 1987, New York)
Relaxation & Breathing Eisenberg D.M. *et al.* "Cognitive behavioral techniques for hypertension: are they effective?" *Annals of Internal Medicine* 1993, 118(12):964–72

HEART DISEASE
Naturopathy Ornish D. *et al.* "Can lifestyle changes reverse coronary heart disease? The Lifestyle Heart Trial" *Lancet* 1990, 336(8708):129–33
Nutritional Therapies Azen S.P., *et al.* "Effect of supplementary antioxidant vitamin intake on carotid arterial wall intima-media thickness in a controlled clinical trial of cholesterol lowering" *Circulation* 1996, 94(10):2369–72
Kushi L. *et al.* "Diet and 20 year mortality from coronary heart disease" *New England J. of Medicine* 1985, 312(13)811–18
T'ai Chi Lai J.S. *et al.* "Two-year trends in cardiorespiratory function among older Tai Chi practitioners and sedentary subjects" *J. of the American Geriatrics Society* 1995, 43(11):1222–7
Osteopathy Morgan J.P. *et al.* "A controlled trial of spinal manipulation in the management of hypertension" *American Osteopathic Association* 1985, 85(5):308–13
Acupuncture Ballegaard S. "Acupuncture in severe, stable *angina pectoris*: a randomized trial" *Actor Medica Scandinavia* 1986; 220(4):307–13
Massage Bauer W.C. *et al.* "Effects of back massage in patients with acute myocardial infraction" *Focus on Critical Care* 1987, 14(6):42–46

Aromatherapy Stevenson C. "The psycho-physiological effects of aromatherapy massage following cardiac surgery" *Complementary Therapies in Medicine* 1994, 2(1):27–35
Psychotherapy & Counseling Linden W. *et al.* "Psychosocial interventions for patients with coronary artery disease: a meta-analysis" *Archives of Internal Medicine* 1996, 156(7):745–52
Visualization Elliott D. "The effects of music and muscle relaxation on patient anxiety in a coronary care unit" *Heart & Lung* 1994, 23(7):27–35
Meditation (*see* High Blood Pressure)

BACK & NECK PAIN
(**Homeopathy, Massage** *see* **Muscle Pain**)
Rolfing Cottingham J.T. *et al.* "Shifts in pelvic inclination angle and parasympathetic tone produced by Rolfing soft tissue manipulation" *Physical Therapy* 1988, 68(9):1364–70
Chiropractic Meade T.W. "Low back pain of mechanical origin: randomised comparison of chiropractic and hospital outpatient treatment" *British Medical J.* 1990, 2;300(6737):1431–37
Meade T.W. *et al.* "Randomised comparison of chiropractic and hospital outpatient management for low back pain: results from extended follow up" *British Medical J.* 1995, 311(7001):349–51
Osteopathy Shekelle P.G. *et al.* "Spinal manipulation for low-back pain" *Annals of International Medicine* 1992, 117(7):590–98
Koes B.W. *et al.* "Spinal manipulation and mobilisation for back and neck pain: a blinded review" *British Medical J.* 1991, 303:1298–303
Acupuncture White A.R., Ernst E. "A systematic review of randomized controlled trials of acupuncture for neck pain" *Rheumatology* 1999, 38:143–47
Ernst. E, White A.R. "Acupuncture for back pain: a meta-analysis of randomized controlled trials" *Archives of International Medicine* 1998, 158:2235–41

OSTEOARTHRITIS
Western Herbalism McCarthy G.M. *et al.* "Effect of topical capsaicin in the therapy of painful osteoarthritis of the hands" *J. of Rheumatology* 1992, 19:604–607
Nutritional Therapies Vaz A. "Double blind clinical evaluation of relative efficiency of ibuprofen and glucosamine sulfate in management of osteoarthrosis of the knee in outpatients" *Current Medical Research Opinion*, 1982, 8:145
Travers R. *et al.* "Boron and arthritis – a double-blind pilot study" *J. of Nutritional Medicine* 1990, 1:127–132
(**Osteopathy** *see* Back Pain)
Yoga Garfinkel M.S. *et al.* "Evaluation of a yoga-based regimen for treatment of osteoarthritis of the hands" *J. of Rheumatology* 1994, 21(12):2341–43
Acupuncture Ernst E. "Acupuncture as a treatment of osteoarthritis: a systematic view" *Scandinavian J. of Rheumatology* 1997, 26:444–47

RHEUMATOID ARTHRITIS
Nutritional Therapies
Kjeldsen-Kragh J. *et al.* "Vegetarian diet for patients with rheumatoid arthritis: two years after introduction of the diet" *Clinical*

Rheumatology 1994, 13(3):475–82
Van de Laar M.A. *et al.* "Food intolerance in rheumatoid arthritis: a double-blind, controlled trial of the clinical effects of the elimination of milk allergens and azo dyes" *Annals of Rheumatic Disease* 1992, 51(3): 298–302
Fortin P.R. *et al.* "Validation of a meta-analysis: the effects of fish oil in rheumatoid arthritis" *J. of Clinical Epidemiology* 1995, 48:1379–90
Gibson *et al.* *British Clinical J. of Pharmacology* 1978, 6:391–95
Massage, Acupuncture (*see* **Muscle Pain**)
T'ai Chi Kirsteins A.E. *et al.* "Evaluating the safety and potential use of a weight-bearing exercise, Tai-Chi Chu'an, for rheumatoid arthritis patients" *American J. Physical Medicine and Rehabilitation* 1991, 70(3):136–41
Psychotherapy & Counseling Bradley L.A. *et al.* "Effects of psychological therapy on pain behaviour of rheumatoid arthritis patients: treatment outcome and six-month follow up" *Arthritis and Rheumatism* 1987, 30:1105–14
O'Leary A. *et al.* "A cognitive-behavioral treatment for rheumatoid arthritis" *Health Psychology* 1988, 7:527–44

PERSISTENT MUSCLE PAIN
Homeopathy Fisher P. *et al.* "Effect of homeopathy on fibrositis (primary fibromyalgia)" *British Medical J.* 1989; 299:365–66
Massage Danneskiold-Samsoe B. *et al.* "Myofascial pain and the role of myoglobulin" *Scandanavian J. of Rheumatism* 1986, 15:175–78
Acupuncture Sprott H. *et al.* *Rheumatology International* 1998, 18:35–36
Hypnotherapy Haanen H.C.M. *et al.* "Controlled trial of hypnotherapy in the treatment of refractory fibromyalgia" *J. of Rheumatology* 1991, 18(1):72–75
Meditation Kaplan K.H. *et al.* "The impact of a meditation-based stress reduction program on fibromyalgia" *General Hospital Psychiatry* 1993, 15(5):284–89

SPORTS INJURIES
Western Herbalism Cichoke A. "The use of proteolytic enzymes with soft tissue athletic injuries" *American Chiropractor* October 1981, 32
Nutritional Therapies Moncada S. *et al.* "Leucocytes and tissue injury: The use of eicosapentenoic acid in the control of white cell activation" *Wien Klinische Wochenschrift* 1986, 98(4):104–106
Homeopathy Bohmer D., *et al.* "Treating sports injuries with Traumeel ointment: a controlled double-blind study" *Biological Medizin* 1992, 21(4):260–68
Chiropractic & Osteopathy (*see* **Back Pain**)
Massage Smith L.L. *et al.* "The effects of athletic massage on delayed-onset muscle soreness, creatine kinase, and neutrophil count: a preliminary report" *Journal of Orthopaedic & Sports Physical Therapy* 1994, 19(2):93–99
Acupuncture Haker E. *et al.* "Acupuncture treatment in epicondylalgia: a comparative study of two acupuncture techniques" *Clinical J. of Pain* 1990 6(3):221–26
Hypnotherapy Achterberg J. *et al.* "Behavioural strategies for the reduction of pain and anxiety associated with acute orthopoedic trauma" *Biofeedback and Self-regulation* 1989, 14(2):101–14

BIBLIOGRAPHY

PREMENSTRUAL SYNDROME
Western Herbalism Dittmar "Premenstrual syndrome: treatment with a phytopharmaceutical" *Therapiewoche Gynakol* 1994, 7:49–52
Nutritional Therapies Abraham G.E. "Nutritional factors in the etiology of the premenstrual tension syndromes" *J. of Reproductive Medicine* 1983, 28: 446–64
Faccinetti F. *et al.* "Magnesium prophylaxis of menstrual migraine: effects on intracellular magnesium" *Headache* 1991, 321:298–301
London R. "Effect of nutritional supplement on PMS symptomatology in women with PMS – a double-blind longitudinal study" *J. American College of Nutrition* 1991, 10(5)494–99
Reflexology Oleson T., Flocco W. "Randomized controlled study of premenstrual symptoms treated with ear, hand, and foot reflexology" *Obstetrics & Gynecology* 1993, 82(6):906–11

MENSTRUAL PAIN
Chiropractic & Osteopathy Kokjohn K. *et al.* "The effect of spinal manipulation on pain and prostaglandin levels in women with primary dysmenorrhea" *J. of Manipulative and Physiological Therapeutics* 1992, 15(5):279–85
Boesler D. *et al.* "Efficacy of high-velocity low-amplitude manipulative technique in subjects with low-back pain during menstrual cramping" *J. of the American Osteopathic Association* 1993, 93(2):203–208, 213–14
Acupuncture Helms J.M. "Acupuncture for the management of primary dysmenorrhea" *Obstetrics and Gynaecology* 1987, 69(1):51–56

INFERTILITY IN WOMEN
Hypnotherapy Quinn P.D.R., Pawson M. "Conceptions of the mind; the role of hypnotherapy interventions in medically unexplained, functional and psychosomatic infertility" *European J. of Clinical Hypnosis* 1994, 1(4)

PREGNANCY
Western Herbalism Fischer-Rasmussen W. *et al.* "Ginger treatment of hyperemesis gravidarum" *European J. of Obstetrics and Gynaecology and Reproductive Biology* 1990, 38:19–24
Nutritional Therapies Zatuchni G.I., *et al.* "Bromelain therapy for the prevention of episiotomy pain" *Obstetrics and Gynecology* 1967, 29(2):275–78
Chiropractic and **Osteopathy** (*see* Back Pain)
Acupuncture De Aloysio D., Penacchioni P. "Morning sickness control in early pregnancy by Neiguan point acupressure" *Obstetrics and Gynecology* 1992, 80:852–54
Cardini F. *et al.* "Moxibustion for correction of breech presentation: a randomised controlled trial" *J. of the American Medical Association* 1998, 280:1580–84
Visualization Feher S.D.K. *et al.* "Increasing breast-milk production for premature infants with a relaxation/imagery audiotape" *Pediatrics* 1989, 83(1):57–60

MENOPAUSE
Western Herbalism Linde K. *et al.* "St John's wort for depression: an overview and meta-analysis of randomised clinical trials" *British Medical J.* 1996, 313:253–58

Nutritional Therapies Adlercreutz H. *et al.* "Dietary phytoestrogens and the menopause in Japan" *Lancet* 1992, 339:1233
Chow R. *et al.* "Effect of two randomised exercise programmes on bone mass of healthy post-menopausal women" *British Medical J.* 1987, 295:1441–44

VAGINITIS
Nutritional Therapies Collins E. "Inhibition of *candida albicans* by *L acidophilus* – experimental study" *J. of Dairy Sciences* 1980, 63:830–32
Aromatherapy Belaiche P. "Treatment of vaginal infections of *Candida albicans* with essential oil of *Melaleuca alternifolia*" *Phytotherapie* 1985, 15

CYSTITIS
Western Herbalism Avorn J. *et al.* "Reduction of bacteriuria and pyuria after ingestion of cranberry juice" *J. of the American Medical Association* 1994, 271(10):751–54
Acupuncture Aune A. *et al.* "Acupuncture in the prophylaxis of recurrent lower urinary tract infection in adult women" *Scandanavian J. of Primary Health Care* 1998, 16:37–39

PROSTATE PROBLEMS
Western Herbalism Wilt T. J. *et al.* "Saw palmetto extracts for treatment of benign prostatic hyperplasia: a systematic review" *J. of the American Medical Association* 1998, 280:1604–609
Shah P.J.R. "The treatment of disorders of the prostate with the rye-grass extract" *Complementary Therapies in Medicine* 1996, 4:21–25

MALE SEXUAL DYSFUNCTION
Western Herbalism Sikora R., *et al.* "Ginkgo biloba extract in the therapy of erectile dysfunction" *J. of Urology* 1989, 141:188

STRESS
Western Herbalism D'Angelo L. *et al.* "Double-blind controlled clinical study of the effect of standardised ginseng extract on psychomotor performance in healthy volunteers" *J. of Ethnopharmacology* 1986. 16:15–22
Aromatherapy Stevenson C. "The psycho-physiological effects of aromatherapy massage following cardiac surgery" *Complementary Therapies in Medicine* 1994, 2(1):27–35
T'ai Chi Jin P. "Efficacy of T'ai Chi, brisk walking, meditation and reading in reducing mental and emotional stress" *J. of Psychosomatic Research* 1992, 36(4):361–70
Meditation Janowiak J.J. *et al.* "Meditation and college students' self-actualization and rated stress" *Psychological Reports* 1994, 75(2):1007–10
Dillbeck M.C. "The effect of the Transcendental Meditation technique on anxiety level" *J. of Clinical Psychology* 1977, 33(4):1076–78

ANXIETY & PANIC ATTACKS
Western Herbalism Kinszler E. *et al.* "Effect of kava extract in patients with anxiety, tension and excitation states of non-psychotic genesis. Double blind study with placebos" *Arzneim Forsch* 1991, 41(6):584–88
Nutritional Therapies King D. "Can allergic

exposure provoke psychological symptoms? A double blind test" *Biological Psychiatry* 1981, 16(1):3–19
Massage Field T. *et al.* "Massage reduces anxiety in child and adolescent psychiatric patients" *J. of the American Academy of Child and Adolescent Psychiatry* 1992, (1):125–31
Therapeutic Touch Simington J.A., Laing G.P. "Effects of therapeutic touch on anxiety in the institutionalized elderly" *Clinical Nursing Research* 1993, 2(4):438–50
Psychotherapy & Counseling Clark D.M. *et al.* "A comparison of cognitive therapy, applied relaxation and imipramine in the treatment of panic disorder" *British J. of Psychiatry* 1994, 164(6):759–69
Meditation Miller J.J. *et al.* "Three year follow up and clinical implications of a mindfulness meditation-based stress reduction intervention in the treatment of anxiety disorders" *General Hospital Psychiatry* 1995, 17:192–200
Hypnotherapy Scott J.A. "A comparison of medical hypnoanalysis and cognitive hypnotherapy for the treatment of anxiety disorders" *Medical Hypnoanalysis J.* 1995 Dec., 10(4):355–81
Visualization Stanton H.E. "Using hypnotic success imagery to reduce test anxiety" *Australian J. of Clinical and Experimental Hypnosis* 1992 May, 20(1):31–37

DEPRESSION
Western Herbalism Linde K. *et al.* "St John's wort for depression-an overview and meta-analysis of randomised clinical trials" *British Medical J.* 1996, 313:253–58
Nutritional Therapies, Massage and **Aromatherapy** Wallcraft J. *Healing Minds* Mental Health Foundation
Acupuncture Luo H. *et al.* "Electro-acupuncture in the treatment of depressive psychosis: a controlled prospective randomised trial using electro acupuncture and amitriptyline in 241 patients" *International J. of Clinical Acupuncture* 1990, I (I):7–13
Exercise Klein M.H. *et al.* "A comparative outcome study of group psychotherapy *vs* exercise treatments for depression" *International J. of Mental Health* 1985, 13(3–4):148–77
Psychotherapy & Counseling Murphy G.E. *et al.* "Cognitive behavior therapy, relaxation training, and tricyclic antidepressant medication in the treatment of depression" *Psychological Reports* 1995, 77(2):403–20
Meditation Smith W.P. *et al.* "Meditation as an adjunct to a happiness enhancement program" *J. of Clinical Psychology* 1995, 51(2):269–73

INSOMNIA
Western Herbalism Lindahl O. *et al.* "Double blind study of a valerian preparation" *Pharmacology, Biochemistry and Behavior* 1989, 32:1065–66
Nutritional Therapies Garfinkel D. *et al.* "Improvement of sleep quality in elderly people by controlled-release melatonin" *Lancet* 1995, 346:541–44
Petrie K. *et al.* "A double-blind trial of melatonin as a treatment for jet lag in international cabin crew" *Biological Psychiatry* 1993, 33(7):526–30
Hypnotherapy Morin C.M., Culber J.P., Schwartz S.M. "Nonpharmacological

interventions for insomnia: a meta-analysis of treatment efficacy" *American J. of Psychiatry* 1994, 151:1172–80
Meditation "Integration of behavioral and relaxation approaches into the treatment of chronic pain and insomnia" *J. of the American Medical Association* 1996, 276:313–18

FOOD SENSITIVITY
Nutritional Therapies Nanda R. *et al.* "Food intolerance and the irritable bowel syndrome" *Gut* 1989, 30(8):1099–104
Environmental Medicine McEwan L.M. *et al.* "Enzyme-potentiated desensitisation: the effect of pretreatment with glucuronidase, hyaluronidase and antigen on anaphylactic sensitivity of guinea-pigs, rats and mice" *International Archive of Allergy* 1972, 42:152–58

HAY FEVER & RHINITIS
Western Herbalism Bellussi L. *et al.* "Evaluation of the efficacy and safety of sobrerol granules in patients suffering from chronic rhinosinusitis" *J. of International Medical Research* 1990, 18:454–59
Homeopathy Taylor Reilly D. *et al.* "Is homoeopathy a placebo response? Controlled trial of homoeopathic potency, with pollen in hayfever as a model" *Lancet* 1986 II(8512):881–85
Wiesenauer M. *et al.* "The treatment of pollinosis with Galphimia glauca D4: a randomized placebo-controlled double-blind clinical trial" *Phytomedicine* 1995, 2(1):3–6
Acupuncture Davies A. *et al.* "The effect of acupuncture on nonallergic rhinitis: a controlled pilot study" *Alternative Therapies* Jan 1988, 4(1):70–74
Hypnotherapy Fry L. *et al.* "Effect of hypnosis on allergic skin responses in asthma and hayfever" *British Medical J.* 1964, i: 1145–48

ASTHMA
Homeopathy Reilly, D. *et al.* "Is evidence for homeopathy reproducible?" *Lancet* 1994, 344:1601–06
Nutritional Therapies Lindahl O. *et al.* "Vegan diet regimen with reduced medication in the treatment of bronchial asthma" *J. of Asthma* 1985, 22(1):45–55
Skobeloff E.M. *et al.* "Intravenous magnesium sulfate for the treatment of acute asthma in the emergency department" *J. of the American Medical Association* 1989, 262:1210–13
Chiropractic Nielsen N.H. *et al.* "Chronic asthma and chiropractic spinal manipulation: a randomized clinical trial" *Clinical & Experimental Allergy* 1995, 25(1):80–88
Acupuncture Linde, K. *et al.* "Evaluation of the effectiveness of acupuncture for the treatment of asthma bronchiale" *The Cochrane Library* 1997, 2
Yoga Nagarathna R., Nagendra H.R. "Yoga for bronchial asthma: a controlled study" *British Medical J. (Clinical Research)* 1985 Oct 19, 291(6502):1077–79
Hypnotherapy Ewer T.C., Stewart D.E. "Improvement in bronchial hyper-responsiveness in patients with moderate asthma after treatment with a hypnotic technique: a randomised controlled trial" *British Medical J. (Clinical Research)* 1986 Nov 1, 293(6555):1129–32

Meditation Wilson A.F. *et al.* "Transcendental meditation and asthma" *Respiration* 1975, 32(1):74–80
Relaxation & Breathing Henry M. *et al.* "Improvement of respiratory function in chronic asthmatic patients with autogenic therapy" *J. of Psychosomatic Research* 1993;37(3):265–70

CANCER
Massage
Corner J. *et al.* "An evaluation of the use of massage and essential oils on the wellbeing of cancer patients" *International J. of Palliative Nursing* 1995, 1(2):67–73
Zanolla R. *et al.* "Evaluation of the results of three different methods of postmastectomy lymphedema treatment" *J. of Surgical Oncology* 1984, 26:210–13
Acupuncture Vickers A.J. "Can acupuncture have specific effects on health? A systematic literature review of acupuncture antiemesis trials" *J. of the Royal Society of Medicine* 1996, 89:303–11
Psychotherapy & Counseling
Spiegel D. *et al.* "Effect of psychosocial treatment on survival of patients with metastatic breast cancer" *Lancet* 1989, 2: 888–91
Greer S. *et al.* "Adjuvant psychosocial therapy for patients with cancer: a prospective randomised trial" *British Medical J.* 1992, 304:675–80
Hypnotherapy Spiegel D. *et al.* "Group therapy and hypnosis reduce metastatic breast carcinoma pain" *Psychosomatic Medicine* 1982, 45:333–39

CHRONIC FATIGUE SYNDROME
Psychotherapy and Counseling Deale A. *et al.* "Cognitive behavior therapy for chronic fatigue syndrome: a randomized controlled trial" *American J. of Psychiatry* 1997, 154:408–14

PERSISTENT PAIN
Western Herbalism Watson C.P.N. *et al.* "Post-herpetic neuralgia and topical capsaicin" *Pain* 1988; 33:333–40
Massage Ferrell-Torry A.T. *et al.* "The use of therapeutic massage as a nursing intervention to modify anxiety and the perception of cancer pain" *Cancer Nursing* 1993, 16(2):93–101
Acupuncture Ter Riet G. *et al.* "Acupuncture and chronic pain: A criteria-based meta-analysis" *J. of Clinical Epidemiology* 1990, 43(11):1191–99
Psychotherapy & Counseling "Treatment of chronic pain and insomnia: integration of behavioral and relaxation approaches into the treatment of chronic pain and insomnia" *J. of the American Medical Association* 1996, 276:313–38
Visualization Albright G.L. *et al.* "Effects of warming imagery aimed at trigger-point sites on tissue compliance, skin temperature, and pain sensitivity in biofeedback – trained patients with chronic pain: a preliminary study" *Perceptual and Motor Skills* 1990, 71:1163–70
Biofeedback Stuckey S.J. *et al.* "EMG biofeedback training, relaxation training and placebo for the relief of chronic back pain" *Perceptual and Motor Skills* 1986, 63:1023–36
Meditation Kabat-Zinn J. "Four year follow-up of a meditation-based program for

the self-regulation of chronic pain: treatment outcomes and compliance" *Clinical J. of Pain* 1986, 2:159–73
Relaxation & Breathing Cappo B. *et al.* "Utility of prolonged respiratory exhalation for reducing physiological and psychological arousal in non-threatening and threatening situations" *J. of Psychosomatic Research* 1984, 28(4)265–73
Healing Sundblom D.M. *et al.* "Effect of spiritual healing on chronic idiopathic pain: a medical and psychological study" *Clinical J. of Pain* 1994, 10(4):296–302

HIV & AIDS
Nutritional Therapies Allard J.P. *et al.* "Effects of vitamin E and C supplementation on oxidative stress and viral load in HIV-infected subjects" *AIDS* 1998, 12(13):1653–59
Massage Scafidi F. *et al.* "Massage therapy improves behaviour in neonates born to HIV-positive mothers" *J. of Pediatric Psychology* 1996, 21(6):889–97
Acupuncture Tindall J. *Complementary Medicine Bulletin* vol 1 (10)4
Stress Management Coates T.J. *et al.* "Stress reduction training in men with HIV" *American J. of Public Health* 1989, 79:885–87
Taylor D.N., "Effects of a behavioral stress-management program on anxiety, mood, self-esteem, and T-cell count in HIV positive men" *Psychological Reports* 1995, 76(2):451–57
McCain N.L. *et al.* "The influence of stress management training in HIV disease" *Nursing Research* 1996, 45(4):246–53
Healing & Therapeutic Touch Sicher F. *et al.* "A randomized double-blind study of the effect of distant healing in a population with advanced AIDS. Report of a small scale study" *Western J. of Medicine* 1998, 169(6):356–63
Ireland M. "Therapeutic touch with HIV-infected children: a pilot study" *J. of the Association of Nurses in AIDS Care* 1998, 9(4):68–77

INCONCLUSIVE TESTS
In the following studies the relevent therapies proved ineffective or inconclusive:

Iridology Diagnosis Knipschild P. "Looking for gall bladder disease in the patient's iris" *British Medical J.* 1988, 297(6663):1578–81
Simon A. *et al.* "An evaluation of iridology" *J. of the American Medical Association* 1979, 242(13):1385–89
Hair Testing Sethi T.J. *et al.* "How reliable are commercial allergy tests?" *Lancet* 1987, 1:92–94
Muscle Testing for Intolerances Rybeck C.H. *et al.* "The effect of oral administration of refined sugar on muscle strength" *J. of Manipulative and Physiological Therapeutics* 1980, 3(3):155–61
Triano J.J. "Muscle strength testing as a diagnostic screen for supplement nutrition therapy: a blind study" *J. of Manipulative and Physiological Therapeutics* 1982, 5(4):179–87
Skin Testing for Food Allergies Jewett D.L. *et al.* "A double-blind study of symptom provocation to determine food sensitivity" *New England J. of Medicine* 1990, 323(7):429–33

USEFUL ADDRESSES

THE ORGANIZATIONS LISTED BELOW range from professional bodies whose members include conventional doctors to those run on a voluntary basis with relatively few members. Contacting an organization is often a good way of obtaining information about a therapy. Many groups provide referrals at little or no cost. Always bear in mind the guidelines for finding a practitioner.

GENERAL

American Association of Oriental Medicine
433 Front Street
Catasauqua, PA 18032
Tel: 888/500-7999
Online: www.aaom.org
E-mail: aaom1@aol.com

American Holistic Medical Association
4101 Lake Boone Trail, Suite 201
Raleigh, NC 27607
Tel: 919/787-5181

American Holistic Health Association
P.O. Box 17400
Anaheim, CA 92817
Tel: 714/779-6152
Online: http://ahha.org

National Health Information Center
P.O. Box 1133
Washington, DC 20013-1133
Tel: 800/336-4797
Online: http://nhic-nt.health.org
E-mail: nhicinfo@health.org

Office of Alternative Medicine
National Institutes of Health
P.O. Box 8218
Silver Spring, MD 20907-8218
Tel: 888/644-6226

National Library of Medicine
8600 Rockville Pike
Bethesda, MD 20894
Tel: 301/496-6095
Online: www.nlm.nih.gov

ACUPUNCTURE

American Academy of Medical Acupuncture
5820 Wilshire Boulevard, Suite 500
Los Angeles, CA 90036
Tel: 213/937-5514
Online: www.acupuncture.com

National Acupuncture and Oriental Medicine Alliance
14637 Starr Road, SE
Olalla, WA 98359
Tel: 253/851-6896
Online: www.acuall.org

National Certification Commission for Acupuncture and Oriental Medicine
11 Canal Center Plaza, Suite 300
Alexandria, VA 22314
Tel: 703/548-9004
Online: www.nccaom.org

ALEXANDER TECHNIQUE

American Society for the Alexander Technique
401 East Market Street
Charlottesville, VA 22902
Tel: 800/473-0620
Online: www.alexandertech.org

AROMATHERAPY

American Alliance of Aromatherapy
P.O. Box 309
Depoe Bay, OR 97341
Tel: 800/809-9850
Online: www.healthy.net/pan/pa/
Aromatherapy/aaat/index.html

National Association for Holistic Aromatherapy
P.O. Box 17622
Boulder, CO 80308
Tel: 800/566-6735
Online: www.naha.org

The Pacific Institute of Aromatherapy
P.O. Box 6842
San Rafael, CA 94903
Tel: 415/479-9121

ART THERAPY

American Art Therapy Association
1202 Allanson Road
Mundelein, IL 60060-3808
Tel: 888/290-0878
Online: www.arttherapy.org

AUTOGENIC TRAINING

Mind Body Health Sciences
393 Dixon Road
Boulder, CO 80302
Tel: 303/440-8460
Online: www.joanborysenko.com

AYURVEDA

The Ayurvedic Institute
11311 Menaul NE
Albuquerque, NM 87112
Tel: 505/291-9698
Online: www.ayurveda.com

BIOFEEDBACK

Association for Applied Psychophysiology and Biofeedback
10200 West 44th Avenue, Suite 304
Wheatridge, CO 80033-2840
Tel: 800/477-8892
Online: www.aapb.org

CHIROPRACTIC

American Chiropractic Association
1701 Clarendon Boulevard
Arlington, VA 22209
Tel: 800/986-4636
Online: www.amerchiro.org

International Chiropractors Association
1110 North Glebe Road, Suite 1000
Arlington, VA 22201
Tel: 800/423-4690
Online: www.chiropractic.org
E-mail: chiro@chiropractic.org

World Chiropractic Alliance
2950 North Dobson Road #1
Chandler, AZ 85224
Tel: 800/347-1011
Online: www.chiropage.com

HEALING

The Barbara Brennan School of Healing
P.O. Box 2005
East Hampton, NY 11937-0903
Tel: 800/924-2564
Online: www.barbarabrennan.com
E-mail: bbshoffice@barbarabrennan.com

Ecumenical Society of Psychorientology
1407 Calle del Norte
Laredo, TX 78044-2249
Tel: 800/545-6463
Online: www.ecumenical.org
E-mail: silvamethod@silvamethod.com

Nurse Healers – Prof. Assoc. Int'l.
11250-8 Roger Bacon Drive, Suite 8
Reston, VA 20190
Tel: 703/234-4149
Online: www.therapeutic-touch.org
E-mail: nh-pai@drohanmgmt.com

HERBALISM

American Botanical Council
P.O. Box 144345
Austin, TX 78714-4345
Tel: 512/926-4900
Online: www.herbalgram.org
E-mail: abc@herbalgram.org

Herb Research Foundation
1007 Pearl Street, Suite 200
Boulder, CO 80302
Tel: 800/748-2617
Online: www.herbs.org

DrinksThatWork
P.O. Box 1528
Santa Cruz, CA 95061-1528
Tel: 888/929-9929
Online: www.drinksthatwork.com

HOMEOPATHY

Homeopathic Educational Services
2124 Kittredge Street
Berkeley, CA 94704
Tel: 800/359-9051
Online: www.homeopathic.com
E-mail: mail@homeopathic.com

The National Center for Homeopathy
801 North Fairfax Street, Suite 306
Alexandria, VA 22314
Tel: 703/548-7790
Online: www.homeopathic.org
E-mail: nchinfo@agc.org

North American Society of Homeopaths
122 East Pike Street, Suite 1122
Seattle, WA 98122
Tel: 541/345-9815
Online: www.homeopathy.org
E-mail: nash@homeopathy.org

HYPNOTHERAPY
American Institute of Hypnotherapy
16842 Von Karman Avenue
Irvine, CA 92606
Tel: 800/63-HYPNO
Online: www.aih.cc
E-mail: aih@hypnosis.com

American Society of Clinical Hypnosis
33 W. Grand Avenue, Suite 402
Chicago, IL 60610
Tel: 312/645-9810
Online: www.asch.net

International Medical and Dental
Hypnotherapy Association
4110 Edgeland, Suite 800
Royal Oak, MI 48073
Tel: 800/257-5467

MASSAGE THERAPY
American Massage Therapy Association
820 Davis Street, Suite 100
Evanston, IL 60201-4444
Tel: 847/864-0123
Online: www.amtamassage.org
E-mail: info@inet.amtamassage.org

MUSIC THERAPY
American Association for Music Therapy
8455 Colesville Road, Suite 1000
Silver Spring, MD 20910
Tel: 301/589-3300
Online: www.musictherapy.org
E-mail: info@musictherapy.org

NATUROPATHY
The American Association of
Naturopathic Physicians
601 Valley Street, Suite 105
Seattle, WA 98109
Tel: 206/298-0126
Online: www.naturopathic.org
E-mail: GartleyMe@compuserve.com

Homeopathic Academy of Naturopathic
Physicians
12132 SE Foster Place
Portland, OR 97266
Tel: 503/761-3298
Online: www.healthy.net/pan/pa/
homeopathic/hanp/index.html
E-mail: hanp@igc.apc.org

NUTRITIONAL THERAPY
American College of Advancement in
Medicine
23121 Verdugo Drive, Suite 204
Laguna Hills, CA 92653
Tel: 714/583-7666
Online: www.acam.org
E-mail: acam@acam.org

American Dietetic Association National
Center for Nutrition and Dietetics
216 W. Jackson Boulevard, Suite 800
Chicago, IL 60606
ADA's Consumer Nutrition Hotline:
800/366-1655
Online: www.eatright.org
E-mail: hotline@eatright.org

The International and American
Associations of Clinical Nutritionists
5200 Keller Springs Road, Suite 410
Dallas, TX 75248
Tel: 972/250-2829
Online: www.iaacn.org

OSTEOPATHY
American Academy of Osteopathy
3500 DePauw Boulevard, Suite 1080
Indianapolis, IN 46268
Tel: 317/879-1881
Online: www.academyofosteopathy.org

American Association of Colleges of
Osteopathic Medicine
5550 Friendship Boulevard, Suite 310
Chevy Chase, MD 20815
Tel: 301/968-4100
Online: www.aacom.org

American Osteopathic Association
142 East Ontario Street
Chicago, IL 60611
Tel: 800/621-1773
Online: www.am-osteo-assn.org
E-mail: info@aoa-net.org

PSYCHOTHERAPY & COUNSELING
American Counseling Association
5999 Stevenson Avenue
Alexandria, VA 22304
Tel: 703/823-9800
Online: www.counseling.org

American Psychological Association
750 First Street, NE
Washington, DC 20002
Tel: 800/374-2721
     202/336-5500
Online: www.apa.org

Association for Humanistic Psychology
45 Franklin Street, Suite 315
San Francisco, CA 94102
Tel: 415/864-8850
Online: www.ahpweb.org
E-mail: ahpoffice@aol.com

QIGONG
East West Academy of Healing Arts
Qi Gong Institute
450 Sutter Street, Suite 2104
San Francisco, CA 94108
Tel: 415/788-2227
Online: http://members.aol.com/eastwestqi
E-mail: eastwestqi@aol.com

REFLEXOLOGY
International Institute of Reflexology
P.O. Box 12642
St. Petersburg, FL 33710
Tel: 727/343-4811
Online: www.reflexology-usa.net

Reflexology Association of America
4012 Rainbow Ste. K-PMB#585
Las Vegas, NV 89103
Online: www.reflexology-usa.org

REIKI
The Intervational Center for Reiki
Training
21421 Hilltop Street, Unit #28
Southfield, MI 48034
Tel: 800/332-8112
Online: www.reiki.org
E-mail: center@reiki.org

SHIATSU
Ohashi Institute, Inc.
12 West 27th Street
New York, NY 10001
Tel: 212/684-4190
Online: www.ohashi.com/institut.html
E-mail: ohashiinst@aol.com

THERAPEUTIC TOUCH
Nurse Healers – Prof. Assoc. Int'l.
11250-8 Roger Bacon Drive, Suite 8
Reston, VA 20190
Tel: 703/234-4149
Online: www.therapeutic-touch.org
E-mail: nh-pai@drohanmgmt.com

TRADITIONAL CHINESE MEDICINE
American Association of Oriental
Medicine
433 Front Street
Catasauqua, PA 18032
Tel: 888/500-7999
     610/266-1433
Online: www.aaom.org
E-mail: aaom1@aol.com

YOGA THERAPY
The American Yoga Association
P.O. Box 19986
Sarasota, FL 34276
Tel: 941/927-4977
Online: http://users.aol.com/amyogaassn
E-mail: YOGAmerica@aol.com

Integral Yoga Institute
227 West 13th Street
New York, NY 10011
Tel: 212/929-0586
Online: http://integralyogaofnewyork.org

International Association of Yoga
Therapists
20 Sunnyside Avenue, Suite A243
Mill Valley, CA 94941-1928
109 Hillside Avenue
Mill Valley, CA 94941
Tel: 415/383-4587

Yogaville
Route 1 Box 1720
Buckingham, VA 23921
Tel: 800/858-9642
Online: www.yogaville.org
E-mail: iyi@yogaville.org

INDEX

A page number in **bold** indicates the main entry on a topic. A main entry for an ailment includes details of the ailment, the factors causing it, the treatment options, and relevant case studies and precautions. A main entry for a therapy includes details of its effects, its history and main principles, its main uses, and a description of what is involved in a treatment session.

ACKNOWLEDGMENTS

Authors' Acknowledgments
We are extremely grateful to those who helped us in various ways with
this book. For their professional advice and wisdom, we would like to
thank psychologist Ashley Conway, acupuncturist Gerry Harris,
osteopath Mark Kane, nutritional therapist Kate Neil, naturopaths Leon
Chaitow and Roger Newman Turner, homoeopath Gabrielle Pinto, and
medical herbalist Julie Whitehouse.

    Many thanks for practical support and general hand-holding to Debbie
Cole and Karen Mayze, and to Mary Bredin and Stephen Claypole for
their considerable qualities of patience, tolerance, and encouragement.

    None of this could be achieved without the good humor, creative
ingenuity, and fortitude of the team at Dorling Kindersley, for which an
enormous thank you to Daphne Razazan and Susannah Marriott, and
especially to David Summers and Penny Warren.

Publisher's Acknowledgments
Dorling Kindersley would like to thank Monica Chakraverty and Tracey
Beresford for editorial assistance, Carol McGlynn and Christa Weil for
proofreading, and Sue Bosanko for the index.

Picture Credits
Picture research: Anna Grapes
Picture library: Melanie Simmonds, Denise O'Brien, Charlotte Oster
The publisher would like to thank the following for their kind
permission to reproduce their photographs: (Abbreviations key: t=top,
b=below, r=right, l=left, c=center, a=above.)
AKG London: 148-149
Science Photo Library: Alfred Pasieka 11tr; Don Fawcett 167; Ed
Young/Agstock 166c
Tony Stone Images: G.W. Willis/BPS 158-159; Ken Fisher 168-169;
Vince Michaels 148cr